Roman Domestic Medical Practice in Central Italy

Roman Domestic Medical Practice in Central Italy examines the roles that the home, the garden and the members of the household (freeborn, freed and slave) played in the acquisition and maintenance of good physical and mental health and well-being. Focussing on the period from the middle Republic to the early Empire, it considers how comprehensive the ancient Roman general understanding of health actually was, and studies how knowledge regarding various aspects of health was transmitted within the household.

Using literary, documentary, archaeological and bioarchaeological evidence from a variety of contexts, this is the first extended volume to provide as comprehensive and detailed a reconstruction of this aspect of ancient Roman private life as possible, complementing existing works on ancient professional medical practice and existing works on domestic medical practice in later historical periods. This volume offers an indispensable resource to social historians, particularly those that focus on the ancient family, and medical historians, particularly those that focus on the ancient world.

Jane Draycott is Lord Kelvin Adam Smith Research Fellow in Ancient Science and Technology at the University of Glasgow, UK. Previously she was Lecturer in Classics at the University of Wales Trinity Saint David, Associate Teacher in Roman Archaeology at the University of Sheffield, all in the UK, and 2011–2012 Rome Fellow at the British School at Rome, Italy.

Medicine and the Body in Antiquity

Series editor

Patricia Baker
University of Kent, UK

Advisory board:

Lesley A. Dean-Jones
University of Texas at Austin, USA

Rebecca Gowland
University of Durham, UK

Jessica Hughes
Open University, UK

Ralph Rosen
University of Pennsylvania, USA

Kelli Rudolph
University of Kent, UK

Medicine and the Body in Antiquity is a series which aims to foster interdisciplinary research that broadens our understanding of past beliefs about the body and its care. The intention of the series is to use evidence drawn from diverse sources (textual, archaeological, epigraphic) in an interpretative manner to gain insights into the medical practices and beliefs of the ancient Mediterranean. The series approaches medical history from a broad thematic perspective that allows for collaboration between specialists from a wide range of disciplines outside ancient history and archaeology such as art history, religious studies, medicine, the natural sciences and music. The series will also aim to bring research on ancient medicine to the attention of scholars concerned with later periods. Ultimately this series provides a forum for scholars from a wide range of disciplines to explore ideas about the body and medicine beyond the confines of current scholarship.

Prostheses in Antiquity
Edited by Jane Draycott

Becoming a Woman and Mother in Greco-Roman Egypt
Women's Bodies, Society and Domestic Space
Ada Nifosi

Roman Domestic Medical Practice in Central Italy
From the Middle Republic to the Early Empire
Jane Draycott

For more information about this series, please visit: www.routledge.com/classical studies/series/MBA

Roman Domestic Medical Practice in Central Italy

From the Middle Republic
to the Early Empire

Jane Draycott

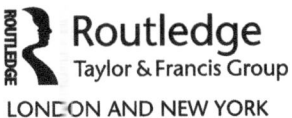

Routledge
Taylor & Francis Group

LONDON AND NEW YORK

First published 2019 by Routledge

2 Park Square, Milton Park, Abingdon, Oxon OX14 4RN
605 Third Avenue, New York, NY 10017

Routledge is an imprint of the Taylor & Francis Group, an informa business

First issued in paperback 2021

Copyright © 2019 Jane Draycott

British Library Cataloguing-in-Publication Data
A catalogue record for this book is available from the British Library

Library of Congress Cataloging-in-Publication Data
A catalog record for this book has been requested

ISBN: 978-1-4724-3396-1 (hbk)
ISBN: 978-1-03-217832-5 (pbk)
DOI: 10.4324/9781315606859

Typeset in Times New Roman
by Apex CoVantage, LLC

For Mark Bradley.
Mentor, friend, inspiration.

Contents

List of figures   viii
Acknowledgements   x
List of abbreviations   xii

Introduction   1

1 Health and well-being in the Roman Republic and Principate   22

2 The Roman house and garden   48

3 The Roman household   94

4 The transmission of medical knowledge   131

Conclusion   154

Bibliography   159
Index   181

Figures

I.1 The funerary relief of Scribonia Attica from Isola Sacra, Ostia, dating from the second century CE. 5

I.2 The funerary relief of Marcus Ulpius Amerimnus from Isola Sacra, Ostia, dating from the second century CE. 6

I.3 A glass bottle that contained expensive oils that could be used for either medical or cosmetic purposes, *circa* 100–500 CE. 9

I.4 A set of instruments; copies of items recovered from Pompeii and currently housed in the Naples National Archaeological Museum and dating from the first century CE. 10

I.5 A bronze medical kit depicting the rod of Aesculapius; a copy of an item recovered from Pompeii and currently housed in the Naples National Archaeological Museum and dating from the first century CE. 11

1.1 A marble statue of the goddess Hygieia, supposedly recovered from Ostia and dating to *circa* 100 BCE–100 CE. 26

2.1 A fresco tondo depicting a seaside villa, *circa* 50–79 CE. 59

2.2 A fragment of a fresco depicting a woman standing on a balcony, *circa* 10 BCE–14 CE. 60

2.3 A frescoed wall with a niche for storage, the Villa of Numerius Popidius Florus, Boscoreale, *circa* 50–70 CE. 67

2.4 A fresco depicting an elaborate garland, Villa of Publius Fannius Synistor, Boscoreale, *circa* 50–40 BCE. 73

2.5 A bronze statuette of a *Lar*, dating to the first or second century CE. 78

2.6 A fresco depicting the *Genius* and the *Juno* sacrificing from the House of Julius Polybius in Pompeii (IX.13.1–3), dating from the first century CE. 80

2.7 A bronze statuette of a *Genius*, dating to the first century CE. 81

3.1 A bronze strigil set; a copy of an item supposedly recovered from Pompeii and currently housed in the Naples National Archaeological Museum and dating from *circa* 199 BCE–79 CE. 106

3.2 A bronze spoon and pick combined, *circa* 199 BCE–500 CE. 107

3.3   A stone funerary relief depicting a woman who has been
      variously identified as a doctor, a pharmacist and a soap-maker,
      dating from the second century CE.   108
3.4   A relief of workers transporting *amphorae*, dating from the
      second century CE.   111
3.5   A scene from the altar of Lucius Minucius Optatus, dating from
      the first century CE.   112
3.6   A fresco depicting cupids and Psyche making perfume, dating
      from the first century CE.   113
3.7   A fresco depicting cupids hanging garlands, dating from the first
      century CE.   114
3.8   A fresco depicting two slaves preparing a meal, dating from the
      early second century CE.   115
3.9   A fresco depicting a woman playing a kithara, Villa of Publius
      Fannius Synistor, Boscoreale, *circa* 50–40 BCE.   119
4.1   A relief of a doctor in his study; a copy.   135
4.2   A fresco fragment depicting two women in conversation,
      first century CE.   139
4.3   A terracotta figurine of a woman nursing a child, third century
      BCE–first century CE.   144
4.4   A marble plaque depicting a woman giving birth, second
      century CE.   146
5.1   A fresco depicting Aeneas being treated by Iapyx, from
      the *triclinium* of the House of Vedius Siricus and Vedius
      Nummianus in Pompeii (VII.1.47), dating from the first
      century CE.   155

Acknowledgements

My research into Roman domestic medical practice in central Italy during the Republic and Empire began as the postdoctoral research project 'The gardens of Hygieia: the role of the Roman *hortus* in domestic medical practice' during my tenure as Rome Fellow at the British School at Rome in the period from October 2011 to June 2012. I would like to thank my fellow award holders, Laura Banducci and Robyn Veal, for the intellectual stimulation that they and their complementary research projects provided over the course of those nine months, and Simon Williams, Laura Bolick and Michael Mulryan for their company over many hours spent in the library, dining room and cortile, and out and about on excursions. I spent two additional periods of time working on this project at the BSR in the summers of 2015 and 2017, and would like to thank all the staff, but particularly Maria-Pia Malvezzi and Stefania Peterlini, who arranged access to numerous museums and archaeological sites and permission to take photographs, and Valerie Scott, who arranged access to numerous academic libraries.

From 2016 to 2018 I was co-investigator on the AHRC Science in Culture Early Career Development Award–funded research project 'From natural resources to packaging, an interdisciplinary study of skincare products over time' (grant ref. 1507EC003/SH11). This meant that I was able to undertake additional research into ancient cosmetics and perfumes that proved extremely useful. I would like to thank the principal investigator, Thibaut Devièse, and the co-investigator, Szu Shen Wong, for providing me with the opportunity to think about ancient health-care from a scientific perspective, and our project partners, Matthew Johnston and John Betts of the Royal Pharmaceutical Society Museum, for providing me with the opportunity to access and examine the objects in their care.

I would like to express my gratitude for the support that I have received from other researchers in the history and archaeology of medicine over the last decade, most notably Ralph Jackson, Patty Baker, Laurence Totelin, Georgia Petridou, Emma-Jayne Graham and Jessica Hughes.

I would like to express my appreciation of and my gratitude to my friends Amy Russell and Liz Gloyn. They were not only the first people to read something resembling a complete draft of this manuscript in the autumn of 2016, but they also provided a considerable amount of emotional support during a particularly difficult period in my life during the spring and summer of 2018. I am also very grateful to the anonymous reader engaged by Routledge for their comprehensive feedback and thoughtful suggestions regarding revisions in the autumn of 2017, and my colleague Sophia Xenophontos for her close and perceptive reading of the final draft.

Finally, I would like to thank the person who has been consistently the most important and influential person in my academic life since I embarked on my doctorate at the University of Nottingham in September 2008, Mark Bradley. In recognition for all that he has done for me, both professionally and personally, over the last decade, I dedicate this book to him.

Abbreviations

AE	L'Année Épigraphique
AJA	American Journal of Archaeology
AJAH	American Journal of Ancient History
AJPA	American Journal of Physical Anthropology
ANRW	Aufstieg und Niedergang der römischen Welt. Rise and Decline of the Roman World
ARG	Archiv für Religionsgeschichte
BMJ	British Medical Journal
CA	Classical Antiquity
CCJ	Cambridge Classical Journal
CIL	Corpus Inscriptionum Latinarum
CJ	Classical Journal
CM	Classica et Mediaevalia
CP	Classical Philology
CQ	Classical Quarterly
ER	European Review
ESM	Early Science and Medicine
G&R	Greece and Rome
GRBS	Greek, Roman and Byzantine Studies
IG	Inscriptiones Graecae
ILS	Inscriptiones Latinae Selectae
JAS	Journal of Archaeological Science
JGH	Journal of Garden History
JHS	Journal of Hellenic Studies
JLA	Journal of Late Antiquity
JRA	Journal of Roman Archaeology
JRS	Journal of Roman Studies
JRSM	Journal of the Royal Society of Medicine
JWH	Journal of World History
MAAR	Memoirs of the American Academy in Rome
NS	Notizie degli scavi di antichità
OLD	Oxford Latin Dictionary
P&P	Past and Present

PBSR	Papers of the British School at Rome
RM	Mitteilungen des Deutschen Archäologischen Instituts, Römische Abteilung
SHA	Scriptores Historiae Augustae
SHM	Social History of Medicine
TAPA	Transactions of the American Philological Association
TPAPA	Transactions and Proceedings of the American Philological Association
VHA	Vegetation History and Archaeobotany

For the most part, I have used the full names of Romans upon their first appearance in the text and their more familiar abbreviated names thereafter, and I have used the Latinised forms of Greek names and words.

Introduction

Approaching ancient Roman medicine

> If your body is seized with a chill and racked with pain, or some other mishap has pinned you to your bed, have you got someone to sit by you, to get lotions ready, to call in the physician so as to raise you up and restore you to your children and dear kinsmen?[1]

Quintus Horatius Flaccus, in his first satire, presents a scenario which, although hypothetical, not to mention satirical, offers an insight into healthcare in the city of Rome during the second half of the first century BCE. Horace, the freeborn son of a Samnite freedman, is nominally addressing his patron Gaius Cilnius Maecenas, a wealthy Etruscan equestrian, *circa* 35–33 BCE, although the point that he is attempting to make by means of the satire is applicable to any reader: that despite the frequency with which people long for wealth and power, these are not necessarily good things to have.[2]

The putative individual under discussion lies bed-ridden at home and requires treatment, and Horace clearly differentiates between the responsibilities of those within and those without the afflicted individual's household. It is the responsibility of a member of the household to sit with them, presumably to keep them company, but perhaps also to attend to any urgent physical needs they might have. It is the responsibility of a member of the household, not necessarily the same one, to get the lotions ready, which implies that the household is in possession of a selection of medicaments in the event of just such an occasion, medicaments which could have been produced on or off the premises but, whatever their origins, were subsequently stored until such time as it became necessary to utilise them. It is the responsibility of a member of the household to send for the physician, who is not, it would appear, a member of the household, but has to come in from outside. Each one of these actions is a necessary part of the potentially extended process of the individual recovering their health after becoming indisposed, but they all take place prior to the intervention of a professional physician, and it is with this part of the process that this study is concerned. Both the individual's acquisition and maintenance of good health and well-being in the first place *and* their restoration and preservation of good health and well-being in the event that they became ill were fundamental parts not only of ancient Roman healthcare, but also of ancient Roman daily life.

In 2006, Fritz Graf observed that research into ancient medicine had split into two fields, one focusing on the medicine of the physician, the other the medicine of the temple, and that this split was by no means a good thing.[3] A decade later, William Harris, though in agreement with Graf, drew attention to what he considered 'a still more serious failing in the study of ancient medicine – namely its pervasive if not unanimous refusal to explore popular medicine in a systematic fashion, which has led to a severely unbalanced narrative about ancient healthcare'.[4] His 2016 edited volume *Popular Medicine in Graeco-Roman Antiquity: Explorations*, the product of a conference at Columbia University's Centre for the Ancient Mediterranean in 2014, sought to begin to address this failing and so rebalance the narrative, but despite observing that 'there must always have been a good deal of self-treatment and treatment within the family (in a wide sense)', neither he nor any of the volume's other contributors chose to explore this aspect of ancient medicine.[5] This relative neglect by scholars of what has been described as 'domestic cultures of health, healing and medical decision making' is not unique to the academic discipline of ancient history, but has also occurred in the fields of medieval, early modern and modern history, although in recent years scholars have been working to address this.[6] It stems in part from the difficulty in defining the household and determining its formal and informal boundaries, and in part from the difficulty of accessing sufficient evidence – whether literary, documentary, archaeological or bioarchaeological – to facilitate the reconstruction of such ephemeral activities as those required for the ongoing process of acquiring, preserving and maintaining a degree of what we would today refer to as health and well-being.[7] Despite recognition of the existence of what has been described as a 'medical marketplace' in Graeco-Roman antiquity, the position of the household within this medical marketplace has been systematically overlooked, if not actively disregarded.[8] This has serious ramifications not only for medical history but also for social and cultural history more broadly.[9] My aim with this monograph, therefore, is to start the process of correcting this oversight in relation to Roman history. I shall examine the role that the household (that is, the house and the garden, and the people that occupy them, broadly defined) played in ancient Roman healthcare in central Italy in the period from the middle Republic to the early Empire. I shall focus primarily, but not exclusively, upon the period of approximately 100 BCE–100 CE, for reasons which will be explained below.

Medical history from below

Whatever the historical period under discussion, it is the 'professional' medical practitioner that has received the lion's share of attention from scholars, and Graeco-Roman antiquity is no exception.[10] It is the professional medical practitioner, after all, that we can frequently put a name to, and on occasion even more than that. For example, thanks to Marcus Tullius Cicero's personal correspondence, we have a considerable amount of information regarding the physicians engaged by him, his family members, friends and acquaintances during the middle of the first century BCE, as well as insight into how these physicians operated in late Republican Roman and Italian society. It would appear that Cicero did not possess a personal physician the way that a number of his contemporaries did, that is, as a slave or freedman living in his household, although whether this was a matter of personal choice or dictated by financial considerations is not explicitly stated.[11] Rather, he employed a physician named Alexio, possibly a freedman or perhaps a freeborn immigrant, for himself, and considered him to be noteworthy for 'his affection for me, his kindness and his charm'.[12] When Alexio died in the May of 44 BCE, Cicero was bereft, and not just because he was placed in the unenviable position of needing to engage a new personal physician. However, even before Alexio's death, Cicero was in the habit of engaging the services of several other physicians when his slave Tiro was ill. In 53 BCE, the physician that he hired to treat Tiro is not named, but in the period 50–49 BCE, when Tiro was ill at Patrae he was left in the care of Marcus Curius, and in 45 BCE, when he was ill at Tusculum, Metrodorus.[13]

While, as far as we can tell, Cicero does not seem to have ever had a physician as a permanent member of his household, many of his contemporaries, both senators and equestrians, did.[14] Thus, we should consider the place of physicians that were formally part of a household, whether slave or freed, and other individuals that were part of the household and whose occupations were related to healthcare, likewise slave or freed, within the Roman medical marketplace. It has been suggested that members of the Roman elite who possessed personal physicians and other types of healthcare practitioner utilised their services for minor ailments while patronising an external healthcare practitioner for more serious health problems.[15] This interpretation of the role of the internal healthcare practitioner rather assumes that they would have been considered inferior to an external one, whether in respect of knowledge, skill or even experience, and this is not necessarily the case. In fact, there is evidence to suggest that individuals in possession of personal physicians and other types of healthcare practitioner actually lent or hired them out to family members, friends and acquaintances on a regular basis, or even made them readily available to the general public in cases of emergency, so clearly their abilities were not in doubt.[16]

We can gain an insight into the positions that such healthcare practitioners held in elite households in the city of Rome thanks to the epigraphic evidence of the epitaphs from *columbaria*, and perhaps attempt to establish the extent to which this was the norm for elite households, at the very least. The *familia urbana* of Livia Drusilla (later Julia Augusta) contained fifteen individuals whose epitaphs attested that their occupations were specifically related to healthcare: eight *medici* (singular *medicus* for a man, *medica* for a woman, 'physician'), two *obstetrices* (singular *obstetrix*, 'midwife'), two *ad valetudinarium* (singular *ad valetudinarium*, 'infirmarian'), one *unctrix* (a female 'anointer') and two *ad unguentum* (singular *ad unguentum*, 'maker of oil, unguents and perfumes').[17] Their titles indicate a high degree of specialisation: of the *medici*, one was the *supra medicos* ('chief physician'), another was the *medicus ocularis* ('eye physician'), a third the *medicus chirurgicus* ('surgical physician').[18] Of the two *ad valetudinarium*, one was male, the other female; their spheres of influence perhaps extended along gender lines.[19]

While it could be argued that, since Livia was the wife of the emperor Augustus and the mother of the emperor Tiberius, her household was atypical, other contemporary elite *columbaria* contain similar numbers of epitaphs attesting occupations relating to some sort of healthcare. The *familia urbana* of the Statilii family included two *medici*, one *obstetrix* and eight *unctores*, that of the Volusii family included two *medici* and one *obstetrix*, and that of the Iunii family included two *medici*. Recognising that many Roman households contained individuals whose roles within the household were specifically related to healthcare, and that these individuals were by no means lacking in knowledge, skills or experience and were even, in some cases, simultaneously operating outside the household in a professional capacity, makes it clear that the Roman household was a place where a range of healers of a variety of sorts could be found. This gives us a feasible place to start the investigation into Roman domestic medical practice, attempt to identify instances of it taking place within the historical record, and come to an understanding regarding its theory, method and practice.

As many as thirty years ago, Roy Porter observed that the history of medicine was, in actuality, the history of physicians, and that this was potentially a major historical distortion.[20] He stated that, since it takes at least two – patient and physician, but perhaps also family and community – to make a medical encounter, an alternative history of medicine written from the patient's perspective is a desideratum, although even using the term 'patient' implies professional medical relations, and so using the term 'sick person' or 'sufferer' is preferable.[21] Thus Porter proposed an alternative approach to the history of medicine: medicine from below.[22] With regard to the history of medicine in ancient Greece and Rome, medicine from below has been slow in occurring.[23] Why has this been the case? Perhaps due to a lack of what Porter denoted 'articulate sufferers'.[24] Whereas later periods of history are redolent with family archives consisting of letters, diaries and other relevant ephemera, ancient Greece and Rome are somewhat lacking. For what has been described as the 'central period' of Roman history (*circa* 200 BCE–200 CE), for articulate suffers of letters about whom we know enough to contextualise their writings we are restricted to the letters of Cicero (106–43 BCE), Lucius Annaeus Seneca (Seneca the Younger) (4 BCE–65 CE), Gaius Plinius Caecilius Secundus (Pliny the Younger) (61–113 CE) and, somewhat later, Marcus Cornelius Fronto (100–late 160s CE), although documentary evidence from the provinces of Egypt and Britain provide fascinating snapshots of individuals and their experiences in this regard.[25] Yet there is much more evidence that has the potential to be utilised in an inquiry of this type. While accessing information about any aspect of Roman domestic medical practice is far from straightforward, since the traces of it are scattered across works of ancient literature from all genres and media, and in the archaeological and bioarchaeological records, it is accessible.[26]

Medical pluralism

Medical anthropologists have long argued for the recognition of medical pluralism, that societies do not only have one healthcare system, rather they have several, and as a result, it is possible for a patient to seek a variety of different types of treatment from a variety of different types of practitioner, whether sequentially or simultaneously. While historians of medicine have certainly acknowledged the ancient world's medical pluralism, they have continued to privilege certain aspects of it.[27] To be sure, as noted above, professional physicians are easier to locate with relative precision in the historical and archaeological records: treatises written by and for them comprise the majority of surviving ancient literary evidence, inscriptions set up by or for them and documents written by or for them comprise the majority of surviving epigraphic and documentary evidence, and *instrumentaria* deposited in graves or recovered from buildings comprise the majority of archaeological evidence for the theory, method and practice of ancient Roman medicine.[28] See for example the epitaph and accompanying funerary reliefs of the married couple Scribonia Attica and Marcus Ulpius Amerimnus from the cemetery at Isola Sacra, which allow us access not only to information about their family, but also their professions, midwife and physician respectively (see Figures I.1 and I.2).[29]

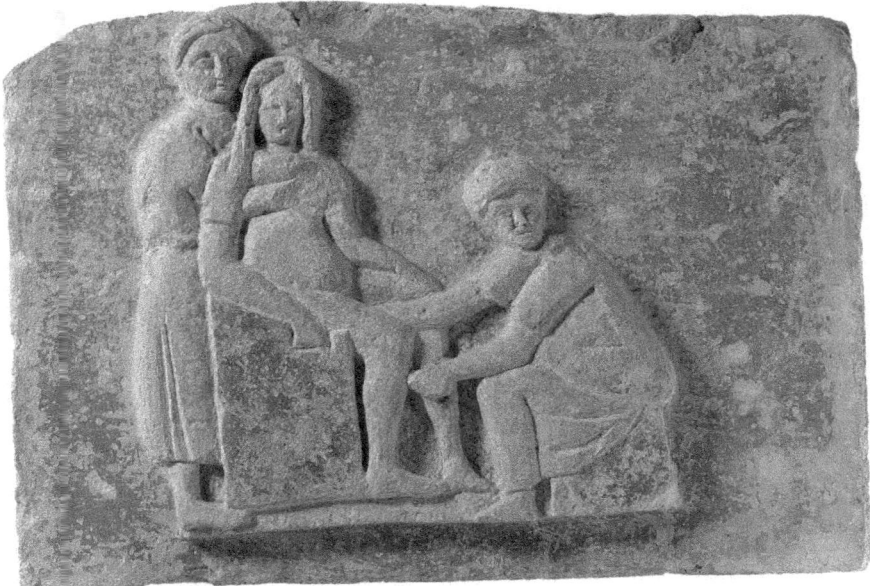

Figure I.1 The funerary relief of Scribonia Attica from Isola Sacra, Ostia, dating from the second century CE.

Source: Image courtesy of the Soprintendenza Archeologica di Ostia.

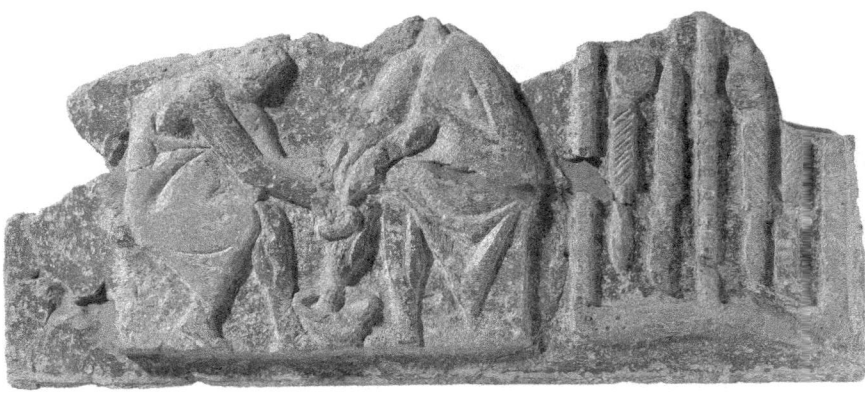

Figure I.2 The funerary relief of Marcus Ulpius Amerimnus from Isola Sacra, Ostia, dating from the second century CE.

Source: Image courtesy of the Soprintendenza Archeologica di Ostia.

Yet academics from a variety of disciplines have proposed models for coming to grips with medical pluralism. To date, two of these models have been utilised in the pursuit of furthering our understanding of the ancient medical marketplace, although I have reservations regarding the suitability of either one for ancient Rome (or ancient Greece, for that matter). The original version of the model was proposed by Arthur Kleinman, who argued that in order to understand patients and healers, it is necessary to study them in particular cultural environments.[30] He put forward a structural model of healthcare as a local cultural system comprising three overlapping parts: the popular sector, the professional sector and the folk sector.[31] In this model, the popular sector incorporates the beliefs and activities of the individual, their family, their social network and their community, and consists of the lay, non-professional, non-specialist, popular culture arena, the context within which health problems are first identified and healthcare activities are first initiated.[32] The professional sector incorporates the organised healing professions, and anyone acknowledged or perceived in a culture as belonging to a professional organisation or group.[33] The folk sector consists of the non-professional non-bureaucratic, specialist arena, its practitioners, whether sacred or secular, having little or no training in professional medicine.[34] This model was developed utilising research from contemporary China, so we do have to consider the extent to which it is appropriate for investigating medical pluralism in antiquity, or any other historical period.[35]

However, David Gentilcore has observed that in early modern Italy medical knowledge was diffused throughout society, with everyone ultimately taking responsibility for their own health, which ensured that a certain amount of medical knowledge was regarded as indispensable, although identifying the forms that this medical knowledge took is not entirely straightforward.[36] Consequently he adapted Kleinman's model and proposed an alternative, albeit one still consisting of three overlapping parts: the popular sector, the professional sector and the ecclesiastical sector.[37] In early modern Italy there were no absolute distinctions between the three sectors, although there was certainly antagonism between their practitioners, and limitations were placed on the activities of certain different types of practitioners. Steven Oberhelman has argued that a version of this model can also be utilised in the study of Greek medicine from antiquity to the twentieth century.[38] This is somewhat more appropriate to the study of Roman medicine in the late Republic and early Empire than Arthur Kleinman's, although still rather too rigidly compartmentalised.

It is certainly necessary to pay attention to the individual, both as a patient and a practitioner, and despite utilisation of binary opposition for convenience of categorisation by scholars (professional and amateur, irrational and irrational, high and low, etc.), ancient Roman healthcare defies such neat and definitive distinctions.[39] It is important to remember that if a healthcare practitioner was engaged, no matter where he or she ultimately came from, the majority of his or her healthcare practice would have been undertaken in the patient's place of residence. While this healthcare practice could have taken place under the healthcare practitioner's personal direction and supervision, it could also have been delegated to members of the patient's household, or even the patient him or herself. Additionally, a healthcare practitioner may not have been engaged at all; rather, one or more members of the household could have played this role either permanently or temporarily, as required. So, we need to consider healthcare that takes place within the household at the recommendation of a healthcare practitioner, and healthcare that takes place within the household but not at the recommendation of a healthcare practitioner. Are these two entirely distinct types of healthcare, are these two types of healthcare with considerable overlap between them or are they to all intents and purposes the same thing? Whatever definitions and categories we might attempt to superimpose upon ancient Roman domestic healthcare practitioners and their practices, the ancient Roman household is where all types of healthcare practitioner and healthcare theory, method and practice intersect, and we see ancient medical pluralism in action. Hence the ancient Roman household is where we should concentrate our attention if we hope to study ancient medicine from below. As a case in point, let us return to the scenario set out in Horace's first satire at the start of this chapter.

Regarding Horace's reference to calling in the physician, an examination of Roman domestic healthcare must certainly acknowledge the roles played by those we might describe as 'professional' healthcare practitioners, such as the physician (*medicus* or *medica*, *iatros* or *iatrinē*), the surgeon (*chirurgus*) and the midwife (*obstetrix*), where relevant. From the early third century BCE onwards, Roman imperial expansion ensured that many non-Romans came to Rome, either involuntarily as slaves or voluntarily as immigrants, and this influx had a significant impact upon healthcare both with relation to practitioners and their practices, although the precise nature of this impact is not always easy to recover in the historical or archaeological record.[40] The epitaph of Gaius Numitorius Nicanor, a freedman whose tomb has been dated to around 47–46 BCE, who states both his place of origin, Thebes, and his occupation, eye doctor (*medicus ocularius*), is unusual.[41] With regard to physicians, only around ten percent of those recorded in inscriptions prior to 100 CE were Roman citizens while over seventy-five percent were slaves or freedmen/freedwomen.[42] Consequently, many of these practitioners were attached to individual households; so while some Romans had personal physicians, surgeons and midwives who, as members of their households, were at their complete disposal, others either relied upon members of their households who were not strictly healthcare practitioners or had to seek out healthcare practitioners as and when the need arose. Depending upon one's circumstances, this might involve having to wait until an itinerant physician happened to be in the area rather than actively seeking one out.[43] We might expect Maecenas, if it is indeed him and his household that Horace is describing, to possess one or more personal physicians as part of his *familia urbana*, as other members of the wealthy senatorial and equestrian elite such as Livia did, yet as we have seen Cicero, clearly somewhat less wealthy than either Maecenas or Livia, did not.[44]

Additionally, regarding Horace's reference to lotions (plural *fomenta*, singular *fomentum*), an examination of Roman healthcare must certainly acknowledge the roles played by what we might describe as medical paraphernalia such as drugs and instruments, although when such items were being utilised for medical practice specifically, as opposed to other domestic purposes, is difficult to identify or even define precisely, whether they are referred to in the literary record or recovered in the archaeological record. A *fomentum* was a warm application such as a poultice, so was presumably prepared, or at least heated up, on the spot. It was, however, a medicament, that is, a substance used for medical treatment. The Latin terms *medicamentum* and *medicamen*, like the Greek *pharmakon*, can be translated as 'a substance administered or applied to produce specific effects upon the body'.[45] Natural substances were utilised because of their perceived properties (for example, hot, cold, wet, dry, etc.), and these properties could be utilised for a variety of purposes. Consequently, they could be used in positive ways or negative ways depending on the context, and such items could be purchased ready-made from a 'professional' healthcare practitioner such as a pharmacist (*seplasarius*), an unguent seller (*unguentarius*) or cosmetic seller (*cosmeticus*) or produced within the household.[46] Likewise, it is difficult to differentiate between instruments used for medical purposes and instruments used for other purposes.[47] It is necessary to consider the context in which these so-called 'drugs' and 'instruments' were being used; while a household might well possess a selection of lotions, ointments and oils that had been either made on the premises or acquired elsewhere, many ordinary foodstuffs were considered to have medicinal properties and could be pressed into service as simple or compound remedies if the need arose, and many medical instruments could double as cosmetic implements, or vice versa (see Figures I.3 and I.4).

Even in cases where the medicinal purpose of an artefact is unequivocal, such as a bronze medicine chest decorated with images of the Graeco-Roman healing

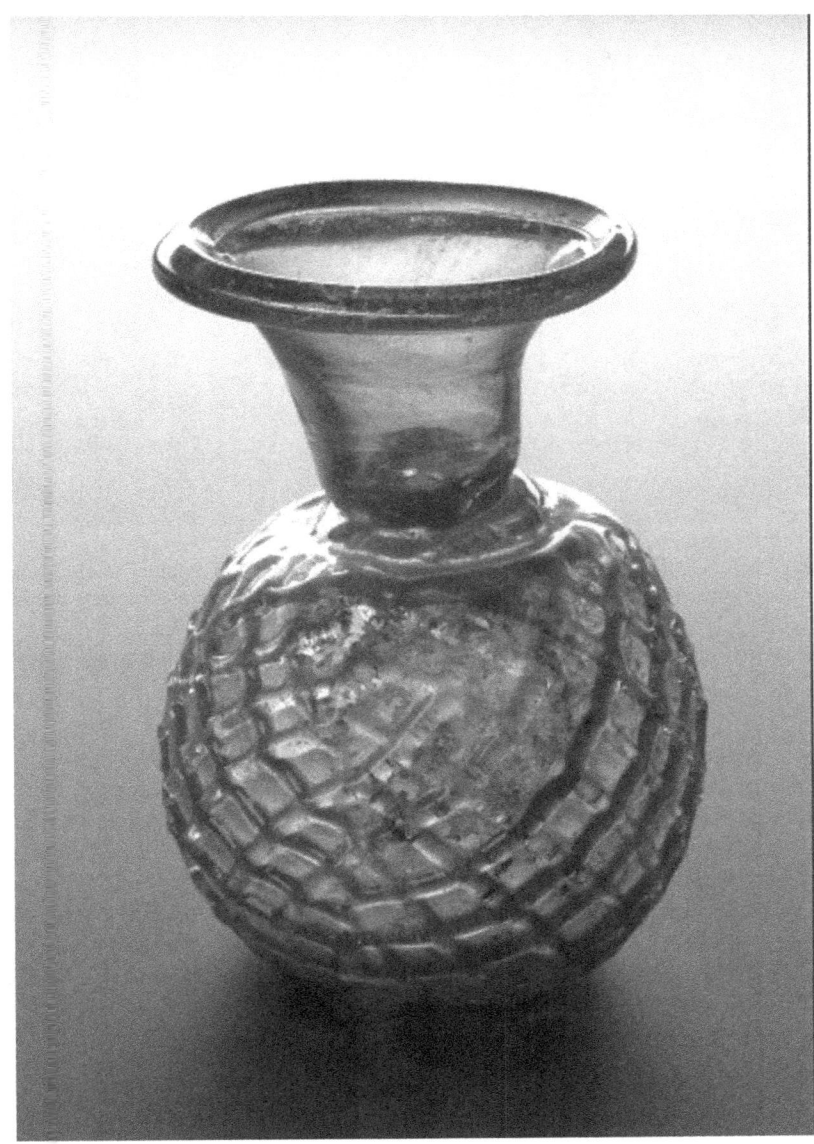

Figure I.3 A glass bottle that contained expensive oils that could be used for either medical or cosmetic purposes, *circa* 100–500 CE.

Source: Image courtesy of the Wellcome Library (Wellcome Collection/Science Museum inv. A608633).

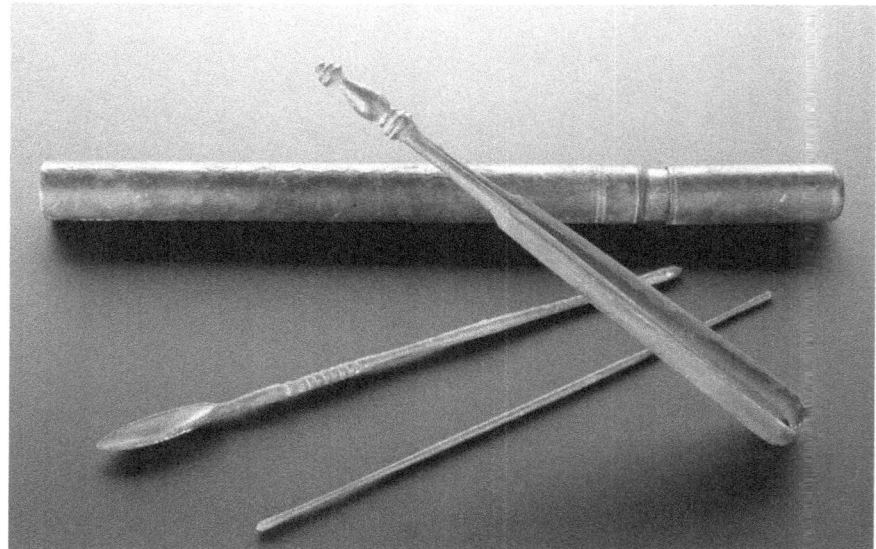

Figure I.4 A set of instruments; copies of items recovered from Pompeii and currently
        housed in the Naples National Archaeological Museum and dating from the
        first century CE.

Source: Image courtesy of the Wellcome Library (Wellcome Collection/Science Museum inv. A156172).

deities Asklepios/Aesculapius and Hygieia/Salus, or the rod of Asklepios/Aescu-
lapius (see Figure I.5), it is necessary to consider whether good-quality medical
equipment found in a domestic context is indicative of the activities of a high
status and wealthy individual taking an active interest in medical practice, or a
physician who is extremely successful or wishes to appear so.[48]

We should bear in mind the potential inherent ambiguity of domestic medical
knowledge: like other types of medical knowledge, it could be used to heal or to
harm, and those who were in possession of it could put themselves at risk by exercising it, particularly if they were women or slaves (whether male or female).[49]

Evidence

So, this is not a study of ancient medicine but rather one of ancient healthcare.
I will argue that concerns over ensuring the acquisition and maintenance of good
health and well-being informed and influenced a considerable amount of daily life
in ancient Rome and the cities and towns of central Italy. My focus, therefore, is
not on the physician but rather on everyone else, the subject under investigation
not the physician's theories, methods and practices but rather, as far as is possible, those of the ordinary person, whether that person was old or young, male

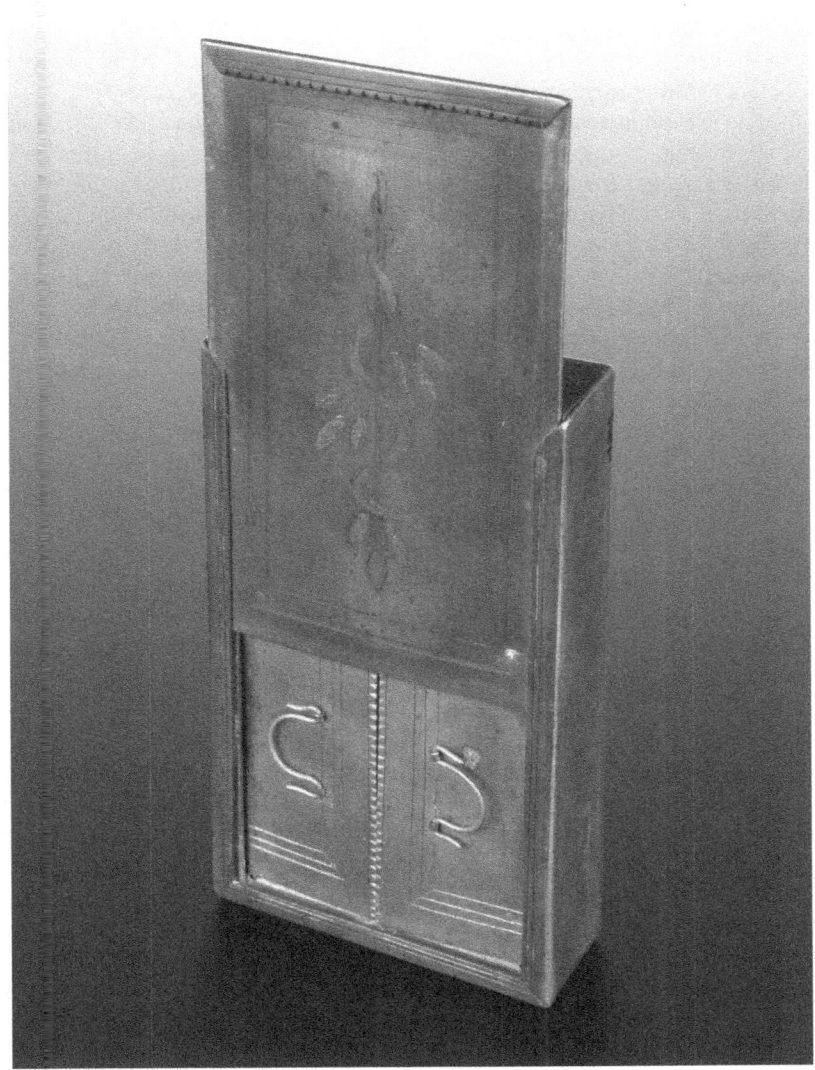

Figure 1.5 A bronze medical kit depicting the rod of Aesculapius; a copy of an item recovered from Pompeii and currently housed in the Naples National Archaeological Museum and dating from the first century CE.

or female, freeborn, freed or slave, senatorial, equestrian, decurion or plebeian, Roman, provincial or other. I will follow the 'mosaicist approach' initially pioneered by historians of culture and excavate information from the extant Latin (and, to a lesser extent, Greek) literary, documentary, archaeological and bioarchaeological evidence, and synthesise information from a variety of different academic disciplines in an attempt to offer a holistic view of this particular aspect of ancient Roman society and culture that is accessible both to ancient historians and to scholars working in other academic disciplines.[50]

Since no surviving ancient treatise contains a detailed explanation of the tenets of ancient Roman domestic healthcare theory, method and practice, it is poorly understood as a social and cultural practice, but this poor understanding can be rectified somewhat if we expand the scope of our investigation and turn our attention away from ancient medical literature and towards other literary genres, while also incorporating other types of evidence such as the documentary, archaeological and bioarchaeological.[51] This is certainly easier for some contexts than for others, such as, for example, Egypt during the Roman period.[52] However, the problematic nature of the evidence for the period from the early first century BCE to the late first century CE necessitates this, as with regard to ancient medical texts written in Latin, only the works of Aulus Cornelius Celsus (*circa* 25 BCE–50 CE), Scribonius Largus (*circa* 1–50 CE) and Gaius Plinius Secundus (Pliny the Elder) (23–79 CE) survive from this period, and these are not necessarily representative of what was going on in households across central Italy (although, in actual fact, they might well be).[53] Just as it is difficult to ascertain what sources ancient medical writers had access to, it is difficult to ascertain what sources everyone else had access to. I shall argue that it is vital to widen the scope of our attention from sickness and therapeutics to health and prevention: as will become clear, concerns over the acquisition and maintenance of good health and well-being were woven into the very fabric of ancient Roman daily life.

Documentary evidence such as epigraphy, *graffiti* and *dipinti* can offer an insight into the sort of economic, social and familial networks that are infrequently or perhaps never mentioned in ancient literature. Inscriptions such as honorific dedications and epitaphs can facilitate a certain amount of reconstruction of the lives of freeborn, freed and slave members of society, while *graffiti* and *dipinti* cannot only do likewise, but also provide access to momentary thoughts, preoccupations and opinions. While ancient literature often records the names of the personal physicians to significant members of the Roman elite, other less illustrious members of the household staff might only be attested in epitaphs in *columbaria*, and others less illustrious still might only attested by the chance survival of one inscription, such as, for example, the otherwise unknown resin worker or seed seller.[54] Yet all these individuals played an important role in the Roman medical marketplace. While admittedly it can be difficult to contextualise random isolated inscriptions beyond attempting to date the style of the letters, and as far as numbers are concerned there is a significant bias in favour of the city of Rome, their contents can illuminate aspects of the medical marketplace otherwise unattested in ancient literature, such as, for example, the frequency with which female physicians were operating in Rome during the late Republic and early Empire.[55] *Graffti* and *dipinti* are somewhat more problematic, due to the relatively recent interest in them and the debate over how to approach them.[56] While examples of both are found throughout the ancient world, as far as numbers are concerned there is a significant bias in favour of Pompeii due to the peculiar nature of the preservation of that site. Yet they can attest behaviour, practices and incidents otherwise unrecorded, such as, for example, the fact that an individual named Chie suffered from painful haemorrhoids.[57]

Archaeological evidence can offer an insight into the day-to-day existence of all levels of ancient society. Particularly useful here are the remnants of buildings, whether residential or industrial, or both simultaneously, and their contents from sites such as Rome, Ostia, Pompeii, Herculaneum and other locations around the Bay of Naples. While it is debatable how representative of Roman society as a whole any of these sites are, they are certainly a useful starting point in any attempt to understand certain aspects of daily life. The ancient literary evidence for housing is biased in favour of the elite and focuses predominantly on imperial, senatorial, equestrian and decurion residences, and while other types of urban and rural residences are described, these descriptions are somewhat manufactured for literary effect. While concerns have been raised over relying on a small selection of sites, the sheer variety of ancient Roman residences found in these places can offer a wide range of information, as can the artefact assemblages often recovered from them, such as medical and surgical instruments, and storage containers and their contents.

Bioarchaeological evidence such as human skeletal remains has the potential to provide extremely detailed information about people and their behaviour through macroscopic, microscopic and chemical analyses.[58] While the remains of specific individuals enable the compilation of osteobiographies and the creation of detailed life stories, sets of remains present the opportunity to track more general trends.[59] Although bioarchaeology is a relatively new development in archaeology it can facilitate understanding of demography, health status and dietary regimes, as well as issues such as migration and urban and rural life.[60] Other types of bioarchaeological evidence such as animal skeletal remains and organic remains such as plants, seeds and pollen are similarly informative not just about diet but also about living situations and the practice of agriculture, horticulture, apiculture and animal husbandry.

Context

This study will concentrate on central Italy – predominantly the city of Rome and the towns of Ostia, Pompeii and Herculaneum – and focus primarily, but not exclusively, on the period from the early first century BCE to the late first century CE. Developments in social and cultural history are harder to pin down precisely than those in political history, so there will be some reference made to evidence spanning the slightly wider chronological period from the early second century BCE to the late second century CE. I have chosen these parameters for two reasons. The first is the sheer amount and variety of evidence that can be utilised in pursuit of information on all aspects of daily life, but particularly healthcare, in this region during this period, thus enabling and facilitating a 'mosaicist' approach. The second is that this region during this period saw a considerable amount of political, social and economic change which had serious ramifications for healthcare. Imperial expansion around the Mediterranean, particularly in Greece and Egypt, saw a huge influx of new people and products into Roman territory.[61] Increasing urbanisation saw a change from agricultural to commercial activities, greater social mobility and the rise of what has been described as 'a multilayered urban society that stood economically between the rich and the poor'.[62]

For sake of ease, the Roman social hierarchy during the Principate has frequently been represented as a pyramid, although despite this, scholars have tended to approach ancient Roman society as if it were polarised between an upper class (senators, equestrians and decurions) and a lower class (plebeians), with little in the way of a middle class.[63] This has had serious ramifications for the study of daily life, particularly issues relating to health and well-being, due to its fostering of the belief that the vast majority of ancient Romans lived at or below subsistence level.[64] However, recent studies have argued that there was, in fact, a considerable middle class, at least in urban settlements.[65] Roman wages were relatively generous and consumers were in a position to exercise choice when making their purchases.[66] These wages were also frequently supplemented by allowances of foodstuffs.[67] This greater distribution of wealth was compounded by social welfare benefits such as the distribution of grain during the Republic and additional commodities such as wine, olive oil and pork in the Principate, as well as occasional gifts and relief from rent and even debts.[68]

If the majority of ancient Romans living in urban areas were better off financially than has previously been recognised, this means that they had a larger disposable income and by implication more purchasing power. As a result, they would have been able to exercise a certain amount of choice with regard to their expenditure, which could affect a variety of aspects of their daily lives that would have impacted either positively or negatively upon their state of health and well-being. They could exercise a certain amount of choice regarding where and how they lived, in the foodstuffs that they consumed and the leisure activities they engaged in. Thus this monograph starts from the premise that Romans from the senatorial, equestrian, decurion and plebeian orders not only cared about acquiring and maintaining good health and well-being, but also that they knew what was necessary to do so, and as a result were significantly more able to do so than has often been assumed.[69] Consequently, Romans were potentially healthier – or at the very least, more interested in the possibility of being healthier – than the majority of scholars have so far given them credit for being.

It is difficult to gauge precisely how healthy the inhabitants of an ancient Roman city or town, particularly the city of Rome itself, were as the evidence is unsatisfactory and contradictory.[70] Depending upon the different types of evidence that are utilised, different conclusions are drawn.[71] Ancient writers observed that people living in urban environments tended to be less healthy than those living in rural environments.[72] However, there is a tendency for studies of health in ancient Rome to be overwhelmingly negative regarding life expectancy, nutrition and hygiene.[73] The life expectancy of the average Roman is assumed to have been low, around twenty to thirty years.[74] There are, however, problems with these estimates due to the fragmentary nature of the evidence utilised.[75] There is also dissent regarding using them, and it has been suggested that a comparative approach that utilises living standards in other historical periods could be more informative.[76]

The study of human skeletal remains and the use of anthropometric data can be used to calculate the mean heights of particular Roman populations, and since height is considered to serve as a barometer of overall health this is potentially very useful for assessing the living standards of ancient Romans.[77] While studies have shown that Roman Italians seem to have been shorter than Italians of either the Iron Age or the Medieval periods, and heights seem to have stagnated somewhat over the course of the Roman period, the inhabitants of Roman Italy had a mean height of over 168 centimetres, indicating good diet and nutrition.[78] Studies focussed on specific areas have been even more precise. At Rome, the mean height was 168.1 centimetres.[79] At Herculaneum, the mean height of men was 169.1 centimetres and the mean height of women was 155.2 centimetres.[80] At Pompeii, the mean height of men was 167.6 centimetres and the mean height of women was 154.7 centimetres.[81] Thus the ancient inhabitants of Pompeii and Herculaneum were slightly taller than contemporary Neapolitans.[82] However, we do need to take care when drawing conclusions based on such specific geographical locations, as the people of Rome, Pompeii and Herculaneum were not necessarily the norm; Pompeii and Herculaneum were particularly privileged due to their situation on the Bay of Naples.[83]

Stable isotope analysis can provide information about paleodiet, and cemetery populations from Rome (Casal Bertone, Castelaccio Europarco, Saint Callixtus, Saints Peter and Marcellinus), Isola Sacra, Velia and Gabii have offered insights not only into the diets of the wealthy elite but also into the diets of other social groups. The implications of this type of bioarchaeological evidence with regards to diet and standards of nutrition are supported by archaeobotanical evidence. Beyond the city of Rome, Roman Latium and Campania were both politically and culturally important in the late Republic and early Principate, so it is not surprising to find them frequently mentioned in the ancient literary evidence produced during this period. Campania was considered to be the most agriculturally fertile region of Italy, although a range of foodstuffs were imported through the port at Puteoli as well.[84] The ancient literary, documentary and archaeological evidence indicate that these regions were focused on market-oriented intensive mixed agriculture, viticulture and arboriculture, and that farming practices were sophisticated and productive. Yet scholars have focussed on reconstructing the diets of the elite and neglected the diets of the rest of the population.[85] However, since Roman farmers seem to have achieved high levels of productivity and produced large surpluses of agricultural produce, it is necessary to factor their success into any discussion of diet. It is often assumed that the standard Roman diet was predominantly vegetarian, but there is a significant amount of evidence for the consumption of meat, fish, game and dairy products, as well as fruits and vegetables.[86] Since people were affluent and staple foodstuffs were cheap, they had more money to spend on products considered luxurious and exotic, such as pepper.[87]

The physical remains of a wide range of foodstuffs have been recovered from Pompeii, Herculaneum and other sites around the Bay of Naples, and indicate that diet in these places was extremely diverse.[88] Herculaneum's Cardo V sewer has been excavated and its contents, the waste from the apartments and shops housed in the Insula Orientalis II, have been analysed.[89] On the ground floor of the Insula Orientalis II were a *taberna*, a wine shop, a bakery and a gem workshop, and the tenants of these shops lived behind and above them. On the upper floors were more apartments. One hundred and fourteen different foodstuffs have been identified, with varying amounts of each.[90] It would appear that the occupants of the Insula Orientalis II enjoyed a diet comprising a few staple foods supplemented by a wide variety of fruits, nuts, seasonings and seafood. Consequently, the middle- and lower-class inhabitants of Herculaneum were eating a more varied, and more expensive, diet than we might have expected.[91]

Structure

In the first chapter, Health and Well-being in the Roman Republic and Principate, I shall investigate not only what, exactly, the Romans perceived health and well-being to be, but also how they sought to acquire it and subsequently maintain it in their daily lives. I shall explore the ancient concept of regimen – diet, physical and mental exercise, personal hygiene – as a means of attaining, ensuring and preserving good health and well-being. I shall assess the accessibility of regimen to social orders other than the senatorial, equestrian and decurion elite through the examination of ancient literary, documentary, archaeological and bioarchaeological evidence. I shall argue that health was considerably more important to the majority of Romans than has heretofore been acknowledged, and in some respects the means of acquiring and maintaining it were more accessible to many of them than has previously been considered to be the case.

In the second chapter, The Roman House and Garden, I shall survey the different types of Roman residence and examine the role that the house played and was perceived to play in the acquisition and maintenance of health and well-being. This includes the location, design and layout of the residence, the facilities and amenities of the residence and the ways in which residents utilised the residence. I shall then focus on one particular – and arguably highly significant – part of the Roman residence, surveying the different types of Roman garden and examining the role that the garden played and was perceived to play in the acquisition, maintenance and preservation of health and well-being. This includes the location, design and layout of the garden, the facilities and amenities of the garden and the ways in which residents utilised the garden. Just as domestic spaces were key sites in the medical marketplace, so were green spaces key sites within domestic spaces, and they provided room for a variety of individual practitioners and a multiplicity of activities related to all aspects of healthcare.

In the third chapter, The Roman Household, I shall build on the findings of the first and second chapters and start from the premise that health was a fundamental concern of the members of the household, as the good health and well-being of the members of the household was necessary if the household was to be as self-sufficient and productive as possible. Consequently, a range of concerns relating to it were factored in to the running of the household. In this chapter, I shall survey the members of the Roman household and examine the roles that each played in the acquisition, maintenance and preservation of good health and well-being. I shall focus particularly on the *pater familias* and the *mater familias*, and their proxies, the estate manager and the housekeeper, as well as consider the contributions of other slave, freed and freeborn members of the household.

Finally, in the fourth chapter, The Transmission of Medical Knowledge, I shall investigate how beliefs, theories and practices relating to the acquisition, maintenance and preservation of health and well-being were acquired, developed and transmitted by members of the Roman household, their friends and their acquaintances. I shall explore transmission through literary means such as the reading of and listening to works of literature, methods of oral communication such as advice, rumour and gossip, and through personal experience such as informal and formal education and training, and socialisation. I shall also consider the fundamental ambiguity of knowledge related to healthcare, with its potential to cure or to kill, and the way that this affected both domestic medical practice, and the way that the Romans perceived domestic medical practice, particularly in relation to female and slave members of the household, and power dynamics. I shall conclude that healthcare knowledge was transmitted between members of the household at all levels and in all directions, rather than simply from the top down, with the *pater familias* dictating, as has often been assumed.

There is one last point to make before we commence, however, and that is that there is an obvious fly in the ointment regarding any discussion of health in antiquity: what the ancients considered to be healthy and unhealthy, and how they recommended ensuring and maintaining good health, were based upon an understanding of the human body and its physiology that is entirely different from the one that we have today. How far does this matter in our attempt to reconstruct attitudes towards health in the Roman Republic and Principate? Not necessarily at all, if our focus is on the ancient Roman individual. If he or she was, as far as he or she was concerned, behaving in a way that was thought to guarantee good health, then he or she was, by the standards of the day, healthy, and it would be somewhat anachronistic to superimpose our contemporary understanding of good health over this and make a judgement to the contrary.

Ultimately, with this monograph I aim to address the concerns of Graf and Harris, open up a new area of study in Roman medicine, and in doing so make a significant contribution to the social and cultural history of the Roman Republic and Empire, and to the medical history of the ancient world.

Notes

1 Horace, *Satires* 1.1.80–83 (trans. H. Rushton Fairclough): *At si condoluit tentatum frigore corpus aut alius casus lecto te adflixit, habes qui adsideat, fomenta pare_ medicum roget, ut te suscitet ac reddat gnatis carisque propinquis?*
2 See Knapp, 1914 for detailed discussion of this satire.
3 Graf, 2006, p. 3.
4 Harris, 2016a, p. vii.
5 Harris, 2016b, p. 36.
6 Bivins et al., 2016, p. 671. In point of fact, Huebner, 2017, p. 3 calls for an increase in comparative work on the Mediterranean household and family through the ancient, medieval and early modern periods as a means of 'mending the academic fragmentation of a subject split between so many different disciplines'.
7 Jackson, 2008, pp. 3–5.
8 Nutton, 1992. That is not to say that this approach to ancient medicine has been adopted uncritically; the concept of the 'medical marketplace' has been criticised as being anachronistic and based on Thatcherite ideas about the market economy, see King, 1997, p. 89. One exception to this general rule of neglect of ancient domestic medical practice and an aspect of ancient medicine that has received a considerable amount of attention from scholars is the relationship between ancient Greek domestic medical practice and the recipes contained in the gynaecological treatises of the Hippocratic Corpus, which are viewed as preserving Greek traditions of healing passed down orally from generation to generation. See Hanson, 1991, 1992; King, 1995, 1998; Totelin, 2009, on this.
9 Harris, 2016b, p. vii, pp. 5–6.
10 For general overviews of ancient Greek and Roman medicine, see for example Nutton, 2013; Cruse, 2004; Jackson, 1988; Scarborough, 1969. While the extent to which it is appropriate to refer to ancient medicine as a 'profession' and ancient medical practitioners as 'professionals' is much debated, by the early imperial period it would appear that both were common parlance in Latin discussions on the subject. See for example Celsus, *On Medicine* Preface 11 (the earliest surviving use of the terms); Scribonius Largus, *Compositions* 17; see also, later, *Digest* 2.13.19.
11 For discussion, see Garland, 1992, p. 166. Varro, *On Agriculture* 1.16.4 states that in rural areas some men prefer to have a standing arrangement with a physician in their neighbourhood rather than have a physician in their household.
12 Cicero, *Letters to Atticus* 377 (15.1) (trans. D. Shackleton Bailey): *Amorem erga me, humanitatem suavitatemque desidero.*
13 Marcus Curius: Cicero, *Letters to Atticus* 125 (7.2), 126 (7.4), 186 (9.17); Metrodorus: Cicero, *Letters to Friends* 220 (16.20).
14 See for example Julius Caesar: Suetonius, *Divine Julius Caesar* 4; Piso: Cicero, *On the Responses of the Haruspices* 35, *Against Piso* 83; Cato the Younger: Plutarch, *Cato the Younger* 70.2; Verres: Cicero, *Verrine Orations* 2 3.54; Antony: Cassius Dio, *Roman History* 53.30, Horace, *Epistles* 1.15.3; Antyllus: Plutarch, *Antony* 28.
15 Treggiari, 1975b, p. 56.
16 *Digest* 38.1.27. See also cases in Cicero, *In Defence of Cluentius* 178; Pliny the Elder, *Natural History* 28.18.67; Tacitus, *Annals* 6.50. See Mouritsen, 2011, pp. 224–227 with specific reference to the *operae* of freedmen who were physicians by trade. See Hasegawa, 2005, p. 50 for the suggestion that elite households contained and monopolised skills and products that were not readily accessible to the general public, but on occasion placed these at the disposal of the public, such as during the aftermath of the amphitheatre collapse at Fidenae in 27 CE, Tacitus, *Annals* 4.62–63 and Suetonius, *Tiberius* 40.
17 Hasegawa, 2005, pp. 38–39; Treggiari, 1975b, pp. 55–56.

18 *Supra Medicos*: *CIL* VI 3982; *Medicus Ocularis*: *CIL* VI 3987; *Medicus Chirurgicus*: *CIL* VI 3986.
19 *CIL* VI 9084, 9085.
20 Porter, 1985a, p. 175.
21 Porter, 1985a, pp. 181–182.
22 This was subsequently put into practice in Porter, 1985b.
23 See also King, 1995, p. 135 for a succinct summary of the problems one encounters when attempting to uncover the ancient patient's perspective. Only very recently, with Israelowich, 2015; Petridou and Thumiger, 2016, have studies in ancient medical history begun to focus their attention explicitly on the patient, but there is still a considerable amount of work to be done in this area.
24 Porter, 1985a, pp. 176–181.
25 On ancient epistolography see Morello and Morrison, 2007. Additionally, Publius Aelius Aristides Theodorus (117–181 CE) offers numerous insights into his health problems over the course of his *Sacred Tales*.
26 Harris, 2016a, p. vii.
27 For the most recent and the most comprehensive survey by far of medicine in Graeco-Roman antiquity see Nutton, 2013. The apparent necessity of privileging certain types of ancient medical theory, method and practice is discussed at the outset, at pp. 1–2.
28 For ancient Greek medical literature, see the *Corpus Medicorum Graecorum*: http://cmg.bbaw.de/publications/publikationen-cmg (accessed July 2018); for Latin medical literature, see the *Corpus Medicorum Latinorum*: http://cmg.bbaw.de/publications/publikationen-cml (accessed July 2018); for epigraphic evidence, see Samama, 2003; for documentary evidence, see *Cedopal*: http://web.philo.ulg.ac.be/cedopal/medicine-in-graeco-roman-egypt/ (accessed July 2018); for archaeological evidence, see Baker, 2013.
29 D'Ambra, 2006.
30 Kleinman, 1980, p. 8. For the possibilities of applying medical anthropological approaches to the history and archaeology of medicine, see Hsu, 2002. For the possibilities of applying medical anthropological approaches to the introduction of Greek medicine to Rome, see Nijhuis, 1995.
31 Kleinman, 1980, pp. 49–50. For a nuanced discussion of the relationship between Hippocratic medicine and folk medicine in ancient Greece, see McNamara, 2003–2004; see also Gordon, 1995.
32 Kleinman, 1980, p. 50.
33 Kleinman, 1980, p. 53.
34 Kleinman, 1980, p. 59.
35 This is discussed by Oberhelman, 2013, p. 5; Israelowich, 2015, adopts this approach.
36 Centilcore, 1998, p. 6.
37 Centilcore, 1998, pp. 22–23.
38 Oberhelman, 2013, pp. 5–6.
39 See for example Riddle, 1996.
40 On the introduction of Greek healthcare to Rome, see Nijhuis, 1995. For migration to the city of Rome, see Tacoma, 2016; Noy, 2000. For forced migration, see Webster, 2010. For medical knowledge following commercial routes around the ancient Mediterranean from prehistory onwards, see Totelin, 2009, p. 189.
41 *AE* 1972 14; see discussion of this issue in Noy, 2010, p. 15.
42 For inscriptions that mention physicians, see Nutton, 1992, pp. 38–39. For inscriptions that mention midwives, see Laes, 2010, pp. 280–284. For inscriptions that mention female physicians and midwives and a discussion of the difference between them, see Parker, 1997.
43 With regard to itinerant physicians, see for example the Lucius Clodius discussed in Cicero, *In Defense of Cluentius* 14. Possible locations for medical practice outside the

home include surgeries, bath-houses and forts; see De Carolis, 2009; Baykan, 2008; Künzl, 1983.

44 Treggiari, 1975b, p. 56.

45 On the meaning of the terms '*pharmakon*' and '*medicamen*', see Artelt, 1968; On the drugs trade and its complexities, see Nutton, 1985; Horstmanshoff, 1999; Retief and Cilliers, 2000.

46 Totelin, 2016; Brun, 2000; Korpela, 1995.

47 Baker, 2004; Bliquez, 2015, p. 109, p. 120.

48 See Martial, *Epigrams* 14.68 for the suggestion of giving someone a medicine chest as a gift; see Lucian, *The Ignorant Book Collector* 29 for the suggestion that certain physicians used gold and silver instruments in an attempt to seem more competent than they actually were.

49 For further discussion of the potential dangers of possessing medical knowledge, see Chapter 4, The Transmission of Medical Knowledge.

50 See Barton 1995; Olson, 2008 for the successful application of a 'mosaicist approach' to certain aspects of ancient Roman social and cultural history.

51 Draycott, 2016; Hillman, 2004, p. 2 on pharmacy in the Roman Republic and Principate; see also Baker, 2002, 2013, for comprehensive instructions on the appropriate use of archaeology by medical historians.

52 Marganne-Mélard, 1996; Hirt Raj, 2006; Draycott, 2012.

53 For a comprehensive summary of surviving medical literature written in Latin, see Langslow, 2000.

54 See for example *CIL* VI 9855, a resin worker from Rome who constructed a tomb for her family; *CIL* XIV 2850, a seed seller from the Porta Triumphalis in Rome who dedicated an inscription to Fortuna at Praeneste.

55 Parker, 1997; Flemming, 2000, pp. 383–391, 2007; Parker, 2012.

56 Baird and Taylor, 2011.

57 *CIL* IV 1820.

58 See Killgrove, 2013 for an overview of Roman bioarchaeology.

59 See for example the osteobiographies of a set of individuals from Herculaneum, at Bisel and Bisel, 2002.

60 For a general survey of the use of osteoarchaeology in classical archaeology, see Mackinnon, 2007.

61 Wallace-Hadrill, 2008.

62 Mayer, 2012, p. 24.

63 Alföldy, 1984, p. 125, 1986, pp. 78–81.

64 See for example Garnsey, 1998, pp. 226–227.

65 Mayer, 2012; Kron, 2014; Scheidel, 2007 for the argument that there was a temporary redistribution of wealth and consequent increase in consumption in the late Republic and early Principate that faltered toward the end of the first century CE.

66 Ray, 2016; Holleran, 2012.

67 Kron, 2014, pp. 126–128. See as a case study the skilled and unskilled workers at Mons Claudianus and Mons Porphyrites in the Eastern Desert of Egypt, at Cuvigny, 1996.

68 Lo Cascio, 1999; Prell, 1997; Erdkamp, 2005.

69 For negative impressions of health in ancient Rome, see Scobie, 1986; Scheidel, 2003; Morley, 2005.

70 Morley, 2005, pp. 192–194.

71 For a recent survey, see Gowland and Garnsey, 2010.

72 Celsus, *On Medicine* 1.2; on urban pollution, see Nutton, 2000; on the relationship between environment and disease, see Horden and Purcell, 2000; on urban and rural mortality differentials, see Woods, 2003.

73 Scobie, 1986.

74 Hopkins, 1966, 1983; Parkin, 1992; Scheidel, 2001a, 2001b; de Ligt and Northwood, 2008; Holleran and Pudsey, 2011.

75 This is acknowledged by Hopkins, 1966; Parkin, 1992, pp. 67–90; Scheidel, 2001a, 2001b.

76 Lo Cascio, 2006; Kron, 2012.

77 There are disagreements regarding which are the best methodologies to utilise for this type of study, see Giannecchini and Moggi-Cecchi, 2008 for discussion of the best way to obtain reliable data from Italian archaeological samples.

78 Giannecchini and Moggi-Cecchi, 2008, pp. 288–289, compare the Romans to the peoples of the Iron Age and the Medieval period; Köpke and Baten, 2003 observes stagnation over the course of two millennia; Borgognini Tarli and Mazzotta, 1986 and Kron, 2005 argue for a mean height of over 168 centimetres indicating good health and nutrition; this was disputed by Scheidel, 2012, p. 327, which stated a mean height of 164 centimetres for males was preferable.

79 Catalano and Minozzi, 2001.

80 Bisel and Bisel, 2002, p. 455; Bisel, 1988.

81 Lazer, 2008, 2016.

82 Lazer, 2008, pp. 182–183.

83 Rowan, 2016, p. 117.

84 Cato the Elder, *On Agriculture* 8; Strabo, *Geography* 5.4.3; Columella, *On Agriculture* 2.10.18, 8.8.8; Pliny the Elder, *Natural History* 18.76–77, Pliny in particular includes a lot of information about Campania in the *Natural History*, mentioning varieties of food and food consumption practices on a number of occasions.

85 André, 1981; Dalby, 2000.

86 Kron, forthcoming.

87 Miller, 1969; pepper is attested 482 times in ancient literature, see Thüry and Walter, 1997, pp. 36–39.

88 Borgongino, 2006; Jashemski and Meyer, 2002.

89 Rowan, 2014; Robinson and Rowan, 2015.

90 Rowan, 2016.

91 This can be compared with the archaeobotanical evidence recovered from the middle-class housing at Pompeii, at Ciaraldi, 2007.

1   Health and well-being in the Roman Republic and Principate

Introduction

> He had always had a sneer for the arts of the physicians, and for men who, after thirty years of life, needed the counsel of a stranger in order to distinguish things salutary to their system from things deleterious.[1]

Publius Cornelius Tacitus, in his *Annals*, recounts the events of the final year of the life of Tiberius Caesar in which the seventy-eight-year-old emperor attempted to disguise his failing health by continuing to behave as he had always done, 'striving to make endurance pass for strength'.[2] While this dissimilation was initially successful, the true state of his health was eventually detected by the physician Charicles, who tricked Tiberius into allowing him to check his pulse.[3] Tacitus states that Charicles was not Tiberius' physician since the emperor had no use for physicians, although whether this was out of disbelief in medicine or distrust of its practitioners – a distrust that does not seem to have been unreasonable under the circumstances – is unclear.[4] Rather, Charicles seems to have been keen to acquire Tiberius' patronage, as he was 'accustomed not to treat the illnesses of the emperor but to offer him opportunities of consulting him'.[5] It would seem that Tiberius, at the advanced age of seventy-eight, felt that he was in a position to monitor his own health and well-being without assistance.[6] According to Gaius Suetonius Tranquillus, this was something that he had apparently been doing since he was thirty years old.[7] Assuming that this story is true, and Tiberius spent almost fifty years taking care of himself without recourse to physicians despite them making no shortage of attempts to solicit him, what was his motivation? It is possible that he inherited his mother Livia's interest in healthy living, but equally his decision to take care of himself could have been rooted in a desire to minimise the chance of information about his health circulating without his express permission, and to avoid relinquishing control of himself to others that he did not necessarily trust.[8]

How typical was Tiberius in this respect? Granted, he was an emperor, and a famously paranoid one with a family whose members were frequently accused of poisoning each other, but similar sentiments are expressed in contemporaneous works of literature. Seneca the Younger (4 BCE–65 CE), himself asthmatic, states that everyone is an authority on the defects of their own body.[9] Pliny the Elder (23–79 CE) opines that everyone (he means Romans) should know what is necessary to maintain their own health and well-being.[10] Plutarch (46–120 CE) went to considerable effort to organise his thoughts on the matter, authoring a treatise entitled *Advice on Keeping Well*:

> Each person ought neither to be unacquainted with the peculiarities of his own pulse (for there are many individual diversities), nor ignorant of any idiosyncrasy which his body has in regard to temperature and dryness, and what things in actual practice have proved to be beneficial or detrimental to it. For the man has no perception regarding himself, and is but a blind and deaf tenant in his own body, who gets his knowledge of these matters from another, and must inquire of his physician whether his health is better in summer or winter, whether he can more easily tolerate liquid or solid foods, and whether his pulse is naturally fast or slow. For it is useful and easy for us to know things of this sort, since we have daily experience and association with them.[11]

It has been observed that moralising rhetoric pervaded the habits of thought of the writers of nearly all the works of Roman literature that survive from antiquity, with vices seen as manifestations of self-indulgence and a lack of self-control.[12] The social elite rationalised their privileged position with reference to their superior morals as their self-control justified their control over the rest of Roman society, since the members of the lower orders were less able to control themselves, and they aimed to set an example for their peers to emulate and surpass, and the lower orders to follow. The focus on self-sufficiency and self-control demonstrated by figures such as Tiberius and espoused by writers such as Seneca, Pliny and Plutarch implies criticism of those perceived to lack these qualities, but we have to wonder how far the concern for health and well-being that is demonstrated in Roman literature extended down the social hierarchy. Certainly, by the latter part of the first century CE there was an expectation within certain circles, but perhaps also extending beyond those, that one should be equipped with both knowledge regarding what constitutes health and well-being, and experience regarding maintaining it. There is clear recognition of the importance of acknowledging the particular strengths and weaknesses of one's individual constitution and acting accordingly.

This chapter will examine the concept of health and well-being in the Roman Republic and Principate, and the ancient literary, documentary, archaeological and bioarchaeological evidence for health and well-being in the city of Rome and central Italy. I propose that Romans from all social classes cared about the acquisition and maintenance of good health and well-being, and were not only in possession of knowledge regarding what was necessary to acquire and maintain it, but were also able to act on this knowledge, with the result that concerns regarding the acquisition and maintenance of good health and well-being were incredibly influential regarding Roman behaviour at all levels of the social hierarchy.

What is 'health'?

In contemporary English, the noun 'health' is understood to refer to the state of being free from illness or injury. This understanding of the term implies a polarity, with health on one side and illness or injury on the other, these states being mutually exclusive: one cannot be or even be considered to be healthy if one is ill or injured. So far, it would seem straightforward. Yet this is not necessarily the case.

Health has been designated an 'abstract concept', something that people find difficult to define.[13] Certainly, it is not a static concept, nor even a stable one, as it is influenced by a variety of things, it changes over time and it changes according to context.[14] Nevertheless attempts to define health have been made. For the World Health Organisation, health is 'a state of complete physical, mental and social well-being and not merely the absence of disease or infirmity'.[15] This definition has been praised for its breadth, and the fact that it recognises that being healthy is not simply about not being ill or injured.[16] Yet it has also been criticised for being absolute and thus ultimately unachievable, and for not only contributing to the medicalisation of society, but also minimising the role of the human capacity to cope autonomously with life's ever-changing physical, mental and social challenges.[17] Additionally, the extent to which it accords with the contemporary twenty-first century understanding of health, let alone the ancient one, has been extensively debated.[18]

Attempts to understand health can be facilitated using theoretical constructs although these, too, are problematic. The medical model views health in terms of pathology, disease, diagnosis and treatment, with the causes of ill health being biological or physiological. However, in its focus on the individual body, the medical model does not take that individual body's context into account, ignoring potentially contributory psychological, social and environmental factors. Conversely, the social model views health as being subject to influence by a range of factors located outside of the physical body, and as being socially constructed, but this in turn ensures that its remit is so broad as to be virtually unusable. The holistic model takes a more integrated approach than either the medical model or the social model, and considers the biological, psychological and social factors, viewing the individual as a whole. The biopsychosocial model is closely related to the holistic model, combining the approaches of the medical and social models and examining the interaction between their components.[19] These theoretical constructs have the potential to help us understand health in antiquity, just as theoretical constructs such as the medical model, the social model, the interactional model and the community model have been helpful in facilitating understanding of disability in antiquity.[20]

Health in Graeco-Roman antiquity

Ariphron's *Hymn to Health*, thought to have been written at the end of the fourth century BCE, offers a useful starting point for considering how health was conceptualised in classical antiquity. The hymn seems to have been well-known and used consistently over a period of several centuries. It was quoted in full by Athenaeus at the end of the second century CE, is referred to by numerous other ancient authors and was even inscribed on stone.[21] It seems to have been particularly popular for toasts in symposia, along with other similarly themed prayers, hymns and drinking songs.[22] Reading these, it is clear that the ancient understanding of 'health' – that is to say, 'good health' – incorporated concern for physical, mental and social well-being, as these were considered necessary prerequisites for living a good life:

> Health, most august of the blessed gods – may I dwell with you for the rest of my life, and may you always willingly remain with me! For if any pleasure can be got from wealth, children, royal power (which human beings regard as almost like a god), or the longings we pursue using Aphrodite's hidden nets, or if the gods have revealed any other pleasure or respite from their labours to human beings, all of these flourish with you, blessed Health, and shine in the Graces' conversation. No one is happy when you are absent.[23]

The fact that this hymn, this prayer, is requesting good health reminds us that this state was not taken for granted, but rather highly sought after. While the goddess Health was not originally a mythological figure, once she was established as such, she became immensely popular and was worshipped over an extended period of time, and her popularity has been attributed to the importance attached to the concept that she embodied (see Figure 1.1).[24] Good health is often referred to as the 'best thing' or the 'prime good', with Health given place of honour amongst the gods.[25] It is considered a fundamental necessity if one wishes to accomplish anything at all: 'wisdom cannot display itself and art is non-evident and strength unexerted and wealth useless and speech powerless in the absence of health'.[26]

How is a state of good health to be acquired in the first place, and how is it to be maintained subsequently? In the twenty-first century, good health is considered to be connected with – if not almost entirely dependent on – an individual's lifestyle, which includes following a balanced diet, undertaking a certain amount of physical and mental exercise and maintaining a high level of personal hygiene. The ancient understanding of good health was not so very far from this. Health was conceived of as a balance between opposing elements in the human body, although theories about what these elements were abounded and conflicted.[27] Humoral theory seems to have been the most prevalent and long-lasting. However, the nature of this balance depended upon the nature of the individual and their constitution, their age and their sex, and was subject to influence from geography, seasonality, climate and weather. The balance was believed to be something controllable by man rather than the gods, and could be achieved by dietetics or regimen (from the Greek *diaita*, literally 'way of living' or 'way of life').[28]

What is regimen? Although regimen is referred to by a variety of authors in the Classical period, it is in the treatises of the Hippocratic Corpus that the concept is outlined most fully. Ideas concerning the validity of regimen for the establishment maintenance and preservation of health are found in a number of treatises

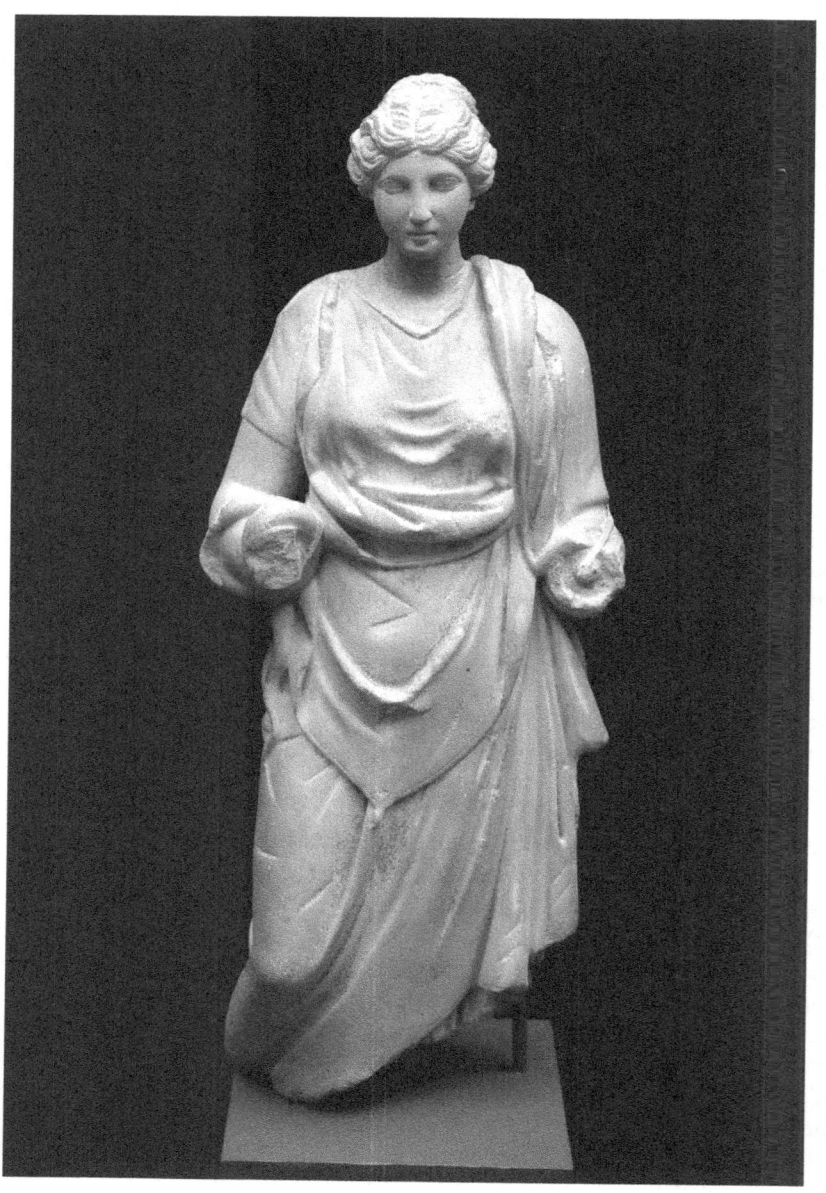

Figure 1.1 A marble statue of the goddess Hygieia, supposedly recovered from Ostia and dating to *circa* 100 BCE–100 CE.

Source: Image courtesy of the Wellcome Library (Wellcome Collection/Science Museum inv. A113241).

included in the Hippocratic Corpus that date to between the end of the fifth and the middle of the fourth centuries BCE, notably *On Regimen, On Airs, Waters and Places, On Regimen in Health, On the Nature of Man, On Regimen in Acute Diseases* and *On Ancient Medicine*. At its most basic, regimen refers to food and drink food being solid and drink being liquid.[29] However, there is also an intermediate stage for the sick, halfway between solid and liquid, that is created by adding liquid to solid in order to dilute the solid and produce gruel.[30] Thus food, drink and gruel serve as the primary elements of regimen, but there are other things, secondary elements, such as active and passive physical and mental exercise, bathing, sleep and sexual activity.[31]

Plato (428/427 or 424/423–348/347 BCE) attributed the invention of regimen to Herodicus of Selymbria (fifth century BCE), who incorporated prescriptions for both diet and exercise, including massage, into his training of athletes.[32] In antiquity Herodicus was believed to have been one of Hippocrates' teachers, and regimen is certainly a prominent feature of a range of Hippocratic treatises, including *Regimen in Health, On Regimen* and *On Regimen in Acute Diseases*. Subsequent authorities such as Diocles of Carystus (*circa* 375–295 BCE), Mnesistheos of Athens, Praxagoras of Cos (*circa* 340 BCE), Phylotimos and Diphilos of Siphos (*circa* 300–250 BCE) also wrote on the subject. References found in contemporary works from other literary genres make it clear that the concept was widely known and understood.[33]

Regimen comprised a personal plan involving diet, physical and mental exercise and personal hygiene. Such a plan was devised specifically for someone to balance their body. Followed diligently, it would ensure and preserve good health and prevent ill health but, in the event of illness, yet another specially devised plan would succeed in restoring the former state of good health, upon which the original plan would be resumed.[34] For success to be assured, a plan required that the patient be considered as an individual with a unique body, mind and spirit, as whatever was making them ill was a result of an imbalance causing disharmony, and the aim of the treatment was to restore balance and ensure harmony. However, it is important to consider the fact that the regimens that survive from antiquity cater to a specific type of constitution: 'discourses both require and create a normative subject: free, male, leisured, in the prime of life, healthy, and native to the geographical zones whose climates uniquely foster Greekness and Romanness. This normative body, while a statistical rarity, is the yardstick of everyone else'[35] It is this, perhaps, that has led to the prevailing scholarly view of health as a luxury, something that only the social elite were concerned with, or able to be concerned with.

Regimen as an approach to ancient healthy living was uncontroversial, even if people differed in their opinions as to precisely which type of regimen was likely to be the most effective. Yet from the earliest days of regimen, there seems to have been tension between physicians and athletic trainers regarding whose recommendations were valid, and competition between individual practitioners regarding the efficacy of their preferred regimen.[36] This competition was a standard feature of professional ancient medical practice, but was it a feature of amateur ancient medical practice, too? Perhaps one of the reasons that Roman domestic medical practice is not comprehensively discussed in ancient literature is because it was not competitive in nature the way that professional medical practice was, and its practitioners were not motivated by public recognition the way that professional practitioners were.

As we have seen, regimen was a Greek medical theory, method and practice, yet there is considerable evidence for the presence of Greek medicine in Italy from at least the early third century BCE, the result of the foundation of Greek colonies in the south of Italy and the gradual Hellenisation of the Italian peninsula.[37] Citing the historian Lucius Cassius Hemina (*circa* 146 BCE), Pliny the Elder describes the introduction of Greek medicine into the city of Rome by the Greek physician Archagathus in 219 BCE, who was set up with a surgery at public expense but alienated people by using cutting and cauterising as methods of treatment, but states that most Romans refused to cultivate the art of medicine themselves, going so far as to state that those who accepted it essentially became Greek themselves.[38] What Pliny does accept, however, is the concept of regimen, although he does attach a list of practices that he considers to be objectionable.[39] However, it is apparent that the type of regimen followed by a citizen of Athens during the Classical period was incompatible with the requirements of and expectations placed upon a citizen of Rome during the Republic and Principate due to the levels of civic activity that he was supposed to engage in on a daily basis.[40] Thus it was necessary for regimen to be adapted according to Roman requirements while bearing in mind the importance of self-control and not becoming a slave to one's own body and devoting oneself entirely to its care. Consequently, we see regimen discussed in moralising literature. There are correct and appropriate amounts of food and drink, exercise and personal hygiene to undertake, and correct and appropriate ways of partaking in them.[41] Ideally, a regimen was developed by a physician and a patient as part of an ongoing collaborative process involving dialogue and consultation.[42]

The increase in prosperity brought about through political, economic and social change such as Roman imperialism and urbanisation over the course of the second and first centuries BCE resulted in the growth of a middle class and the spread of power and prosperity down the social ladder, blurring the lines and distinctions between the different social classes.[43] Consequently, any regimen followed by a Roman citizen, whether senator, equestrian, municipal decurion or plebeian, needed to take into account the limited time available once sufficient time had been set aside for the pursuit of political, economic and social endeavours, whatever those might be. Thus during the late Republic we see the rise of the practice of *otium* juxtaposed with that of *negotium*, and the distinction between a life of leisure and a life of labour with a balance between the two considered desirable and aspirational.[44] During the transition from Republic to Principate over the course of the period from the mid-first century BCE to the mid-first century CE, the members of the Roman senatorial elite were gradually denied their traditional position of political authority and increasingly turned their attention to *otium* as a means of distinguishing themselves from their peers.[45] Thus the maintenance of health and well-being became a conspicuous and prominent part of *otium* for the senatorial order, and to a lesser extent, the equestrian, decurion and plebeian orders as well. The type of *otium* that we hear the most about is that of the senatorial and equestrian elite that takes place on their estates, *villae suburbanae, maritimae* and *urbanae*.[46] However, everything that these individuals did there was accessible to others, albeit on a smaller (that is, less extravagant) scale. After all, everyone had some degree of free time and a certain amount of personal autonomy regarding how they spent it.[47] The activities the Romans undertook during their leisure time contributed directly to the acquisition and maintenance of good health and well-being: food and drink, physical and mental exercise, personal hygiene.[48] While individual aspects of ancient Roman leisure have been studied in relation to health and well-being, the role that each of these activities played in relation to regimen as a whole and the possibility that Romans from a range of social classes were following some sort of regimen has not been explicitly stated.

Regimen in the Roman republic

A variety of different terms could be utilised to refer to matters relating to health in the Latin of the middle and late Republic and Principate. *Salus* encompasses a range of meanings relating to the safety of both individuals and things, which includes physical well-being and health. *Sanus* refers to the state of being of individuals and things, the extent to which someone or something is sound and thus in a good or healthy condition. *Valetudo* is qualified by adjectives, and consequently can be employed in a positive, neutral or negative sense. It is clear that both physical and mental health and well-being were cause for concern.[49] In the *Tusculan Disputations*, Cicero explicitly discusses physical and mental health, and recognises the same tendency toward problems in the health of the body with the health of the mind:

> Disease is the term applied to a break-down of the whole body, sickness to disease attended by weakness, defect when the parts of the body are not symmetrical with one another and there ensue crookedness of the limbs, distortion, ugliness. And so the first two, disease and sickness, are a result of shock and disorder to the bodily health as a whole; defect, however, is discernible of itself, though the general health is unimpaired. But in the soul we can only separate disease from sickness theoretically. Defectiveness, however, is a habit or a disposition which is throughout life inconsistent and out of harmony with itself. So it comes that in the one perversion of beliefs the result is disease and sickness, in the other the result is inconsistency and discord. For not every defect involves equal want of harmony, as for instance the disposition of those who are not far off wisdom is indeed out of harmony with itself, as long as it is unwise, but it is not distorted or perverse. Disease, however, and sickness are subdivisions of defectiveness, but it is a question whether disorders are subdivisions of the same class. For defects are permanent dispositions, but disorders are shifting, so that they cannot be subdivisions of

permanent dispositions. Moreover as in evil the analogy of the body extends to the nature of the soul, so it does in good. For the chief blessings of the body are beauty, strength, health, vigour, agility; so are they of the soul. For as in the body the adjustment of the various parts, of which we are made up, in their fitting relation to one another is health, so health of the soul means a condition when its judgments and beliefs are in harmony.[50]

The earliest work of Latin prose to survive, Marcus Porcius Cato's (Cato the Elder) *On Agriculture*, acknowledges the importance and necessity of good health for the successful running of an estate on several occasions, but does not go into detail about what, precisely, Cato considers good health to consist of. Rather, in relation to the estate manager's responsibilities to the other members of the household, Cato states that 'the household should not be in poor condition, or sick, or hungry', and then subsequently in relation to the estate manager himself, that 'he must ensure that he knows all the work of the farm and must do it himself often, but not so much as to tire himself out. . . . If he does this he will be less inclined to go about, will keep healthier, and will sleep better'.[51] So Cato certainly highlights diet and rest as important factors.

Although no treatises dealing specifically with regimen survive from the middle or late Republic, there is a significant amount of ancient literary evidence indicating that the belief in and the practice of regimen was widespread. Two regimens will be examined here, those of Cato the Elder (234–149 BCE) and Asclepiades of Bithynia (late second century BCE) respectively. Although the literary evidence for them is fragmentary, and attest to very different approaches, their regimens do have certain elements in common, and both are notable for their focus on the individual and the home.

First, we will examine the regimen of Cato the Elder. At some point during his long life, Cato wrote – or, alternatively, and perhaps more accurately, compiled – a work addressed to his eldest son, Marcus Porcius Cato Licinianus. It was certainly produced after 192 or 191 BCE – when Cato's eldest son was likely born – and a date during the 170s BCE has been suggested on the grounds that it would have been considered by Cato to be the most use to Licinianus as he was approaching adulthood. Known today by the title *To His Son* (*Ad filium*), this work seems to have consisted of a selection of precepts, exhortations and observations on a variety of subjects that Cato considered it appropriate for Licinianus to familiarise himself with, such as medicine, agriculture, military matters and rhetoric, with the emphasis placed firmly on the successful practical application of such knowledge.[52] The work seems to have been circulated either by Cato or Licinianus and was known to writers in the Republic and early Empire. While the text no longer survives in its entirety, fragments of it can be found in the works of Pliny the Elder and Plutarch. In his discussion of the history of medicine in the city of Rome, Pliny quotes from *To His Son* directly:

I shall speak about those Greek fellows in their proper place, son Marcus, and point out the result of my enquiries at Athens, and convince you what benefit comes from dipping into their literature, and not making a close study of it. They are a quite worthless people, and an intractable one, and you must consider my words prophetic. When that race gives us its literature it will corrupt all things, and even all the more if it sends hither its physicians. They have conspired together to murder all foreigners with their physic, but this very thing they do for a fee, to gain credit and to destroy us easily. They are also always dubbing us foreigners, and to fling more filth on us than on others they give us the foul nickname of Opici. I have forbidden you to have dealings with physicians.[53]

Much has been made of Cato's apparent prejudice against the Greeks in general and their medicine in particular.[54] However, considering that Cato was writing in the wake of the Greek physician Archagathus' arrival in Rome and thus would have been well-acquainted with his controversial methods and resultant notoriety, this prejudice is not entirely unreasonable.[55] In all likelihood, Cato was not alone among Romans in preferring to rely upon what he perceived to be traditional Italian healthcare theory and practice.[56] Pliny is keen to make it clear that Cato practised what he preached in this regard, and goes on to explain that, rather than be a hypocrite and patronise either Greek physicians or those Roman physicians that came to model themselves on Greek ones, Cato monitored his own health, and that of his family members, and treated any illnesses with the aid of a notebook (*commentarius*) of prescriptions.[57] While none of the prescriptions from *To His Son* survive, in all likelihood they were very similar to those found in Cato's later work *On Agriculture*.[58]

Unlike Pliny, Plutarch does not quote from *To His Son*, but he does paraphrase some of its contents, and this information is extremely helpful in establishing what, exactly, Cato recommended as an alternative to engaging a Greek or Greek-style physician:

> [Cato] himself, he said, had written a book of recipes, which he followed in the treatment and regimen of any who were sick in his family. He never required his patients to fast, but fed them on greens, on bits of duck, pigeon, or hare. Such a diet, he said, was light and good for sick people, except that it often causes dreams. By following such treatment and regimen he said he had good health himself, and kept his family in good health.[59]

Cato's exhortation to Licinianus to follow in his footsteps in avoiding physicians and – presumably – utilising his father's collections of prescriptions to maintain health and diagnose and treat illness locates Cato's healthcare theory, method and practice squarely within his home. As *pater familias*, Cato had legal authority not only over his son but also over the other members of his *familia*, and so was in a position to dictate an entire regimen, which would have incorporated a prescribed diet, physical and mental activity, personal hygiene and rest periods.[60] Cato's regimen is notable for its rejection of fasting, and prescription of greens, duck, pigeon and hare, all of which would have been near to hand on an agricultural estate in central Italy. With regard to prescribed diet, hare was believed to promote sleep, which would certainly have been appropriate to a period of convalescence.[61] To what extent can we reconstruct Cato's regimen for members of his household that were not sick? There is detailed information regarding the rations that he allotted.[62] His slaves received grain, wine, olives, oil and salt at various points in the year, and the size of those rations varied according to status and duties within the household. Here we see an acknowledgement that diet was varied and individualised.

Second, we will examine the regimen of Asclepiades of Bithynia.[63] Although it is difficult to date Asclepiades' tenure in Rome precisely, his death can be dated to shortly before 91 BCE.[64] While not subscribing to humoral theory, Asclepiades' corpuscular theory of physiology, which argued for a body composed of small units, spaces or pores, likewise sought the correct balance between these elements, and this balance could be achieved through diet, exercise and bathing.[65] To what extent can we reconstruct Asclepiades' regimen? Later commentators make a point of differentiating his therapeutics from those of his predecessors, which per-haps goes some way towards explaining their popularity with his patients.[66] How-ever, he was apparently also a very effective self-publicist, being a particularly good public speaker, and so able to promote his therapeutics through lectures.[67] Asclepiades sought to restore harmony to the body and did so by recommend-ing the regulation of the intake of food and drink, particularly wine; massage; active exercise, such as walking; passive exercise, such as rocking in an appli-ance; and hydrotherapy through bathing in both hot and cold waters. His works were an important source for Celsus' *On Medicine*. Since hot water was already used in Roman bathhouses, it was his cold water cure that seems to have been truly revolutionary.[68] While he preferred gentle remedies, he did have recourse to more drastic ones such as drugs, emetics and clysters, venesection, tapping and pharyngotomy.[69] In his work *Preparations*, he criticises physicians who do not have remedies prepared for any ailment, and one of his remedies for troubles of the arteries survives in Scribonius Largus' *Compositions*.[70] It is also important to consider the influence that Asclepiades' therapeutics had on his pupils and their own works. Themison of Laodicea further developed Asclepiades' regimen and wrote on diet, before founding the Methodist system of medicine.[71]

Regimen in the Principate

For the belief in and practice of regimen in Rome during the Principate and early Empire, we have rather more definitive ancient literary evidence. Celsus' *On Med-icine* is the earliest surviving medical treatise written in Latin, and since Celsus and his works are referred to by Pliny the Elder (23–79 CE), Marcus Fabius Quin-tilianus (*circa* 35–100 CE) and Lucius Junius Moderatus Columella (*circa* 70 CE), they have been dated to the reign of the emperor Tiberius. Despite the fact that *On Medicine* was not originally a self-contained piece of work but rather comprised the second part of a six-part encyclopaedia (the other five parts covering agricul-ture, military arts, rhetoric, philosophy and jurisprudence), interpretations of *On*

Medicine have ranged from its being a compilation of material from a Hellenistic original, to a Latin translation of a Greek original, to the work of a Roman medical professional.[72] In point of fact, Pliny the Elder refers to Celsus as an *auctor* rather than a *medicus* in his *Natural History*, Quintilian discusses Celsus in the context of his philosophical writings in *Institutes of Oratory* and Columella defers to him on the subject of agriculture frequently in *On Agriculture*. The opening of the proem of *On Medicine* indicates that it followed directly on from the part of the encyclopaedia concerned with agriculture, and also gives the impression that, in Celsus' opinion at least, agriculture and medicine were directly connected: 'just as agriculture promises nourishment to healthy bodies, so does the healing art promise health to the sick'.[73] There is no indication that knowledge of either of these subjects is restricted in any way. While Quintilian states that Celsus wrote with elegance and polish, he refers to him as 'a man of very ordinary ability'.[74] The choice of words has been much debated.[75] It is not necessarily a criticism, but rather a statement of fact regarding breadth of Roman education. So, the contents of the first book offer us an invaluable insight into what, exactly, the Roman view of good health was, and perhaps more importantly, how it could be maintained at this time.

The first book opens with a general description of the life that a healthy man (*sanus homo*) should aim to lead, and this is elaborated upon over the course of the book. This life should be varied but balanced, and attention should be paid to exercise (both physical and mental), diet (both food and drink), personal hygiene (bathing, massage and anointing), sexual activity and bodily functions (vomiting and defecating). Care should be taken with regard to seasonality, as some seasons are high risk and others low risk, and physical location, as some locations are healthier than others. Celsus asserts that human constitutions come in a variety of different types and emphasises how important it is that an individual should be familiar with their own, thus indicating a certain amount of personal autonomy was expected with regard to healthcare:[76]

> A man in health, who is both vigorous and his own master, should be under no obligatory rules, and have no need either for a medical attendant or for a rubber and anointer. His kind of life should afford him variety; he should now be in the country, now in town, and more often about the farm; he should sail, hunt, rest sometimes, but more often take exercise; for while inaction weakens the body, work strengthens it; the former brings on premature old age, the later prolongs youth. It is well also at times to go to the bath, at times to make use of cold waters; to undergo sometimes inunction, sometimes to neglect the same; to avoid no kind of food in common use; to attend at times a banquet, at times to hold aloof; to eat more than sufficient at one time, at another no more; to take food twice rather than once a day, and always as much as one wants provided one digests it. . . . Physical intimacy indeed is neither to be desired overmuch, nor overmuch to be feared; seldom used it braces the body, used frequently it relaxes. Since, however, nature and not number should be the standard of frequency, regard being had to age and constitution, physical

intimacy can be recognised as harmless when followed neither by languor nor by pain. The use is worse in the day time, and safer by night; but care should be taken that by day it be not immediately followed by a meal, and at night not immediately followed by work and watching. Such are the precautions to be observed by the strong, and they should take care that whilst in health their defences against ill-health are not used up.[77]

While the prologue of *On Medicine* offers a brief history of the art of medicine, and the following six books each focus on a separate aspect of this art, both the inclusion of a book on health and its placement at the beginning of the treatise proper emphasise the importance of good health. Celsus' hypothetical subject is the *sanus homo qui et bene valet et suae spontis est*. Who, exactly, does he imagine he is addressing his recommendations to? As above, *sanus homo* can be translated as 'a man in health', or simply 'a healthy man', but equally *homo* can be used to indicate 'man' in the sense of 'human being' or 'person' rather than simply just 'male person'. If Celsus had wanted to be gender specific, he could have used *vir*, 'man' as in 'adult male' or 'male person'. Likewise, *suae spontis* can be translated as 'his own master', but also, potentially, 'their own master'. Thus, this does not necessarily preclude women from utilising the treatise and following the recommendations, providing that they are in good health, physically capable and have a certain amount of personal autonomy. This does, however, potentially preclude slaves from doing so, and as we read further, it is clear why this is the case. Celsus is directing his recommendations to those who are in a position to decide how exactly they spend their time and are thus able to allocate sufficient time for both *negotium*, 'business affairs', and *otium*, 'leisure pursuits': 'he who has been engaged in the day, whether in domestic or on public affairs, ought to keep some portion of the day for the care of the body'.[78]

So how did healthy, capable and autonomous Romans spend their time? To a degree, it is possible to reconstruct the ancient Roman daily routine. The Roman day lasted for twelve hours, beginning when the sun rose and ending when it set. The daylight was divided up into twelve sections of equal length, thus ensuring that the days were longer in summer than winter, and in the middle of summer each hour was approximately seventy-five minutes long, while in the middle of winter it was forty-five minutes. Marcus Valerius Martialis gives us an indication of how people spent this time: the working day lasted for the first five hours of the day and ended at noon and was then followed by an hour or two of rest before people went to the baths and then had dinner.[79] What the working day consisted of and how long it lasted obviously depended upon an individual's social status. For senators, equestrians and decurions who were patrons and clients, the first few hours of the working day were when the *salutatio* took place, followed by political and legal business transacted in the forum and basilica, but this came to a halt at midday.[80] For the urban plebs, shopkeepers and food sellers were open for most of the day.[81] For slaves, how they spent their time was up to their master or mistress.

With regard to the portion of the day conventionally set aside for care of the body, Celsus' first recommendation is that light exercise should be taken, and his definition of light exercise encompasses both physical and mental exercise. Particular physical exercises include weapons training, hand-ball, running and walking; mental exercises include reading aloud.[82] Theoretically, the opportunity to undertake these was available to everyone, no matter what their social or financial status, as while some venues charged an entrance fee, many others were free of charge.[83] Weapons training, hand-ball and running could be undertaken in the palaestra, the gymnasium or in other rooms at public bathhouses, facilitating working up a sweat prior to bathing. Walking could be undertaken in a variety of locations, both public ones such as parks and porticoes, and private ones such as in the garden. Rome was well-equipped with public amenities from the middle of the first century BCE onwards. The Portico of Pompey, built by Gnaeus Pompeius Magnus in 55 BCE, adjoined his theatre and was originally intended to provide shelter to the spectators in case of rain, but its central area included a garden space that was suitable for shady walks.[84] Also popular were the Portico of Agrippa, also known as the Portico of the Argonauts, built in 25 BCE, the Portico of Vipsania, began by Marcus Vipsanius Agrippa's sister Vipsania Pollia and finished by Augustus, the Portico of Livia, begun by Augustus in 15 BCE and completed in 7 BCE, and the Portico of Octavia, built by Augustus and dedicated to Octavia after 27 BCE.[85] The porticoes offered the residents of Rome the opportunity not just to walk, but to appreciate beautiful works of art, view instructive displays such as Agrippa's map of the Roman world and read Greek and Latin literature in their associated libraries. Similarly, the pleasure gardens of members of the senatorial and equestrian elite could be accessed by the general public, such as the Gardens of Agrippa on the Campus Martius (like the Baths of Agrippa, left to the Roman people in Agrippa's will), the Gardens of Caesar on the right bank of the Tiber (left to the Roman people in Caesar's will) and the Gardens of Sallust (seemingly at least part of the time open to the public).[86] Additionally, some types of manual labour were considered to be good exercise.[87] Marcus Vitruvius Pollio (*circa* 80–70–*circa* 15 BCE), writing in the late first century BCE, claimed that palaestra and gymnasia, the buildings in which the Greeks undertook the activities necessary for their regimen, were not common in Italy.[88] They could, however, be found in the urban centres of Campania, southern Italy and Sicily.[89] For example, Pompeii boasts the Samnite Palaestra and the Great Palaestra, in addition to the combination of the palaestra and the bathhouse, with the Republican Baths, the Stabian Baths, the Forum Baths and the Central Baths.[90] Also worth considering is the fact that there is a significant amount of evidence that not only was exercise undertaken by both men and women, but that men and women exercised in the same ways, in the same places, at the same times.[91]

Celsus' second recommendation regarding care of the body follows on naturally from exercising, and involves bathing, anointing with oil and massage.[92] Such practices could be undertaken at a public bathhouse or at a private one. In an urban centre, bathhouses were accessible to everyone, no matter what their social status or wealth: while some bathhouses charged entrances fees, others were free. Both men and women bathed, although seemingly in different parts of the bathhouse and at different times of day, and there does not seem to have been a prohibition on slaves going to public bathhouses.[93] Agrippa built a bathhouse with an adjacent garden on the Campus Martius in 25 BCE, and upon his death in 12 BCE he left the complex to the Roman people for their free use.[94] Over the course of the following two centuries, Roman emperors built increasingly large and luxurious complexes in the city of Rome. Nero built a bathhouse in conjunction with a gymnasium in 62 CE, and although the complex burned down later that year, it was extremely popular while it lasted.[95] Titus built a bathhouse that was opened in tandem with the Colosseum in 79 CE.[96] Trajan built a bathhouse alongside Titus', a project perhaps originally planned by Domitian, which was apparently used by women.[97] In addition to the grand imperial complexes, there were also numerous smaller bathhouses, such as that built by Gnaeus Domitius Ahenobarbus on the *Via Sacra*, that built by Claudius Etruscus on either the Quirinal or the Pincian and that of Licinius Sura on the Aventine.[98] Even provincial towns were well served. Pompeii possessed six substantial public bathhouses, and a number of private ones.

Celsus' third recommendation involves the amount and type of food and drink to be taken during the evening meal. He encourages savoury foodstuffs and discourages sweet, and recommends his patients eat first light items such as salads, then either roasted or boiled meat. He also advises the use of purgatives and emetics under certain circumstances. As far as food was concerned, there were two main categories: foodstuffs that could be eaten fresh or with minimal preparation such as washing, cutting or cooking, so wild and cultivated plants, fruits, vegetables, nuts, animal by-products and so on, and foodstuffs that necessitated processing of some kind before they could be eaten, such as cereals and meat.[99] Consequently, these foodstuffs can be considered as being either stable or unstable, with fresh foodstuffs necessitating rapid consumption due to their tendency to go off, and processed foodstuffs lasting longer. Foodstuffs were not necessarily readily available to all people in all places all year-round; we have to consider where people acquired their foodstuffs, and what they did with them prior to eating. Rome has been described as a 'consumption city' or a 'consumer city', and other cities and towns such as Ostia, Pompeii and Herculaneum can be considered in this way too, as they do not produce the foodstuffs necessary to maintain their populations themselves.[100]

Celsus' fourth recommendation involves sexual activity, and the assumption is that this will take place at home and involve other members of the household. Sex was considered to have many benefits for health and well-being, and was believed to be both preventative and therapeutic, but it could also be dangerous. For men, sexual intercourse involved ejaculation, which resulted in the loss of a vital fluid. Since men needed to generate heat to produce sperm and were thought to put more physical effort into sex due to the necessity of them being the active partner, sex was potentially dangerously exhausting. Consequently, men were advised to have sex infrequently and, when they did have sex, to do so with a woman.[101] However, sex was thought to confer different benefits on men and women due to their different physiologies and constitutions. For those who followed the Hippocratic humoral theory, regular sex was particularly beneficial to women, ensuring that their bodies, considered colder and wetter than those of men, remained sufficiently cold and wet. Once a girl had gone through puberty, menstruation, sexual intercourse, pregnancy and childbirth were all considered necessary, and a well-regulated reproductive cycle was indicative of female health and well-being.[102] Consequently, recreational sex that utilised contraception and/ or methods of non-productive sexual intercourse were considered deleterious to women's health. Such considerations may, in fact, have dictated when men and women had sexual intercourse. It has been suggested that paintings of sexual intercourse found in public bathhouses, such as those at the Suburban Baths in Pompeii, served as warnings of the dangers of deviant sexual activity and aimed to reinforce correct behaviour.[103]

Throughout *On Medicine*, Celsus incorporates not only the advice of professional medical practitioners, but also that of lay medical practitioners, and repeatedly recommends remedies that are practical, inexpensive and easily obtainable.[104] All the same, we do have to wonder how relevant Celsus' recommendations were for the majority of Romans, assuming they were even aware of them. We have already established that Pliny the Elder, Columella and Quintilian were familiar with Celsus' works to the point of being able to utilise them as sources for their own literary endeavours, but what about others lower down the social scale? It is possible that this type of information was disseminated through public lectures, at least in Rome and other urban centres.[105]

It is notable that Celsus does not specify an age; it is clear that his subject is an adult, but beyond that, he simply has to be *bene valet*, 'vigorous', 'strong', or even just 'able'. In fact, following this sort of guidance was thought to preserve one's youth and vitality, thus rendering age irrelevant. According to Cicero, it was one's duty to 'resist old age, to compensate for its defects by a watchful care; to fight against it as we would fight against disease; to adopt a regimen of health; to practice moderate exercise; and to take just enough food and drink to restore our strength and not to overburden it'.[106]

To what extent did individuals follow this sort of regimen? Pliny the Younger writes of his friend Titus Vestricius Spurinna:

> He stays in bed in the morning, asks for his shoes at the second hour, takes a walk for three miles, and exercises his mind as well as his body. If friends are with him, he discusses matters of serious interest; if not, he is read to – sometimes he is read to when friends are present, if they do not mind. Then he seats himself, and the reading or (preferably) the conversation continues. Later he gets into his carriage together with his wife (a wonderful lady) or one of his friends – recently it was me . . . when the time for his bath is announced (at the ninth hour in winter, and at the eighth in summer), he will walk in the sun without his clothes, if there is no breeze. Then he plays ball energetically and for quite a long time; this is another of the exercises with which he struggles against old age. After the bath he sits down, but puts his meal off for some time; in the meantime he listens to a reading of something light and agreeable.[107]

The fact that Pliny troubled to write to his friend Calvisius Rufus and describe Spurinna's regimen in such detail indicates that there was a general interest in the subject, and that certain individuals could been seen as inspirational. If, as was the case with Spurinna, one reached old age having retained a high level of physical and mental acuity, it would serve as a ringing endorsement of the regimen followed. Pliny focuses an equal amount of attention on the things that Spurinna does to maintain both his physical and mental health and makes it clear that Spurinna does not undertake these activities in isolation but rather in company. While regimen is individualised, it also has a social component.

When Pliny the Younger's friend Gnaeus Pedanius Fuscus Salinator asked for details of Pliny's summer regimen, he responded in considerable detail:

> I wake when I like, usually about sunrise, often earlier but rarely later. . . . Three or four hours after I first wake (but I don't keep to fixed times) I betake myself according to the weather outside either to the terrace or the covered arcade, work out the rest of my subject, and dictate it. I go for a drive, and spend the time in the same way as when walking or lying down; my powers of concentration do not flag and are in fact refreshed by the change. After a short sleep and another walk I read a Greek or Latin speech aloud and with emphasis, not so much for the sake of my voice as my digestion, though of course both are strengthened by this. Then I have another walk, am oiled, take exercise, and have a bath. If I am dining alone with my wife or with a few friends, a book is read aloud during the meal and afterwards we listen to a comedy or some music; and then I walk again with the members of my household, some of whom are well-educated. Thus the evening is prolonged with varied conversation, and, even when the days are at their longest, comes to a satisfying end.[108]

It would appear that Pliny's regimen was open to adaptation depending on the circumstances, but that it comprised an equal amount of physical and mental activity. It was focused primarily upon him, but open to the participation of others.

Archaeological and bioarchaeological evidence

Ancient literary evidence is a useful starting point when attempting to establish the parameters of what ancient authors considered to be healthy and unhealthy, and the ways in which they recommended attaining and maintaining good health. It is, however, only a starting point. For one thing, ancient literary evidence, no matter what the genre, tends to be primarily ideological, idealising and moralising rather than realistic. There are, however, indications, particularly regarding works of medical literature, which tend to be prescriptive rather than descriptive, and frequently passes comment, either in a positive or negative way, on contemporary practices.[109] In practice, of course, things were not quite so straightforward. Ancient literary evidence is heavily biased in favour of the Roman elite, whether imperial, senatorial or equestrian. In order to devise a regimen, an individual had to either be cognisant of how to devise one for themselves, or to be in a position to hire someone to devise one for them. Subsequent to this, the same individual had to be in a position to implement and follow it. Any mention of regimen as a sure-fire way of ensuring good health is being made by an individual with sufficient resources to put theory into practice. It is also worth noting that the majority of surviving ancient regimens are addressed to men, with those few that are addressed to women, infants and children are contingent on certain conditions being met, such as pregnancy.[110] Therefore we have to consider the extent to which such a regimen-based approach to health and well-being was even relevant to the members of the lower social orders. It would be absurd to suggest that members of the lower social orders, or even those members of the imperial, senatorial and equestrian orders that were not catered to by the mainstream regimen, had no concern for their health and well-being at all. However, the extent to which they were in a position to act on that concern is eminently debateable.

With reference to the city of Rome, it has been suggested that approximately ninety-eight percent of the city's estimated one million inhabitants were non-elite and so were classed as poor, although there were different levels of poverty: temporary and permanent.[111] The temporary poor would have consisted of artisans and shopkeepers, generally in possession of a reasonably high social and economic status but ever vulnerable and liable to slip into poverty during times of shortage or at difficult points in their life cycles.[112] The permanent poor comprised the ordinary poor and the very poor. The ordinary poor would have consisted of those who lived at the edge of subsistence, providing unskilled part-time or seasonal labour.[113] The very poor would have consisted of those who were truly destitute and consequently lacking in shelter, work and even food.[114] Each one of these groups would have had different capabilities as far as the possibility of following a regimen was concerned. Their diets would have varied according to their purchasing power, their dependent relationships and social networks, and their exercise regimes and personal hygiene would have varied according to their access to appropriate facilities.

Archaeological evidence is potentially more representative of society at large and can offer an insight into a far wider range of both individual and collective experiences, not only from the city of Rome, but also from a variety of other sites in central Italy. Bioarchaeology, the study of skeletal remains from archaeological sites, offers an insight into the health and ill health, diet and nutrition. The human skeleton can be macroscopically and microscopically examined, it can be chemically analysed, with isotope and DNA analyses used to provide information regarding demography, health status and dietary regime that are otherwise unrecoverable.[115] While an enormous amount of human remains dating to the Roman Republic and Empire have been excavated from a variety of sites in Italy, very few of these have been studied comprehensively. However, the studies that have been done can offer us interesting insights into health in this period. What is clear is that there was considerable variation in health across geographical location, age, sex and social class. There was also considerable variation in diet. There are a variety of possible reasons for this variation but one might well have been consumers exercising choice informed by the requirements of their particular regimen.

Osteological evidence indicates that immigrants to the city of Rome changed their diets significantly upon arrival in the city, although whether this change was voluntary and due to a desire to assimilate and acculturate or involuntary and due to food availability is unfortunately unknown.[116] Skeletons excavated from periurban and suburban cemeteries indicate that there could be considerable variation in diet even within the city of Rome itself. The Casal Bertone and Castellaccio Europarco cemeteries, dating from the first to the third centuries CE, demonstrate significant variation in diet. The Casal Bertone cemetery was located just outside the city walls, while the Castellaccio Europarco was associated with a large agricultural area, and the two populations were utilising different foodstuffs, with the inhabitants of the former eating more marine resources and less millet than the latter.[117]

Outside of Rome, it would appear that there was considerable diversity of diet, not only in different communities within a comparatively small geographical area, but also within the same communities. For example, the osteological evidence from the necropolis of Isola Sacra, which served the inhabitants of Portus Romae between the first and third centuries CE, indicates that the local population were predominantly middle class, likely administrators, traders and merchants.[118] Their diet consisted of a mixture of terrestrial and marine resources, unsurprising in a coastal settlement.[119] Conversely, osteological evidence from a contemporaneous cemetery located slightly further inland, perhaps serving an agricultural community, attested a diet consisting of predominantly terrestrial resources. This difference could be attributed to geography with those living nearer the coast in a better position to access fresh fish and seafood, but it could also be attributed to social status with those employed in Portus Romae more affluent and therefore better able to afford more expensive foodstuffs than those farming inland. However, there was also considerable variation between individuals within these two communities. The inhabitants of Portus Romae seem to have differentiated diet according to sex and age, with men eating different foodstuffs from women and children.[120] Archaeobotanical evidence from Pompeii and Herculaneum indicates that the communities on the Bay of Naples had access to a considerable variety of foodstuffs.[121]

Also worth considering are potential health problems that would have occurred and needed to be addressed no matter what explanation was given for them. Conditions such as periostitis and osteoarthritis, caused by trauma or strenuous physical activity, would have caused swelling, pain and made movement difficult.[122] Fractured bones would have needed setting.[123] The vast majority of Romans were affected by all manner of physical impairments and difficulties.[124] Ancient literary evidence tells us what specific individuals such as Cicero and Seneca the Younger did regarding their chronic health problems; we can surmise that others did likewise as far as they were able.

While the purpose of regimen was to ensure the establishment and preservation of good health and well-being, it is indisputable that some types of regimen, notably those devised for pregnant and lactating women, infants and children were actually detrimental to health.[125] Text-based research into nutrition and malnutrition in antiquity has been supported by these human skeletal remains, which indicate that pregnant and lactating women, and infants and children were particularly at risk from malnutrition, and that poor maternal health during pregnancy and poor health during infancy and childhood created problems for individuals later in life, leaving them prone to certain medical conditions that would require regular treatment.[126]

Whether or not a regimen was followed, health problems would still arise and need to be dealt with. While members of the social elite could afford to engage a physician, it is evident from ancient literary evidence that they also possessed a certain amount of medical knowledge themselves, so were potentially in a position to make a choice regarding the approach to take in dealing with health problems. Depending on their situation at any given point in time, the temporary poor might well be able to afford to engage a physician or patronise another type of healthcare practitioner such as an apothecary. The ordinary poor might be prepared to make sacrifices in order to afford to engage a physician or patronise another type of healthcare practitioner such as an apothecary. The very poor were likely not in a position to do anything.

Conclusion

There is a significant amount of literary evidence that suggests that the attainment, maintenance and preservation of health and well-being was something of a preoccupation of the Roman senatorial and equestrian elite in the middle and late Republic and early Principate. This preoccupation is not only expressed in medical and associated philosophical literature, but also technical literature such as agricultural treatises. However, it is unlikely that it was only the members of the elite social orders that cared about their health and well-being or were in a position to do anything about it. While it is true that certain aspects of regimen were more likely to have been the preserve of the social elite who were in possession of the leisure time and financial resources necessary to allow them to devote a significant amount of effort to the cultivation of good health and well-being, others were more readily accessible to those lower down the social hierarchy. While this is not readily attested in ancient literature, bioarchaeological evidence indicates that there was considerable variation in general health, in part a result of the considerable variation in diet. This is not to say that the Romans did not suffer from serious health problems, as it is clear that they did. Rather, they managed these health problems. For some the way to do this was through engaging a physician or other type of healthcare practitioner, while for others alternative strategies were developed and utilised.

Yet it is important to remember that, no matter who was responsible for devising and prescribing a regimen, it was up to the individual for whom it had been devised and prescribed to follow it. The vast majority of a regimen would be undertaken at the individual's discretion and, for the most part, in their own household, which in turn locates healthcare theory, method and practice firmly in the household.[127] With regard to diet, in antiquity people ate food and drink consisting of items they had either produced or purchased themselves, which were prepared by themselves or by members of their household under their direction and were, on the whole, consumed at home. Likewise, with regard to physical and mental exercise, a substantial amount of it was undertaken either at home or in an environment of the individual's choosing, such as a palaestra, a gymnasium or a park. While certain aspects of maintaining personal hygiene such as bathing might have to be undertaken out with the home, the environment in which they took place was one of the individual's choosing.

The attainment, maintenance and preservation of health and healthiness through regimen involved a considerable amount of personal autonomy and was situated firmly within the domestic sphere, and this will be examined in the subsequent chapters.

Notes

1 Tacitus, *Annals* 6.46 (trans. J. Jackson): *Solitusque eludere medicorum artes atque eos qui post tricesimum aetatis annum ad internoscenda corpori suo utilia vel noxia alieni consilii indigerent.*

2 Tacitus, *Annals* 6.46 (trans. J. Jackson): *In patientia firmitudinem simulans.*

3 Tacitus, *Annals* 6.50; Suetonius, *Tiberius* 72.3.

4 Alternatively, Cassius Dio, *Roman History* 58.28.1 attributes this refusal to consult a physician to Tiberius' misplaced faith in a prophecy that he would live another ten years. Whatever the reason, and whatever the truth of this story, while the *columbaria* of Livia and other members of the Julio–Claudian family attest personal physicians of Livia (as discussed in the Introduction), Augustus (*CIL* VI 8656), Marcella (*CIL* VI 4452), Livia Drusi (*CIL* VI 8899) and Livilla (*CIL* VI 8711), they do not attest any personal physicians of Tiberius.

5 Tacitus, *Annals* 6.50 (trans. J. Jackson): *Non quidem regere valetudines principis solitus, consilii tamen copiam praebere.* Perhaps he had in mind the success of Antonius Musa once he had come to the attention of the emperor Augustus, detailed at Suetonius, *Divine Augustus* 81; Cassius Dio, *Roman History* 53.30; Pliny the Elder, *Natural History* 29.6.

6 This is supported by an anecdote incorporated into Plutarch's, *Advice on Keeping Well* 26.1 (trans. F. C. Babbitt): '*I have heard that the Tiberius Caesar once said that a man over sixty who holds out his hand to a physician is ridiculous*': Ἤκουσα Τιβέριόν ποτε Καίσαρα εἰπεῖν ὡς ἀνὴρ ὑπὲρ ἑξήκοντα γεγονὼς ἔτη καὶ προτείνων ἰατρῷ χεῖρα καταγέλαστος ἐστιν. The seemingly did not apply while on campaign, see Velleius Paterculus, *Roman History* 2.114.1–3, indicating the demarcation between the acquisition and maintenance of health and well-being and the treatment of trauma.

7 Suetonius, *Tiberius* 68.4.

8 On Livia Drusilla's interest in physical and mental health and well-being, see Barrett, 2002, pp. 108–112. For further discussion of this issue and its potential effects on Roman domestic medical practice, see Chapter 4, The Transmission of Medical Knowledge.

9 Seneca the Younger, *Moral Epistles* 1.68.

10 Pliny the Elder, *Natural History* 29.8.

11 Plutarch, *Advice on Keeping Well* 26.1 (trans. F. C. Babbitt): τὸ δεῖν ἕκαστον αὑτοῦ μήτε σφυγμῶν ἰδιότητος εἶναι ἄπειρον (πολλαὶ γὰρ αἱ καθ' ἕκαστον διαφοραί) μήτε κρᾶσιν ἀγνοεῖν ἣν ἔχει τὸ σῶμα θερμότητος καὶ ξηρότητος μήθ' οἷς ὠφελεῖσθαι χρώμενον ἢ βλάπτεσθαι πέφικεν. αὐτοῦ γὰρ ἀναίσθητός ἐστιν καὶ τυφλὸς ἐνοικεῖ τῷ σώματι καὶ κωφὸς ὁ ταῦτα μανθάνων παρ' ἑτέρου καὶ πυνθανόμενος τοῦ ἰατροῦ πότερον μᾶλλον θέρους ἢ χειμῶνος ὑγιαίνει, καὶ πότερον τὰ ὑγρὰ ῥᾷον ἢ τὰ ξηρὰ

προσδέχεται, καὶ πότερον φύσει πυκνὸν ἔχει τὸν σφυγμὸν ἢ μανόν· καὶ γὰρ ὠφέλιμον εἰδέναι τὰ τοιαῦτα καὶ ῥᾴδιον, ἀεί γε δὴ πειρωμένους καὶ συνόντας. For a slightly later work on a similar subject, see Galen, *Hygiene*.

12 Edwards, 1993, p. 2, p. 5. On this in relation to therapy specifically, see Xenophontos, 2014.

13 Earle, 2007, p. 38.

14 Eergdolt, 2008, pp. 1–6.

15 WHO, 1948, cited in WHO, 2006.

16 Warwick-Booth et al., 2012, p. 8.

17 Lucas and Lloyd, 2005; Godlee, 2011.

18 King, 2005, pp. 1–11.

19 Warwick-Booth et al., 2012, pp. 13–17.

20 See most recently Riddle, 2013, p. 25 for a summary of the medical and social models and his proposed 'interactional' model of disability; see also Edwards, 1997, p. 35, for her proposed 'community' model of disability.

21 Ariphron, *Fragment* 813, at Athenaeus, *Dinner Sophists* 15.702a–b; see also Lucian, *The Lapse* 6; Plutarch, *On Moral Virtue* 450b; Maximus of Tyre, *Dissertations* 7.1; Sextus Empiricus, *Against the Ethicists* 11.49; Stobaeus, *Anthology* 4.27.9. For inscriptions, see *IG* II² 4533 (Athens); *IG* IV² 1,132 (Epidauros).

22 Wilkins, 2005, pp. 137–138.

23 Athenaeus, *Dinner Sophists* 15.702 (trans. S. D. Olson, with alterations): Ὑγίεια, πρεσβίστα μακάρων, μετὰ σεῦ ναίοιμι τὸ λειπόμενον βιοτᾶς, σὺ δέ μοι πρόφρων ξυνείης· εἰ γάρ τις ἢ πλούτου χάρις ἢ τεκέων ἢ τᾶς ἰσοδαίμονος ἀνθρώποις βασιληίδος ἀρχᾶς ἢ πόθων οὓς κρυφίοις Ἀφροδίτας ἕρκεσιν θηρεύομεν, ἢ πόνων ἀμπνοὰ πέφανται, μετὰ σεῖο, μάκαιρ᾽ Ὑγίεια, τέθαλε πάντα καὶ λάμπει Χαρίτων ὀάροις· σέθεν δὲ χωρὶς οὔτις εὐδαίμων. This hymn is discussed at Stafford, 2000, p. 150, 2005.

24 Stafford, 2000, p. 167.

25 Theognis, *Elegies* 1.255–256; Aristotle, *Nicomachean Ethics* 1099a.27–28; Plato, *Gorgias* 451e3; Lucian, *The Lapse* 6–7; Alexander, *Problems and Solutions* 1.9; Sextus Empiricus, *Against the Ethicists* 11.49.

26 Sextus Empiricus, *Against the Ethicists* 50 (trans. R. G. Bury): Ἡρόφιλος δὲ ἐν τῷ διαιτητικῷ καὶ σοφίαν φησὶν ἀνεπίδεικτον καὶ τέχνην ἄδηλον καὶ ἰσχὺν ἀναγώνιστον καὶ πλοῦτον ἀχρεῖον καὶ λόγον ἀδύνατον ὑγείας ἀπούσης.

27 Craik, 1995, pp. 346–347.

28 For discussion of the term *diaita*, see Jouanna, 2015, pp. 210–214.

29 *Regimen in Acute Diseases* 38; *Ancient Medicine* 3.

30 *Ancient Medicine* 5.

31 *Regimen in Acute Diseases* 18.68; *Airs, Waters, Places* 1.

32 Plato, *Republic* 406 A–C. This belief is also found in the works of later writers such as Soranus and Porphyrius.

33 Alcaeus 61.12; Pindar, *Olympian Odes* 265 and *Pythian Odes* 1.93; Aeschylus, *Prometheus Unbound* 490; Sophocles, *Electra* 1073 and *Oedipus at Colonus*, 352, 751; Euripides, *Fragments* 21.4, 812.6, 525.5, 759.2, 917.2; Aristophanes, *Wasps* 624, *The Assemblywomen* 673, 1103, 1112, *Peace* 572, *Birds* 413, *Frogs* 114.

34 There does not seem to have been a clear separation between physical and mental health problems in classical antiquity. It is only relatively recently that scholarly attention has turned to the subject of the latter, and as a result the study of mental disorder and mental illness in the ancient world is one of the fastest growing fields in ancient medicine. See as a starting point Harris, 2013a; Thumiger and Singer, 2018.

35 Holmes, 2010, p. 161.

36 König, 2005.

37 For a general summary, see Nutton, 2013, pp. 160–173; for more detail, see the earlier work Nutton, 1993; Scarborough, 1993.

38 Pliny the Elder, *Natural History* 29.6.

39 Pliny the Elder, *Natural History* 29.8.

40 Edelstein in Temkin and Temkin, 1967, p. 308; Rousselle, 1988, p. 8.
41 See for example Seneca the Younger, *Moral Epistles* 90.19.
42 Gautherie, 2014; on the Roman physician's relationships with patients, see Mudry, 1980.
43 Toner, 1995, p. 8.
44 Cicero, *On Duties* 3.1. On *otium*, see André, 1966.
45 Sallust, *On the Jurgurthan War* 4.4; for Cicero's specific complaints regarding this, see *Letters to Friends* 254.2 (IX.8.2), *On Duties* 2.2, *Orations* 148, *Tusculan Disputations* 3.83. On *otium* during the Principate, see Seneca the Younger, *On Otium*; Pliny the Younger, *Letters* 1.22.11, 5.6.45.
46 See for example Pliny the Younger, *Letters* 2.17, 5.6; Statius, *Silvae* 1.3, 2.2. See this discussed with reference to particular villas on the Bay of Naples in Zarmakoupi, 2014.
47 Cicero, *In Defence of Archias* 13; Columella, *On Agriculture* 1.8.2.
48 See Gill, 2013, p. 340 for a description of ancient regimen as 'lifestyle management' and p. 341 as 'care of the self'.
49 See Gill, 2013, 2018 for discussion of the use of philosophy as a preventative measure for the maintenance of good mental health and 'therapy for the emotions' which did not necessarily involve a healthcare practitioner in antiquity.
50 Cicero, *Tusculan Disputations* 4.13.28–30 (trans. J. E. King): *Morbum appellant totius corporis corruptionem, aegrotationem morbum cum imbecillitate, vitium, cum partes corporis inter se dissident, ex quo pravitas membrorum, distortio, deformitas. Itaque illa duo, morbus et aegrotatio, ex totius valetudinis corporis conquassatione et perturbatione gignuntur; vitium autem integra valetudine ipsum ex se cernitur. Atque ut in malis attingit animi naturam corporis similitudo, sic in bonis. Sunt enim in corpore praecipua, pulchritudo, vires valetudo, firmitas, velocitas, sunt item in animo. enim corporis temperatio, cum ea congruunt inter se e quibus constamus, sanitas, sic animi dicitur, cum eius iudicia opinionesque concordant.*
51 Cato the Elder, *On Agriculture* 5.2 (trans. A. Dalby): *Familiae male ne sit, ne algeat, ne esuriat.* Cato the Elder, *On Agriculture* 5.4–5 (trans. A. Dalby): *Opus rusticum omne curet uti sciat facere, et id faciat saepe, dum ne lassus fiat . . . si hoc faciet, minus libebit ambulare et valebit rectius et dormibit libentius.*
52 Astin, 1978, p. 183.
53 Pliny the Elder, *Natural History* 29.7.14 (trans. W. H. S. Jones): *Dicam de istis Graecis suo loco, M. fili. quid Athenis exquisitum habeam et quod bonum sit illorum litteras inspicere, non perdiscere, vincam. Nequissimum et indocile genus illorum, et hoc puta vatem dixisse: quandoque ista gens suas litteras dabit, omnia corrumpet, tum etiam magis, si medicos suos hoc mittet. Iurarunt inter se barbaros necare omnes medicina, et hoc ipsum mercede faciunt ut fides is sit et facile disperdant. Nos quoque dictitant barbaros et spurcius nos quam alios opicon appellatione foedant. Interdixi tibi de medicis.*
54 Most recently, see Nutton, 2013, pp. 165–167; von Staden, 1996, pp. 375–394; Gruen, 1992, pp. 52–83.
55 Pliny the Elder, *Natural History* 29.12; see also Polybius, *Roman Histories* 12.25d for a contemporary assessment of Greek medicine in this period.
56 For the extent to which so-called Roman medicine had already undergone a certain amount of Hellenisation see von Staden, 1996, pp. 387–394.
57 Pliny the Elder, *Natural History* 29.15.
58 On these, see Draycott, 2016.
59 Plutarch, *Cato the Elder* 23.4 (trans. B. Perrin): αὐτῷ δὲ γεγραμμένον ὑπόμνημα εἶναι, καὶ πρὸς τοῦτο θεραπεύειν καὶ διαιτᾶν τοὺς νοσοῦντας οἴκοι, νῆστιν μὲν οὐδέποτε διατηρῶν οὐδένα, τρέφων δὲ λαχάνοις ἢ σαρκιδίοις νήσσης ἢ φάσσης ἢ λαγώ· καὶ γὰρ τοῦτο κοῦφον εἶναι καὶ πρόσφορον ἀσθενοῦσι, πλὴν ὅτι πολλὰ συμβαίνει τοῖς φαγοῦσιν ἐνυπνιάζεσθαι· τοιαύτῃ δὲ θεραπείᾳ καὶ διαίτῃ χρώμενος ὑγιαίνειν μὲν αὐτός, ὑγιαίνοντας δὲ τοὺς ἑαυτοῦ διαφυλάττειν.

60 See Holmes, 2010, p. 163 on the master using regimen as a means to control his inferiors.
61 Pliny the Elder, *Natural History* 28.79.
62 Cato the Elder, *On Agriculture* 56–58.
63 On the life of Asclepiades, see Green, 1955; Rawson, 1982.
64 Cicero, *On Oratory* 1.62, discussed by Rawson, 1982, pp. 360–361.
65 On the theories of Asclepiades, see Vallance, 1990, 1993.
66 See for example Celsus, *On Medicine* preface 11; Pliny the Elder, *Natural History* 25.12–20; Apuleius, *Florida* 19. However, he was apparently a follower of the third-century BCE physician Cleophantus, who treated fevers by prescribing wine, see Celsus, *On Medicine* 3.14.1.
67 Cicero, *On Oratory* 1.62. Asclepiades was so renowned as a physician that Mithridates VI issued an invitation to his court at Pontus, see Pliny the Elder, *Natural History* 7.124.
68 Pliny the Elder, *Natural History* 26.14. For discussion, see Fagan, 1999a, pp. 98–99.
69 Celsus, *On Medicine* 3.4.2 and 3.18.13; Pliny the Elder, *Natural History* 26.12–20, 25.6; Scribonius Largus, *Compositions* 3H.
70 Scribonius Largus, *Compositions* 3H, 75.
71 Celsus, *On Medicine* preface 11; Caelius Aurelianus, *Chronic Diseases* 1.1.50, 2.1.57.
72 Spencer, 1935, pp. xi—xii.
73 Celsus, *On Medicine* proem 1; see also 5.28.16; this is also mentioned by Columella, *On Agriculture* 1.1.14; Pliny the Elder, *Natural History* 14.33; Celsus, *On Medicine* proem 1 (trans. W. G. Spencer, with adjustments): *Ut alimenta sanis corporibus agricultura, sic sanitatem aegris Medicina promittit.*
74 Quintilian, *Institutes of Oratory* 10.1.124 (trans. J. S. Watson): *Non sine cultu ac nitore*; Quintilian, *Institutes of Oratory* 12.11.24 (trans. J. S. Watson): *Vir mediocri ingenio.*
75 Brand, 2008, pp. 31–32.
76 Celsus, *On Medicine* 1.2.4; 1.3.13.
77 Celsus, *On Medicine* 1.1.1–4 (trans. W. G. Spencer, with adjustments): *Sanus homo, qui et bene valet et suae spontis est, nullis obligare se legibus debet, ac neque medico neque iatroalipta egere. Hunc oportet varium habere vitae genus: Modo ruri esse, modo in urbe, saepiusque in agro; navigare, venari, quiescere interdum, sed frequentius se exercere; siquidem ignavia corpus hebetat, labor firmat, illa maturam senectutem, hic longam adulescentiam reddit. Prodest etiam interdum balineo, interdum aquis frigidis uti; modo ungui, modo id ipsum neglegere; nullum genus cibi fugere, quo populus utatur; interdum in convictu esse, interdum ab eo se retrahere; modo plus iusto, modo non amplius adsumere; bis die potius quam semel cibum capere, et semper quam plurimum, dummodo hunc concoquat. Sed ut huius generis exercitationes cibique necessariae sunt, sic athletici supervacui: nam et intermissus propter civiles aliquas necessitates ordo exercitationis corpus adfligit, et ea corpora, quae more eorum repleta sunt, celerrime et senescunt et aegrotant. Concubitus vero neque nimis concupiscendus, neque nimis pertimescendus est. Rarus corpus excitat, frequens solvit. Cum autem frequens non numero sit sed natura aestimandus, habita ratione aetatis et temporis, scire licet eum non inutilem esse, quem corporis neque languor neque dolor sequitur. Idem interdiu peior est, noctu tutior, ita tamen, si neque illum cibus, neque hunc cum vigilia labor statim sequitur. Haec firmis servanda sunt, cavendumque ne in secunda valetudine adversae praesidia consumantur.*
78 Celsus, *On Medicine* 1.2.5 (trans. W. G. Spencer): *Quem interdiu vel domestica vel civilia officia tenuerunt, huic tempus aliquod servandum curationi corporis sui est.*
79 Martial, *Epigrams* 4.8.1–6.
80 Juvenal, *Satires* 3.184–189, 5; Martial, *Epigrams* 10.10; Seneca the Younger, *On the Shortness of Life* 14.3–4; Martial, *Epigrams* 8.44.8.
81 Holleran, 2012.
82 Celsus, *On Medicine* 1.2.6. See also Galen, *On Exercise with a Small Ball.*

83 See for example the Baths of Agrippa; according to Cassius Dio, *Roman History* 54.29.4, upon Agrippa's death in 12 BCE he left them to the Roman people in perpetuity.

84 Vitruvius, *On Architecture* 5.9.1; Propertius, *Elegies* 2.32.11–12.

85 Portico of Agrippa: Cassius Dio, *Roman History* 53.27; Martial, *Epigrams* 2.14.6, 3.20.11, 11.1.12. Portico of Vipsania: Cassius Dio, *Roman History* 55.8.3–4; Pliny the Elder, *Natural History* 3.17; Martial, *Epigrams* 1.108.1. Portico of Livia: Cassius Dio, *Roman History* 54.23, 55.8; Suetonius, *Divine Augustus* 29; Ovid, *Fasti* 6.639. Portico of Octavia: Suetonius, *Divine Augustus* 29; Cassius Dio, *Roman History* 49.43.

86 Agrippa: Cassius Dio, *Roman History* 54.29.4; Ovid, *Letters from Pontus* 1.8.37–38. Caesar: Horace, *Satires* 1.9.18; Cicero, *Philippics* 2.109; Suetonius, *Divine Julius Caesar* 83; Appian, *Civil War* 2.143; Cassius Dio, *Roman History* 44.35; DeLaine, 2018, p. 169 on the healthiness and health benefits of baths and palaestras.

87 Varro, *On Agriculture* 2.2; Martial, *Epigrams* 3.58.

88 Vitruvius, *On Architecture* 5.11.1.

89 Livy, *From the Founding of the City* 29.19.12–13; Suetonius, *Divine Augustus* 98.3; Strabo, *Geography* 5.4.7.

90 Yegül, 1992, pp. 55–66.

91 Martial, *Epigrams* 7.67; Juvenal, *Satires* 6.421.

92 On the role of bathing in the maintenance of health, see Fagan, 2006; on the role of anointing in the maintenance of health, see Bond, 2015.

93 Fagan, 1999b.

94 Cassius Dio, *Roman History* 53.27.1. The bathhouse subsequently burned down in 80 CE, but was restored by Titus or Domitian: Cassius Dio, *Roman History* 66.24; SHA *Hadrian* 19; *CIL* VI 9797.

95 Suetonius, *Nero* 12; Aurelius Victor, *Epitome of the Caesars* 5; Eutropius 7.15; the complex's popularity: Martial, *Epigrams* 2.14.13, 2.48.8, 3.25.2, 7.34.5 and 9, 12.83.5.

96 Suetonius, *Divine Titus* 7; Cassius Dio, *Roman History* 66.25.1.

97 Pausanius, *Description of Greece* 5.12.6; Cassius Dio, *Roman History* 69.4.1.

98 Ahenobarbus: Seneca the Elder, *Controversiae* 9.4.18; Etruscus: Statius, *Silvae* 1.5 and Martial, *Epigrams* 6.42; Sura: Martial, *Epigrams* 6.64.12–13.

99 Curtis, 2008, p. 370.

100 Morley, 1996, p. 5, p. 13. For further discussion of food and drink, see Chapter 3, The Roman Household.

101 Rousselle, 1988, pp. 5–23.

102 See Caldwell, 2015, pp. 79–104 on the use of regimen during puberty as a means of preparing Roman girls for marriage; see Harlow and Laurence, 2002, pp. 54–64 on female adolescence as part of the life course.

103 Koloski-Ostrow, 2015, p. 117.

104 Brand, 2008, pp. 35–36.

105 Rawson, 1985, pp. 51–53; Scarborough, 1993, pp. 27–28. For further discussion of formal and informal ways in which information about health was disseminated, see Chapter 4, The Transmission of Medical Knowledge.

106 Cicero, *On Old Age* 35–36 (trans. W. A. Falconer): *Resistendum, Laeli et Scipio, senectuti est eiusque vitia diligentia ompensanda sunt, pugnandum tamquam contra morbum sic contra senectutem, habenda ratio valetudinis, utendum exercitationibus modicis, tantum cibi et potionis adhibendum, ut reficiantur vires, non opprimantur.* On the maintenance of health in old age, see Cokayne, 2007; on old age as part of the Roman life course, see Harlow and Laurence, 2002, pp. 117–131; on Roman old age, see Cokayne, 2003; Parkin, 2003. Conversely, on the regimen of youths, see Eyben, 1993, pp. 124–127.

107 Pliny the Younger, *Letters* 3.1.3–8 (trans. B. Radice): *Mane lectulo continetur, hora secunda calceos poscit, ambulat milia passuum tria nec minus animum quam corpus*

exercet. Si adsunt amici, honestissimi sermones explicantur; si non, liber legitur, interdum etiam praesentibus amicis, si tamen illi non gravantur. Deinde considit, et liber rursus aut sermo libro potior; mox vehiculum ascendit, adsumit uxorem singularis exempli vel aliquem amicorum, ut me proxime. . . . Ubi hora balinei nuntiata est (est autem hieme nona, aestate octava), in sole, si caret vento, ambulat nudus. Deinde movetur pila vehementer et diu; nam hoc quoque exercitationis genere pugnat cum senectute. Lotus accubat et paulisper cibum differt; interim audit legentem remissius aliquid et dulcius.

108 Pliny the Younger, *Letters* 8.36.1–5 (trans. B. Radice): *Evigilo cum libuit, plerumque circa horam primam, saepe ante, tardius raro . . . emendantique similis, nunc pauciora nunc plura, ut vel difficile vel facile componi tenerive potuerunt. Notarium voco et die admisso quae formaveram dicto; abit rursusque revocatur rursusque dimittitur. Ubi hora quarta vel quinta (neque enim certum dimensumque tempus), ut dies suasit, in xystum me vel cryptoporticum confero, reliqua meditor et dicto. Vehiculum ascendo. Ibi quoque idem quod ambulans aut iacens; durat intentio mutatione ipsa refecta. Paulum redormio, dein ambulo, mox orationem Graecam Latinamve clare et intente non tam vocis causa quam stomachi lego; pariter tamen et illa firmatur. Iterum ambulo ungor exerceor lavor. Cenanti mihi, si cum uxore vel paucis, liber legitur; post cenam comoedia aut lyristes; mox cum meis ambulo, quorum in numero sunt eruditi. Ita variis sermonibus vespera extenditur, et quamquam longissimus dies bene conditur.* See also Pliny the Younger, *Letters* 8.40 for Pliny's winter regimen, very similar to his summer one.

109 Garnsey, 1999, p. 84.
110 Garnsey, 1999, pp. 100–112.
111 Garnsey, 1998, p. 226. However, for a nuanced discussed of whether it is appropriate to speak of poverty in ancient Rome, see Morley, 2006; Scheidel, 2006.
112 Garnsey, 1998, p 227.
113 Garnsey, 1998, p. 227.
114 Garnsey, 1998, p. 227; unfortunately, their experiences are difficult to recover from Roman literature, as portrayals of poverty were written by the elite, in addition to being highly fictionalised, see Woolf, 2006.
115 Killgrove, 2013.
116 Killgrove and Montgomery, 2016, p. 22.
117 Killgrove and Tykot, 2012, p. 9.
118 Prowse et al., 2004.
119 Prowse et al., 2004, p. 270.
120 Prowse, 2011, p. 420.
121 Rowan, 2014.
122 See Henneberg and Henneberg, 2002, p. 176 for evidence of chronic systemic infection from Pompeii.
123 See Henneberg and Henneberg, 2002, p. 174 for evidence for bone setting and surgery from Pompeii; bioarchaeological evidence attests that some people received medical attention and their fractures healed well, others did not.
124 Graham, 2013.
125 On regimen for infants, see Harlow and Laurence, 2002, pp. 41–43; see also Carroll and Graham, 2014 for comprehensive discussion of literary, documentary and archaeological evidence for infant health. On regimen for girls and women, see Caldwell, 2015.
126 Garnsey, 1998, pp. 226–252; Garnsey, 1999.
127 See Harlow and Laurence, 2002, pp. 20–33 for the acknowledgement that the Roman house is a crucial part of the Roman life course.

2 The Roman house and garden

Introduction

I have run off to my *villa* at Nomentum, for what purpose, do you suppose? To escape the city? No; to shake off a fever which was surely working its way into my system. It had already got a grip upon me. My physician kept insisting that when the circulation was upset and irregular, disturbing the natural poise, the disease was under way. I therefore ordered my carriage to be made ready at once, and insisted on departing in spite of my wife Paulina's efforts to stop me; for I remembered master Gallio's words, when he began to develop a fever in Achaia and took ship at once, insisting that the disease was not of the body but of the place. . . . As soon as I escaped from the oppressive atmosphere of the city, and from that awful odour of reeking kitchens which, when in use, pour forth a ruinous mess of steam and soot, I perceived at once that my health was mending. And how much stronger do you think I felt when I reached my vineyards! Being, so to speak, let out to pasture, I regularly walked into my meals! So I am my old self again, feeling now no wavering languor in my system, and no sluggishness in my brain. I am beginning to work with all my energy.[1]

On numerous occasions in ancient literature, the state of an individual's health, whether good or bad, is explicitly linked with the specific geographical location that they happen to be in at that particular moment in time. In this passage, Seneca the Younger writes that he has removed himself from the city to the country for the sake of his health, juxtaposing his city and country residences and stating that he is not attempting to escape the city *per se*, rather he is attempting to escape certain aspects of being in the city that are having a deleterious effect on his state of health.[2] He makes a point of differentiating the air that he breathes in the city from the air that he breathes in the country.[3] This encourages a complete change of lifestyle, and the consequence of this is an overall improvement in both his physical and his mental health and well-being. It is notable that while Seneca's physician made the initial diagnosis regarding his physiology, it is his brother Lucius Junius Gallio that first offered him a prescription, recommending treating a fever by changing location, a treatment whose efficacy he could personally vouch for, and now that Seneca can personally vouch for this treatment, he is recommending it to his friend Lucilius. Health was a popular topic of conversation between family members, friends and acquaintances, and healthcare knowledge acquired through a variety of means and media was readily disseminated, and we have a clear case of both of these in action here.[4] But just how easy was it to change one's physical location in order to treat a health problem? How accessible, and thus feasible, a prescription was this?

Travelling for the express purpose of improving health was common in antiquity, and here wealthy individuals in possession of multiple residences had an obvious advantage, as they could choose where they resided, when and for how long.[5] They were also well-equipped in other ways, such as in respect of their household staff or, if in possession of multiple residences, staffs. For those who were not so fortunate themselves, they might have recourse to others who were through family ties, patron and client relationships or social networks. Pliny the Younger writes to his friend Gaius Valerius Paulinus concerning his freedman Zosimus:

> Some years ago he was exerting himself during a passionate performance when he began to spit blood. I then sent him to Egypt, and after a long stay there he recently returned with his health restored. Now after demanding too much of his voice for several days on end he has had a slight return of his cough as a reminder of the old trouble, and once again has brought up blood. So I think the thing to do is to send him to your place at Forum Julii [in Gallia Narbonensis, modern Fréjus], for I have often heard you saying that the air is healthy there and the milk excellent for treating this kind of case. Please write to your people and ask them to receive him on the estate and in your home, and to meet the expenses of anything he may need.[6]

Pliny writes that he sent Zosimus to Egypt some years ago, but presumably either does not consider this relapse serious enough to warrant such a drastic intervention, or, since the original trip to Egypt seems to have provided only a temporary respite, has decided to try an alternative.[7] Knowledge of this alternative has come about from Valerius Paulinus sharing his personal experiences of the healthy air and produce of Forum Julii with Pliny, leading to Pliny considering it a suitable place for Zosimus to convalesce as a result. Here we see Pliny acting as patron to his client and utilising his own social networks on his client's behalf. Zosimus therefore benefits not only from the advice that Valerius Paulinus gave to Pliny, but also from Pliny's ability to use his connections to provide suitable accommodation, complete with all necessary components.

These two examples demonstrate the important link between geographical location and health and well-being in ancient thought. Certain places were widely considered to have beneficial effects, and theoretically one could choose to visit them in order to access these. Provided one had complete flexibility regarding where and how they lived, they could go out of their way to accommodate their health and well-being and the requirements of their specific regimen. However, how many people did have complete flexibility regarding where and how they lived? The extent to which an ordinary Roman could change their geographical location in the service of their health is debateable. Members of the social elite, yes. Everyone else, not necessarily. Wealthy plebeians and freedmen and women, yes. Plebeians and freedmen and women that were not wealthy and slaves lived where they were required to live according to circumstance and sought to make the best of it. Under those circumstances, shortcomings in accommodation could be ameliorated, at least on a temporary basis, by the open-air lifestyle facilitated by ancient Roman cities and towns, and civic amenities such as public bathhouses and latrines, porticoes and parks.[8]

It is clear that for the Romans location had an important role to play not only in acquiring and maintaining health and well-being in the first place, but also, if at any point one's health happened to decline, regaining it. The aim of this chapter, therefore, is to examine the extent to which concerns about acquiring and maintaining good health informed not only the location but also the design, layout and usage of the ancient Roman house and garden, thereby contextualising Roman domestic healthcare practice.

The role of the environment in the acquisition and maintenance of health and well-being

The idea that the natural environment has a formative influence on peoples, and thus by implication their civilisations, has been an important theme in intellectual history for the last two and a half millennia.[9] The Hippocratic treatise *Nature of Man* sets out the theory of the four humours (that an individual's constitution is composed of a combination of blood, phlegm, yellow bile and black bile), before acknowledging that these humours fluctuate according to the changing of the seasons.[10] Another Hippocratic treatise, *Airs, Waters, Places*, takes this further by arguing that while the health of an individual depends upon their constitution and the manner in which they live, up to a point, it is also affected by a range of other factors, and it is these factors that will ultimately prevail:

> Whoever wishes to pursue properly the science of medicine must proceed thus. First he ought to consider what effects each season of the year can produce; for the seasons are not at all alike, but differ widely both in themselves and at their changes. The next point is the hot winds and the cold, especially those that are universal, but also those that are peculiar to each particular region. He must also consider the properties of the waters; for as these differ in taste and in weight, so the property of each is far different from any other.[11]

Part of the environment that needs to be understood is the heavens, and the treatise encourages the physician to study astronomy in order to facilitate his (or perhaps her) understanding and interpretation of the stars.[12] Astronomy informed meteorology, which in turn informed medicine, and precision in its application was considered to be extremely important.[13] Additionally, since it was not just human beings that are affected by their environment, but also animals and plants, this ensured that the tenets of the treatise could potentially be applied to animal husbandry, agriculture and horticulture as well as to medical practice, and these disciplines could inform each other in turn.[14]

While *Airs, Waters, Places* was written to cater to the specific needs of an itinerant physician, providing the physician with the knowledge necessary to evaluate unfamiliar settlements and design a course of treatment for their inhabitants accordingly, it is hardly surprising that in time its tenets found favour with those responsible for planning settlements.[15] Plato utilised them hypothetically in his writing of the treatise *Laws*.[16] Vitruvius, author of the only treatise dedicated to architecture to survive from antiquity and himself an architect and engineer, was in the enviable position of being able to utilise them not only in theory but also in practice.[17]

Designing a Roman house

Generally, the primary concerns of an architect in the early phases of design and planning a building are use and utility, with not only the projected use of the proposed building, but also the possibility of maximising its utility.[18] It is clear from ancient Roman technical literature that, no matter what the intended use and utility of a proposed building, one of the fundamental considerations of the Roman architect was its potential healthiness (or unhealthiness, for that matter). According to Vitruvius, architecture was a discipline that required familiarity with a number of different types of knowledge, one of which was medicine.[19] Medical knowledge was necessary to assess the salubriousness of the location chosen for building, particularly its climate, air and water.[20] He goes so far as to state 'no building will be healthy without attention to these points', indicating that buildings were supposed to be healthy and that considerations regarding the healthiness of a building were incorporated into its very inception.[21] That is not to say that architects were expected or required to be practising physicians, but we might imagine a sliding scale of healthcare knowledge going from a general acquaintance with some aspects of some of the treatises of the Hippocratic Corpus to something akin to Celsus' familiarity with diet, drugs and surgery, and the difference between theory and practice.[22] Additionally, the extent to which healthiness was born in mind by an architect (or their patron) might well vary depending on the intended use of the building once its construction was completed.

Vitruvius proceeds logically through offering advice on siting cities and towns, planning the layout of cities and towns and the placement of public and private buildings, and considerations over healthiness are evident throughout.[23] A city or town should be situated in a certain type of location, taking advantage of light, air and water.[24] Civic amenities can, up to a point, help with this. Water quality is acknowledged to be variable depending on its source, but the provision of works, reservoirs, fountains and water-basins makes for a cleaner city, with purer air and the unwholesome atmosphere removed.[25] A building should be designed in accordance with its projected use.[26] Thus a temple dedicated to Aesculapius, Hygieia or any other deity concerned with healing that receives visits from individuals seeking cures for chronic health problems and expecting to see a demonstrable improvement in their conditions should be situated in a location that offers good air and water.[27] A theatre should be situated in a location that is as healthy as possible since men, women and children spend a considerable amount of time there and 'the pores of their bodies being opened by the pleasure they enjoy, are easily affected by the air, which, if it blows from marshy or other noisome places, infuses its bad qualities into the system'.[28] A theatre should be surrounded by porticoes, and each portico should contain a central space large enough to accommodate displays of greenery as well as space for walking. This benefits both the eyes and the body since

> the air from green plants being light and volatile, insinuates itself into the body when in motion, clears the sight, removing the gross humours from the eyes, leaves the vision clear and … when the body is heated by the exercise of walking, the air, extracting its humours, diminishes corpulency, dissipating that which is superabundant in the body.[29]

We see these tenets carry over into private – that is, domestic – architecture. There is considerable variety in Roman private building, with numerous adaptations made according to the requirements of the geographical location.[30] While Vitruvius only discusses elite housing in urban and rural locations, he does state that a residence should be designed with the specific requirements of its residents in mind, and he gives examples, such as an individual of the middle rank not requiring a substantial vestibule, *atrium* or *tablinum* due to them not serving as a patron to significant numbers of clients, or an individual who relies upon the produce from their estate requiring storage space for this produce, or advocates and literary figures requiring space for meetings and performative displays.[31] We can potentially apply this rationale to the types of resident and residence that he does not mention, at least as far as purpose-built accommodation, or the original phase of occupation of accommodation that is subsequently changed, is concerned.

Central Italy was viewed by some ancient authors as having been particularly blessed in relation to its geography and climate, and these blessings were thought to extend to its people.[32] In Strabo's *Geography*, two books out of seventeen are devoted to the Italian mainland and the associated islands, and specific regions and the settlements within them are noted for their health. In the north, Ravenna is particularly healthy, the explanation given for this is that the surrounding rivers wash away dirt and cleanse foul air.[33] In the south, Croton is famous for its healthfulness, fame which is reflected in the proverb 'more healthful than Croton', and the explanation given for this is that the god Apollo granted Croton health at the request of the city's founder Myscellus upon his visit to the Oracle at Delphi.[34] The superlative healthfulness of Ravenna and Croton was actively utilised; gladiators were trained in the former, athletes in the latter.[35] Similarly, Neapolis was considered particularly good for rest and relaxation, and provided a refuge for those who wished to withdraw from the hustle and bustle of Rome.[36] What of the places with which this study is primarily concerned: Rome, Ostia, Pompeii and Herculaneum? Rome itself was not considered particularly healthy, and certainly the city had not originally been sited or planned according to the sort of architectural ideals espoused by Vitruvius.[37] The provision of city amenities such as sewers and aqueducts was one means of attempting to rectify the site's deficiencies.[38] Another was co-ordinated rebuilding after disastrous fires, such as the one that occurred during the reign of Nero and destroyed or seriously damaged ten of Rome's fourteen regions. Tacitus explicitly compares the rebuilding efforts in the wake of this fire with those of an earlier one:

> The districts spared by the palace were rebuilt, not, as after the Gallic fire, indiscriminately and piecemeal, but in measured lines of streets, with broad thoroughfares, buildings of restricted height, and open spaces, while colonnades were added as a protection to the front of the tenement-blocks. . . . These reforms, welcomed for their utility, were also beneficial to the appearance of the new capital. Still, there were those who held that the old form had been the more salubrious, as the narrow streets and high-built houses were not so easily penetrated by the rays of the sun; while now the broad expanses, with no protecting shadows, glowed under a more oppressive heat.[39]

There seems to have been debate among medical practitioners as to whether narrow or wide streets were healthier.[40] Herculaneum was considered a healthy place to live due to its promontory that extended out into the sea and caught the southwest wind, and Ostia and Pompeii were likewise coastal towns and theoretically healthy as a result.[41]

The belief that certain geographical locations are inherently healthy or unhealthy fundamentally underpins the contents of not only Vitruvius' *On Architecture*, but also works belonging to other literary genres that contain extensive sections on architecture, such as Cato's *On Agriculture* (*circa* 160 BCE), Marcus Terentius Varro's *On Agriculture* (mid-first century BCE) and Columella's *On Agriculture* (mid-first century CE), particularly in relation to private architecture. It would appear that, in cases where houses were built from scratch, concerns regarding acquiring and preserving good health and well-being did, in fact, inform not only the location, design and layout of the Roman house and garden but also the ways in which they were subsequently used.[42]

For the earliest Roman treatise that deals with the Roman house at length, we have to look back to the middle Republic (*circa* 274–148 BCE), more specifically the period immediately following the Second Punic War (218–201 BCE). Cato the Elder was born in Tusculum in Latium in 234 BCE. The earliest surviving source for his life is Cornelius Nepos' first-century BCE work *Cato*, while the most detailed is Plutarch's second-century CE work *Cato the Elder*.[43] According-ing to Cato himself, his early years were spent labouring on his father's farm in Sabine territory: 'I spent all my boyhood in frugality, privation and hard work, reclaiming Sabine rocks, digging and planting those flinty fields'.[44] There is ample evidence to suggest that this was not simply aristocratic self-fashioning, as Cato's agricultural knowledge and experience was expressed at length in *On Agriculture*, the first such work to be written in Latin, and one that was subsequently utilised (not always uncritically) by a range of Roman writers, not least Varro, Columella and Pliny the Elder, whom we shall examine in their turn.[45]

Cato's reputation as an agriculturalist remained prevalent long after his death; Cornelius Nepos not only considered it worth referring to in the brief sketch of Cato's life contained in his work *On Great Generals*, but also went so far as to list it first among his many achievements: 'In all lines he was a man of extraordinary activity; for he was an expert husbandman, an able jurist, a great general, a praiseworthy orator and greatly devoted to letters'.[46] The treatise, very much a product of its time both with regard to its style and its content, was directed at a very specific audience: young men who, thanks to Rome's victory in the Second Punic War, were in a position to purchase agricultural land in Latium, Campania or Samnium, along with sufficient slaves to enable them to cultivate grapes and olives in order to produce wine and oil for sale, but were not in possession of sufficient knowledge or experience as to how to proceed beyond that.[47] Thus the extent to which it can be used as a source for information on farming in other regions is questionable.[48] The priority is economic self-sufficiency and investment potential.[49]

Cato begins *On Agriculture* with a list of points that, in his opinion, those thinking of acquiring a farm should consider; chief among them is the recommendation that the farm should be 'in a healthy position'.[50] The land is fundamental: 'it must have good weather; it must not be liable to storms. It must thrive from its own excellence and from its good location: if possible, it should be at the root of a mountain, south-facing . . . and a good water supply'.[51] However, just as the possession of a farm situated on a piece of land in a salubrious location is not on its own enough to make one a successful farmer, the possession of a farm on a piece of land in a less than salubrious location does not automatically guarantee failure. Although Cato begins his treatise with advice for those considering acquiring a farm and makes the assumption that if a farm is less than ideal, his reader will not purchase it, he does also include instructions for purifying the land through a religious ritual known as the *suovetaurilia*, which involved the sacrifice of a pig, a sheep and a cow.[52]

Our second source for the Roman house dates to the Late Republic (147–30 BCE). Varro (116–27 BCE) was born in Reate in the Sabine territory north-east of Rome, and, like Cato, he grew up in a land-owning family so had firsthand experience of agriculture. However, the extent to which his own personal knowledge and experience informed his writing, as opposed to simply extensive reading and paraphrasing of appropriate authorities such as Aristotle and Theophrastus, has been queried.[53] After all, Varro was a polymath who wrote on a variety of subjects – Quintilian declared him 'the most learned of all Romans' – so is it feasible that all of his writings were inspired by his own personal experience, as opposed to diligent research?[54] Yet, at least superficially, Varro's *On Agriculture* is rather more personal than Cato's *On Agriculture*. The first book of the three-volume work was dedicated to Varro's wife Fundania, who at the time he was writing had just purchased a farm herself, while the second was dedicated to his friend Turranius Niger, a cattle-breeder from Mutina, and the third was dedicated to his friend Quintus Pinnius, whom Varro feels could make use of his advice regarding expanding his *villa* through the production of luxury goods.[55] All three dedicatees are thus in a position to benefit from Varro's work and the advice contained within it. Unlike Cato, Varro was familiar with the work of the Carthaginian agricultural writer Mago, and more than fifty Greek agricultural treatises, and was not aiming to produce a didactic handbook.[56] Rather, his aim with *On Agriculture* was to demonstrate the real possibility of the rural way of life, following the physical and moral annihilation of Italy during the course of the Civil Wars (49–30 BCE).[57]

Varro takes his discussion of the healthiness of the farm's position one step further than Cato. Using the festival of Sementivae at the Temple of Tellus (a celebration of sowing that was sacred to Tellus, Mother Earth and Ceres, the goddess of agriculture) as the setting for an encounter between himself, his father-in-law Gaius Fundanius and two friends named Gaius Agrius and Publius Agrasius (although genuine Roman *nomena*, it is clear that they are used here because they derive from *fundus*, 'a piece of land, a farm, an estate' and *ager*, 'productive land, a field, farm, estate, arable land, pasture'), he has Agrasius open the conversation with a question: 'You have all travelled through many lands; have you seen any land more fully cultivated than Italy?'.[58] Agrius' reply explicitly links the 'healthfulness' of land with not only the possibility of successfully cultivating it, but also the results of said cultivation:

> I think there is none which is so wholly under cultivation. Consider first: Eratosthenes, following a most natural division, has divided the earth into two parts, one to the south and the other to the north; and since the northern part is undoubtedly more healthful than the southern, while the part which is more healthful is more fruitful, we must agree that Italy at least was more suited to cultivation than Asia.[59]

In Varro's discussion of what, precisely, makes a piece of land healthy, he goes so far as to introduce the character of Scrofa, loosely based on Gnaeus Tremelius Scrofa, apparently 'the Roman most skilled in agriculture' into his circle of friends at the Temple of Tellus in order to address this specific issue.[60] According to Scrofa:

> Especial care should be taken, in locating the steading, to place it at the foot of a wooded hill, where there are broad pastures, and so as to be exposed to the most healthful winds that blow in the region. A steading facing the east has the best situation, as it has the shade in summer and the sun in winter.[61]

If one was not building a farm from scratch, Varro has different advice. This is perhaps the result of his stated motivation for writing *On Agriculture* in the first place: that his wife Fundania had recently purchased a farm and wished to make it profitable, thus providing for herself after Varro's death, but had yet to do anything with it and so needed guidance prior to commencing. Consequently, although Varro's Agrius states that if you find yourself the owner of a farm on unhealthy land, you should either sell it or abandon it, his Scrofa offers an alternative course of action:

> Granting that healthfulness, being a product of climate and soil, is not in our power but in that of nature, still it depends greatly on us, because we can, by care, lessen the evil effects. For if the farm is unwholesome on account of the nature of the land or the water, from the miasma which is exhaled in some spots; or if on account of the climate, the land is too hot or the wind not salubrious, these faults can be alleviated by the science and the outlay of the owner.[62]

Our third – and most extensive – source dates to the first century CE. Little is known of Columella (4–70 CE) beyond that which is included in his treatise *On Agriculture*.[63] He was born in Gades in the province of Baetica, where his uncle owned a substantial amount of land and, rather than being an absentee landowner or landlord, the elder Columella was directly involved in what transpired on his estates, going so far as to experiment with cross-breeding African and Spanish sheep.[64] The younger Columella subsequently acquired several estates near Rome at Ardea, Carseoli and Alba, and thus had firsthand knowledge of agriculture in Italy and a number of Roman provinces, including Spain, Cilicia and Syria, and in addition to this was well-acquainted with Carthaginian, Greek and Roman agricultural writing, and combined extensive firsthand experience of agriculture with extensive research into theories, methods, and practices.[65] Consequently, his work is not only more extensive, comprehensive and systematic, but also more general, and thus – for our purposes – more broadly applicable, than either Cato's or Varro's.[66]

Columella goes further than either Cato or Varro in relation to the importance of the healthiness of the land. He not only connects the health of the land with the success or failure of efforts made to cultivate it, but also, ultimately, with the health of the land's owner:

> In an unhealthy climate, no matter how fruitful and rich the soil, the owner cannot live to the harvest; for where the reckoning must be made with Orcus, not only the harvesting of the crops but also the life of the husbandmen is uncertain, or rather death is more certain than gain.[67]

Columella's ideal farm is one 'with fertile soil, partly level, partly hills with a gentle eastern or southern slope; with some parts of the land cultivated, and other parts wooded and rough; not too far from the sea or a navigable stream, by which its products may be carried off and supplies brought in'.[68]

For those who, unlike Vitruvius, Cato, Varro and Columella, were not in a position to build their home from scratch or divest themselves of a property that had proved to be unsuitable, all was not necessarily lost. Varro uses Scrofa to present an example of a case in which altering existing buildings proved beneficial to health:

> The situation of the buildings, their size, the exposure of the galleries, the doors, and the windows are matters of the highest importance. . . . Did not

our friend Varro here, when the army and fleet were at Corcyra, and all the houses were crowded with the sick and the dead, by cutting new windows to admit the north wind, and shutting out the infected winds, by comrades and his servants in good health?.[69]

Certainly, there is a considerable amount of literary evidence for homes having been renovated.[70] Cicero writes to his brother Quintus regarding the latter's property portfolio, and the changes that have already been, or are in the process of being, made.[71] Pliny the Younger writes on a number of occasions of changes he has made to his various properties.[72] Additionally, numerous surviving *villae*, *domus* and *insulae* show evidence of having been renovated at various times during their period of occupation. Such renovation might occur because of changes in fashion but also because of changes in the nature of occupation, with a larger residence split up into smaller ones, smaller residences combined to form a larger one or portions of a residence being turned over to economic activity.

How a building's physical situation plays to its residents or regular users is location, and how it plays to everyone else, is context.[73] As we have seen, ancient architects seem to have had similar concerns. Vitruvius states that Roman residential buildings should be designed and planned according not only to where they are to be located, taking the country and its climate into account, but also who is going to be occupying them and how they were going to be utilising them.[74] The healthiness of the residence impacts upon the healthiness of its occupants, and is therefore fundamental in ensuring not just survival but also success. Vitruvius highlights the contribution to health and well-being made by the climate and the quality of light, air and water, and recommends taking these into account when designing, planning and building an urban residence. This contribution is also noted by Cato, Varro and Columella when designing, planning and building a rural residence. Judging solely from the information contained in their writings, it seems that a patron and the architect take into account concerns over the climate and the quality of light, air and water in selecting an ideal location for building a residence, whether urban or rural, and that these concerns in turn inform the design, layout and subsequent usage of the ideal home. However, this material is not without its problems. The four treatises are didactic works of technical literature, and all four were written with an agenda.[75] Each has a significant moral component and aims to impart information regarding what is necessary to be a good Roman.[76] So how far can we trust that these qualities were commonly recognised as being important when it came to someone choosing where to live?

While the terms used by Roman writers to refer to private buildings are relatively few in number, they are anything but straightforward. The literary genre and context in which they are used has considerable influence over how each term should be interpreted.[77] We can distinguish several different types of Roman residence: *villa*, *domus*, *insula* and *casa*.[78] All of these designations are problematic to some degree. In central Italy in the period from the early third century BCE to the late first century CE, social and cultural developments arising from Roman imperialism, Hellenisation and urbanisation ensured that significant changes to Roman living situations occurred, and as a result the terms used to describe ancient Roman residences can to mean different things at different times. There was a wide range of different types of accommodation, and also a wide range of different qualities of accommodation, a sliding scale of quality. At least in urban areas, the vast majority of Romans rented their primary residence, whether that residence was a *domus* or a *cenaculum* or taberna in an *insula*. The section of the rental market utilised depended upon social status and wealth. We know more about elite living situations than we do non-elite, but it is important to remember that members of the elite – whether socially, financially or both – frequently possessed multiple residences of varying different types, rotating both their period and manner of occupation.[79] We have far less information about those lower down the social scale, and virtually nothing about the peasantry.[80] In the case of the living situations of the lower classes, we are dependent on the writings – not always serious and probably not always accurate either – of members of the elite. These tend to be not only idealising, but also moralising, explicitly juxtaposing the sophisticated but dissolute urban elite with the ignorant but noble country dwellers.[81] Also worth noting is that, whatever the type of residence, those occupying it could potentially experience it very differently. Owners of multiple residences could only occupy one residence at a time, and the way that they used that residence could differ considerably from the way that household staff, whether free or slave, used it, whether they were occupying it simultaneously or not. How the household staff behaved when the master or mistress was not present was a source of considerable anxiety. There is evidence to suggest that, at least in larger residences, the slave members of the household occupied certain areas of the residence.

Sizeable agricultural estates had existed in Italy since the sixth century BCE.[82] For Cato, a *villa* was a farmstead devoted to agricultural production.[83] However, from the second century BCE such estates began to incorporate not only agricultural production but also luxurious leisure, peaking in the late first century BCE and the first century CE, particularly in the area around Rome and on the Bay of Naples.[84] Consequently for Varro, there were two types of *villa*: the *villa urbana*, a luxurious estate devoted to leisure pursuits, and the *villa rustica*, a frugal estate devoted to agricultural production, such as Cato's.[85] For Columella, a *villa* was an estate in which different parts had different functions: the *pars urbana*, where the *dominus* resides, the *pars rustica*, the part of the estate devoted to agricultural activities, and the *pars fructaria*, the part of the estate devoted to storage of what is produced.[86] These distinctions are perhaps too absolute, and have their origins in ideology rather than typology, the dichotomy between work and leisure, frugality and luxury. Perhaps the most flexible way of describing a *villa* is that it is an elite estate, whether located in a rural setting or on the coast, which is simultaneously used for economic activities and leisure pursuits, elite referring to those who possessed a prominent status in society due to either social position or wealth (see Figure 2.1).[87]

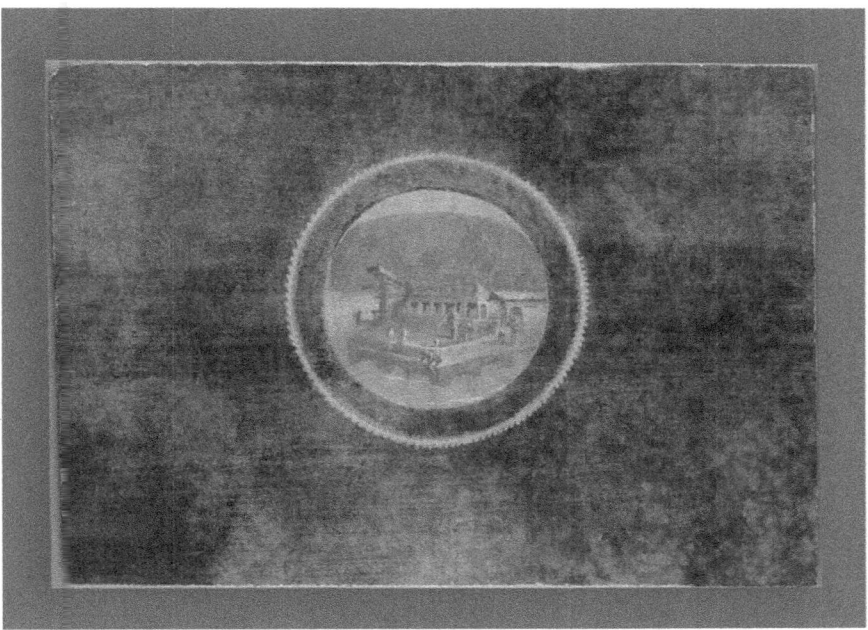

Figure 2.1 A fresco tondo depicting a seaside villa, *circa* 50–79 CE.

Source: Image courtesy of the J. Paul Getty Museum Open Content Program (J. Paul Getty Museum inv. 72.AG.84).

Publius Papinius Statius (45–96 CE) is the first to describe elite *villae* in detail and devotes entire poems to individual examples. In his description of Manlius Vopiscus' *villa* at Tivoli, he makes the point that this *villa* has been designed, planned and built in such a way that climate and weather have no effect on it, and this in turn is beneficial to health, preventing seasonal illnesses such as fevers.[88] In fact, a stay at the *villa* bestows a 'glow of health' (*nitor sanus*), cleanses and contributes to a long life.[89] Pliny the Younger describes his own *villae* at length in letters to his friends and acquaintances. When describing his *villa* at Laurentium to a friend who wonders why he likes the residence so much, he begins with emphasising three key things about the estate, 'the attractions of the house itself, the amenities of its situation, and its extensive sea-front'.[90] Another of Pliny's *villae* is not so fortunately situated, and he spends the first paragraph of the letter in which he describes this *villa* defending it:

> I am touched by your kind concern when you try to dissuade me from my intention of staying in Tuscany in summer. You think the place is unhealthy, but while it is perfectly true that the Tuscan strip of sea-coast is relaxing and dangerous to health, my property is some distance away from the sea, and is

in fact at the foot of the Apennines, which are considered the healthiest of mountains.[91]

Pliny again emphasises the climate, the surrounding countryside and the situation of the residence, and offers support for his claims by saying that the *villa* is so healthy that even his slaves benefit from staying there.[92]

Over time the term *domus* ceased to be used to indicate a 'home' in the general sense and instead came to be used to refer to a particular type of residence, one that was located in an urban setting and was entirely self-contained.[93] Such

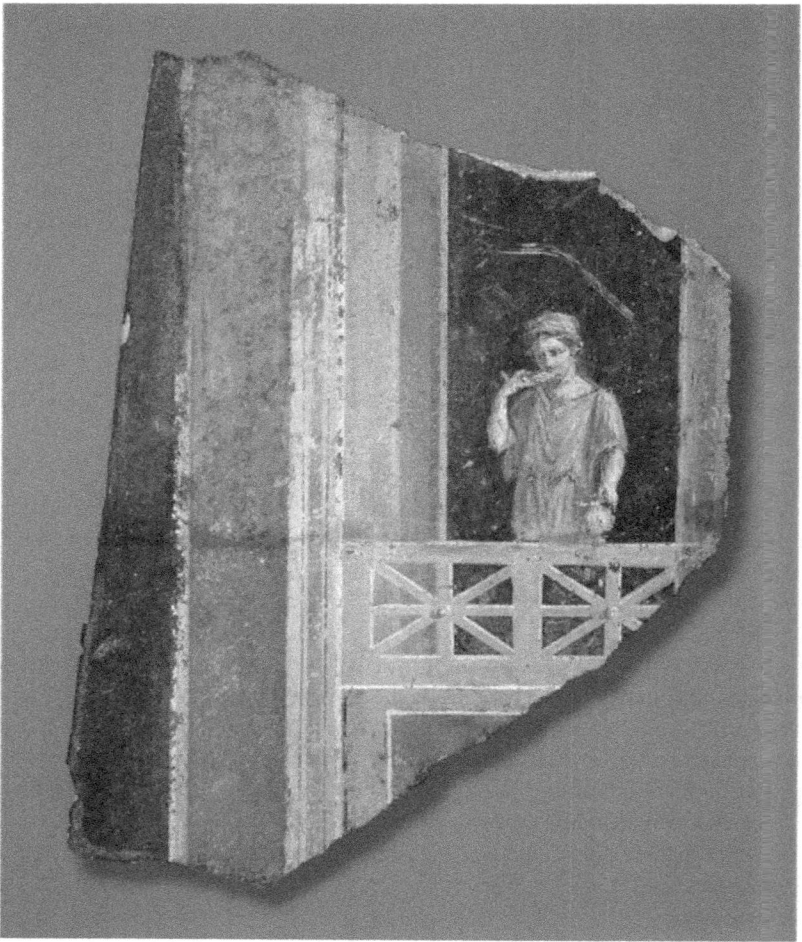

Figure 2.2 A fragment of a fresco depicting a woman standing on a balcony, *circa* 1C BCE–14 CE.

Source: Image courtesy of the J. Paul Getty Museum Open Content Program (J. Paul Getty Museum inv. 96.AG.172).

a residence was usually situated on the ground floor of an *insula*, and was occupied by one relatively well-to-do household, whether its inhabitants were owner-occupiers or simply renting the accommodation. Generally, two types of *domus* are recognisable: the first is the *atrium* house, in which the *atrium* was the centre of the residence and provided the residents with light, air and water, in use from the third century BCE onwards; the second is the *atrium/peristyle* house, in which use of the *atrium* was supplemented by the *peristyle*, in use from the late third century BCE onwards, with the addition of the *peristyle* at the rear of the house increasing the amount of light, air and water that was available to the residents. However, there is also archaeological evidence for numerous other small houses that do not conform to either of these types, have irregular layouts and indicate experimentation and individualisation on the part of those who occupied them.[94]

The term *insula*, quite literally 'island', was used to refer to high-rise tenements containing multiple storeys composed of *cenacula*, sets of rooms that were usually rented and where individual households resided, built around a central space that served to emit a certain amount of light and air.[95] The facilities tended to be fairly limited, with residents having to go outside for water and toilet facilities. These were found in densely populated urban environments such as Rome and Ostia and enabled the housing of large numbers of people in relatively small spaces. *Insulae* such as the *Insula* of Arriana Paulina and the Praedia of Julia Felix in Pompeii contained a variety of accommodation options available for rent, including *tabernae* ('shops, work-shops or taverns') and *cenacula* ('upstairs flats').[96] The most common type of *cenaculum* found in Ostia comprises rooms on three sides of a central room, with the fourth side facing the street or the courtyard.[97] Some upper stories might even include balconies, such as the *Insula Romana* at the base of the Capitoline Hill in Rome (see Figure 2.2).

The term *casa* can be used to refer to any one of a wide range of simple buildings from 'cottage' to 'hut' to 'hovel', depending on the context. There is rather more literary than archaeological evidence for this type of residence and its occupants.

Designing a Roman garden

Like the ancient Roman homes of which they were integral components, ancient Roman gardens came in a variety of shapes and sizes. While by no means all homes were equipped with a garden, archaeological excavation has shown that a significant proportion of them were.[98] Although the majority of ancient Roman literature privileges certain specific 'types' of gardens, archaeological and bioarchaeological evidence indicates that, in actuality, there were many different types of gardens, and these gardens in turn could serve multiple purposes simultaneously.[99]

The writers of the Roman agricultural treatises recommended that an agricultural estate set aside a portion of land for the purpose of cultivating a garden. Cato had firm opinions on the subject:

> If you ask me what is the best kind of farm, I should say: a hundred iugera of land, comprising all sorts of soils, and in a good situation; a vineyard comes first if it produces bountifully wine of a good quality; second, a watered

garden; third, an osier-bed; fourth, an oliveyard; fifth, a meadow; sixth, grain land; seventh, a wood lot; eighth, an arbustum; nine, a mast grove.[100]

Both Varro and Columella likewise recommend planting gardens.[101]

Comprehensive information regarding the practical aspects of horticulture is presented across a range of genres.[102] While a considerable amount of this information was directed at the owners of agricultural estates of which the garden was only one small part, to a degree the fundamentals would have remained the same no matter what the size or context of the garden space.[103] First and foremost, it was important to situate the garden in the best possible spot, preferably on level ground in a spot that could catch the sun.[104] Whether the garden was outside or inside the residence, practicalities were important: the domestic water supply, convenience and access.[105] Security was also a factor, as garden produce was highly desirable.[106] It was also important to consider what produce was going to be grown in the garden, as depending on whether plants were wild or cultivated, domestic or foreign, they would have different needs with regard to planting and maintenance such as irrigation and fertilisation.[107] Seasonality was more relevant to rural gardens than urban ones.[108] In Campania, it was theoretically possible to harvest multiple crops per year and produce crops all year round.[109] No matter how small or large the cultivated space, its productive potential could be maximised by intercultivation. People exercised personal choice in their planting, both with regard to personal preference and taste, and with regard to economic considerations.[110] It is also necessary to consider the contribution made by wild plants (*silvestris*) in addition to cultivated ones (*sativus*). The term *silvestris* refers to the place where the plant grows rather than the plant itself.[111] Consequently, to the Romans there seem to have been three types of 'wild' plants: the first grew outside the bounds of cultivation, fallow land or pasture; the second grew on land used for pasture; and the third grew on fallow land.[112] Thus a 'wild' plant was not necessarily one found out in the woods or on the side of a mountain, but rather one that was not being deliberately cultivated, what we might consider a weed, so could be present in a garden of any size or location. Likewise, such plants could be utilised by the affluent as garnishes or by the less affluent as staples. Seneca the Younger makes the point that Fabricius, a former triumphator, dines on roots and herbs that he has foraged for himself during the process of tilling his own fields and is just as happy doing so as he would be with a feast of exotic foodstuffs.[113] However, wild plants, once gathered, could be transplanted into a garden and henceforth cultivated, although this could be a difficult process.[114]

As stated by Cato and Varo, on a large estate, the garden enabled the cultivation of fruit, vegetables, herbs and flowers that could supplement the grain, wine and oil, and thus could either be consumed by those living on the estate or be sold and the money earned utilised for purchasing items that could not be produced.[115] On a small-holding, the fruit, vegetables, herbs and flowers produced by the garden could be crucial to survival.[116] Historically, the *heredium*, the portion of land allotted to each Roman citizen by Romulus, consisted of two *iugera*, what a man could reasonably be expected to plough in a day, which comprised both agricultural and horticultural land (*ager* and *hortus* respectively).[117] The *Twelve Tables* recognised the garden as the family estate, and so it was the garden that was responsible for the maintenance, survival and continuity of the family from one generation to the next.[118] Simulus, a farmer whose day is described in the poem *Moretum*, cultivates just such a garden:

> Adjoining the cottage was a garden, sheltered by a few osiers and the slender stalks of reeds which he used as a fence; it was small in extent, but rich in various herbs. Naught did it lack that a poor man's need demands; at times a wealthy neighbour would turn to the poor man's stock for more. Nor did his little property cost him anything but his labour: if ever rainy weather or a holiday kept him idle in his cottage, if by any chance there was respite from the task of ploughing, that time was given to the garden. He knew how to set out the various plants, to entrust seeds to the hidden soil, and to lead nearby streams as required around the crops. Here flourished cabbage, here beets, their arms far outspread, with sorrel in profusion, mallows, and elecampane; here skirret and leeks, that owe their name to the head, and lettuce that brings pleasing relief to rich meals: here the roots of spiky asparagus which grow into spearpoints, and the heavy gourd that swells into its broad belly. But this crop was not for the owner (for who more frugal than he?) but for the people; and every ninth day over his neck he would carry his bundles to town for sale. Thence he would return home, with shoulders light but with heavy pockets, and seldom accompanied by purchases from the market. It was red onion that tamed his hunger, and his plot of chives, and watercress which with its sharp taste screws up the face, and rocket which revives a man's flagging potency.[119]

While a garden might reasonably be defined as a cultivated space found in a domestic context, a wide range of Greek and Latin terminology is utilised by ancient authors to refer to variations on this theme, and this is somewhat problematic when it comes to attempting to translate descriptions and discussions of ancient gardens into contemporary English.[120] Additionally, it is tempting to excerpt the sections of ancient Latin literature that deal with horticulture.[121] However, contextualising these discussions within the genres in which they appear – whether technical treatise, bucolic poem, epistle, etc. – is of crucial importance for understanding not only the relationship between the Roman home – whether *villa, domus, insula* or *casa* – and its garden, but also the relationship between both of these and domestic medical practice. It is also necessary to move beyond the ancient literature and incorporate archaeological and bioarchaeological evidence.[122] Recent studies concentrating on specific sites have shown precisely how integrated into their architectural surroundings gardens were.[123] Gardens were created to take advantage of their surroundings, so it is important to consider the context. Rural residences might have extensive land dedicated to cultivation, while urban residences might be more pressed for space. The occupants of an agricultural estate might cultivate a kitchen garden adjacent to the *villa rustica*, such as at the Villa Regina at Boscoreale, while the occupants of a *domus* might cultivate a kitchen garden at the rear of the house, such as in the House of the Surgeon at Pompeii. The occupants of a *cenaculum* in an *insula* might utilise the space afforded by their windowsill for a window box or their balcony for potted plants, while the interior courtyard might be dedicated to some sort of garden space, such as in the Praedia of Julia Felix at Pompeii or the Garden Houses at Ostia.[124] Some residences, whether rural or urban, might boast multiple garden spaces, each with a different purpose, such as Pliny the Younger's *villa* at Laurentum, or the House of the Faun at Pompeii, with its kitchen garden and peristyle garden.[125]

Regarding cultivated spaces found in domestic contexts, three specific manifestations are particularly relevant to our investigation of the role of the garden in Roman domestic medical practice and will be examined here: *hortus*, *peristyle* and *viridarium*.[126] The *hortus*, the Latin term used most frequently and, as a result, most problematically, was initially what we might describe as a kitchen garden, a garden used to cultivate herbs and vegetables, perhaps also containing fruit- or nut-bearing trees, although by the middle of the first century BCE the term had come to be used to refer to an entire elite estate, particularly one that was utilised for *otium* as well. The *peristyle*, the term borrowed from the Greek *peristulos*, was composed of three or even four colonnades surrounding a central garden space, and facilitated walking. The *viridarium* (*viridiarium* was also used) was a space – not a *peristyle* – that displayed deliberately arranged specimen plants through agricultural features such as windows and doors; numerous examples are found in the *villa* at Oplontis.[127] This has been interpreted as being for the purpose of juxtaposing the best of horticulture with the amenities of the indoors, in a rather different way than the *peristyle* did.[128] There are indications of other rather unusual types of gardens: Martial refers twice to greenhouses, and there are also references to roof gardens, and evidence for them on the southern and western walls of Pompeii.[129]

Using a Roman house

The *atrium* was the principal room of the Roman *villa* or *domus*.[130] It was thought to have once been the main living space of the Roman family, the term *atrium* perhaps deriving from *ater*, 'black', due to the room's roof beams being blackened by smoke from the hearth fire which burned below.[131] This belief in the smokiness of the *atrium* is found elsewhere, particularly in relation to the objects that were kept there such as family trees and ancestor masks and busts, emphasising the longevity of some families' occupation of their houses.[132] While there may originally have been a hole in the ceiling of the *atrium* directly over the hearth fire to let the smoke out, by the middle of the Republic the centre of the ceiling was entirely open, which facilitated light and air entering the building, and when it rained water likewise entering the building and collecting in a shallow pool directly below. Varro connects the names of both of these features, the *compluvium* and the *impluvium*, with *pluvia*, 'rain', indicating the importance of the *atrium* facilitating the provision of water for the household.[133] While it was possible for private households to pay to be connected to aqueducts, or even connect themselves illegally, for those households lacking such a connection, having an *impluvium* meant that at least some water was on hand.[134] One outlet led from the *atrium* to the cistern so that the water could be stored, another led to the street outside to ensure that any overflow ran out into the street. In Pompeii and Herculaneum around forty percent of houses had an *impluviate atrium*, but these houses tended to be the larger and grander ones, indicating that these houses were occupied by members of the towns' social elite.[135]

As a space, the *atrium* served as a reception room in which the *dominus* acting as patron received his clients during the daily *salutatio*.[136] For a long time, study of the *atrium* focused on the use of the space by the *dominus*, but more recently attention has turned to the use of the space by other members of the household, and also the use of the space for commercial activities.[137] The *atrium* was flanked by smaller rooms, and according to Varro these served a variety of purposes, depending upon what was required.[138] These rooms might serve as storerooms (*cella* from *celare*, 'to conceal'), pantries (*penaria*, from *penus*, 'food') or bedrooms (*cubicula*, from *cubare*, 'to lie down').

The *culina* can be defined as an area of the house, or – in the case of houses large enough to allow subdivision into functionally defined spaces – a specific room, where cooking was meant to be carried out on a regular basis.[139] According to Publius Ovidius Naso (43 BCE–17/18 CE), the hearth was originally located at the front of the house, and Publius Vergilius Maro (17–19 BCE) associates the hearth and its fire with the threshold and its doorposts, and this may well have been the case in smaller houses that lacked an *atrium* with a *compluvium*, thus allowing the smoke to escape through the front door, rather than billowing back into the house.[140] Much later, Servius quotes Cato as claiming that cooking used to be done in the *atrium*, and a hearth has been found in the *atrium* of House I.6.13 at Pompeii.[141] Varro is of the opinion that in *villae* the *culina* should be located at the front of the building so that food can be prepared and eaten before dawn, thus facilitating the working day.[142] Unlike the *dominus* and *domina*, who ate in a *triclinium* – the particular *triclinium* used depending upon the time of year on formal occasions and other rooms of the house on informal ones – it seems that slaves ate in the *culina* all year round.[143]

If an area of the house, the placement of the *culina* varied. Cooking facilities have been found in *peristyles*, no doubt taking advantage of the light and air of the space. Seneca the Younger recounts that in his day it was fashionable to cook in the *triclinium* so that the food stayed hot, while Decimus Junius Juvenalis (*circa* late first century/early second century CE) claims that people were in the habit of taking slaves and cooking equipment around with them.[144] In the limited space of the *cenacula* in *insulae*, people would cook on a transportable brazier or oven. If a specific room, the placement of the *culina* depended to a degree on the availability of the necessary amenities such as a water source, drainage, heat, light, ventilation, storage and potentially also proximity to the latrine or the bathhouse. It also depended on what was considered *not* appropriate to have in proximity, such as animals.[145] Whether the *culina* was a specific room or simply a space, cooking was a potentially hazardous activity. Steps were taken during construction to make purpose-built *culina* safe so as to avoid fires.[146] The use of charcoal for fuel reduced the amount of smoke produced during the process of cooking, but there was still a need for ventilation, see for example the perforated roof tiles found in the House of the Ephebe at Pompeii. Cooking requires water, which could be obtained from any one of a number of sources. Some residences were in possession of a private well, others benefitted from a *compluvium, impluvium* and perhaps also a cistern, others were connected to aqueducts.[147] However, for residences that lacked water supplies of their own, there was also the possibility of accessing water from a public well or fountain supplied by an aqueduct.

Latrines were frequently located in or adjacent to the *culina*, whether for the purposes of taking advantage of the water supply or to provide a convenient means of disposing of all kinds of household waste.[148] Most consisted of cesspits dug into bedrock rather than connections to sewer systems, necessitating their being cleaned out periodically.[149] Residences without latrines managed with chamber pots, and emptied the contents into the street.[150]

Bathing was considered to be good for health, to the extent that a detailed regimen of bathing in hot, warm and cold water in order to treat various ailments existed in antiquity. The origin of Roman bathing has been traced to the traditions of folk medicine in central Italian villages.[151] The basic private baths of the late third to the early second century BCE were located close to the kitchen in order to share heat and water, and contained the equivalent of the *caldarium, tepidarium* and *frigidarium* found in the public baths of later periods. More elaborate examples of private baths dating from the first century CE can be found at the House of the Labyrinth and the House of the Faun at Pompeii, and the Villa of Poppidius Florus at Pisanella and the Villa at Boscoreale.

The acquisition, provision and preparation of resources was crucial to ancient Roman domestic healthcare, and it is clear that a considerable amount of these resources were acquired, provided and prepared in advance, in anticipation of their use. The Roman agricultural treatises not only provide comprehensive instructions regarding the processes by which this was accomplished, but also information on how to store the products afterwards. With regard to olive oil and wine, Cato, Varro and Columella make similar recommendations regarding their storage. Cato gives a detailed list of the equipment required for cultivating olive groves, harvesting the olives and processing them into oil and amurca, and both he and Columella recommend that the pressing room and the storeroom or cellar (*cella olearia*) be located close together for the sake of convenience, but far away from the kitchen, bathhouse or other potential sources of foul odours.[152] Vitruvius and Columella make similar recommendations regarding the storage of wine in a storeroom or cellar (*cella vinaria*).[153] Both oil and wine should be stored in *dolia*. Arrangements similar to the ones described have been identified at Settefinestra, and at the Villa della Pisanella at Boscoreale.[154] With regard to legumes, once threshed and dried these were stored in *amphorae*.[155] Root vegetables could be subjected to dry storage, brine storage or pickled.[156] However, these methods were not necessarily appropriate to smaller rural residences such as *casae* or urban residences such as *domus* and *cenacula*. The Appendix Vergiliana's *Moretum* depicts the humble farmer Simulus simply piling his foodstuffs on the ground.[157] Vitruvius describes the type of storage that he considers necessary in a *domus*:

Those who depend upon country produce must have stalls for cattle and shops in the forecourt, and within the main building, cellars, barns, stores and other apartments are for the storage of produce rather than for an elegant effect.[158]

There are numerous parallels in the archaeological record from Pompeii and Herculaneum. Penelope Allison's analysis of the contents of thirty Pompeian *atrium* houses has shown that the fronts of the houses, particularly the rooms located off the front halls and the *atria*, generally known as *ala*, contained shelves, indicating that they were used for the storage of household goods.[159] Elisabetta Cova has studied these areas in more detail, analysing the seventy-nine *alae* in the forty-eight houses of *Regio* VI, and observed that storage practices changed over time, with modifications being made to create permanent storage installations.[160] There were a number of different methods of storage: built-in cupboards, walk-in closets, wall cupboards with shelves and wooden doors, open shelves, racks, freestanding cupboards, storage chests, loft space and subterranean space (see Figure 2.3).[161] In House VI.xiii.13 at Pompeii, the entire *ala* was turned into a cupboard and the five *amphorae* found inside it indicate that it was used to store food.[162]

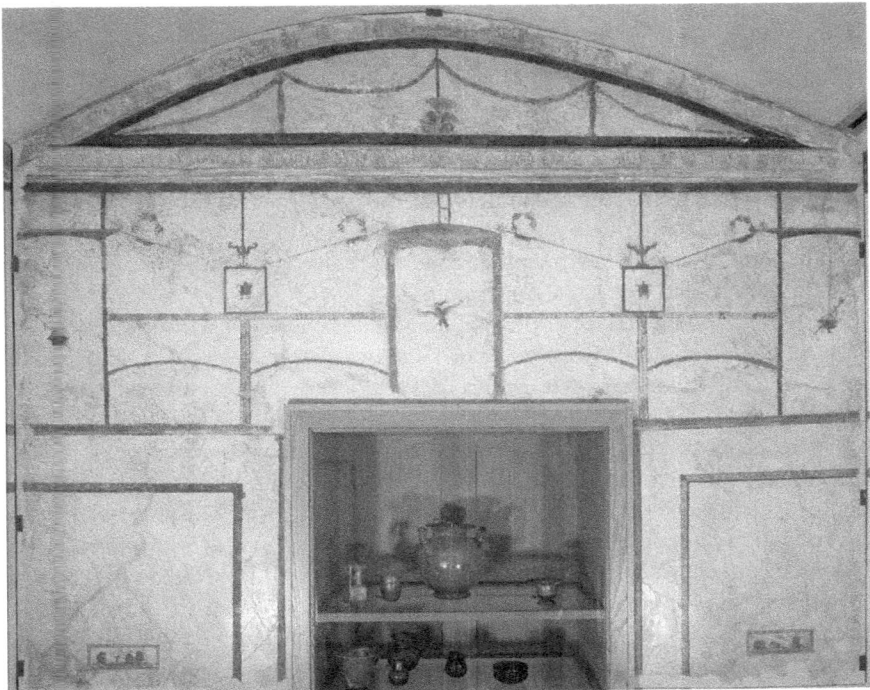

Figure 2.3 A frescoed wall with a niche for storage, the Villa of Numerius Popidius Florus, Boscoreale, *circa* 50–70 CE.

Source: Image courtesy of the J. Paul Getty Museum Open Content Program (J. Paul Getty Museum inv. 70.AG.89).

The artefact distribution at the front of the house suggests that this area was used for a wide range of domestic activities.[163] While the *atrium* is often associated with the *salutatio*, it appears that an important part of the reception of visitors involved not only the display of the occupants of the household, chiefly the *pater familias* or *dominus* in his role as patron to his clients, and their religious institutions, such as the household shrine and the *imagines*, but also the household's wealth in the form of its resources.[164] This display of household wealth not only indicated the household's current prosperity, but also its future prosperity. Most foodstuffs were stored in purpose-built vessels: *incitegae* were used for spices and dried goods, *lagoenae* and *amphorulae* stored, measured and dispensed liquids such as wine, oil and sauces, *dolia* and *amphorae* held sizeable quantities of either dry or liquid goods including wine, oil, garum, grain, olives, dried fruit and preserved fish. Other small rooms at the front of the house, generally known as *cubicula*, were frequently found to contain small storage chests that stored objects relating to personal rather than communal domestic activities.

Using a Roman garden

From the early first century BCE the Romans began to link the natural world and health and well-being in a much more fundamental way than they had done previously.[165] They believed that the humans of prehistory had been close to nature, living off the land without the assistance of any type of technology beyond primitive tools and weapons, and that they were stronger and more resilient as a result.[166] They were able to do this because nature provided everything that they needed.[167] While different philosophies underpin the writings of Titus Lucretius Carus (98 or 97–55 BCE) and Pliny the Elder, and they present nature in very different ways, they both emphasise nature's role as the provider for and the nurturer of humankind.[168] Nature was personified as female since the noun *natura* is gendered female and presented as a maternal figure.[169]

Perhaps it should not be surprising, then, that a liking for garden space seems to have been common; it has even been claimed that gardens were fundamental to the ancient Roman psyche.[170] Certainly gardens occupy prominent places in ancient Roman mythology and historiography. Roman writers depict kings, generals and other influential citizens as having been avid cultivators in addition to the demands placed upon them by their political and military careers, in sharp contrast with the situation in the second century BCE and onwards, where this sort of activity has devolved onto slaves.[171] Pliny the Elder traces the high esteem in which gardens were held all the way back to the days of the Homeric heroes.[172] Prominent figures in Rome's early history were associated with and situated in gardens at crucial moments. The encounter between Numa Pompilius, the second king of Rome, and Jupiter reportedly took place in Numa's garden. Tarquinius Superbus, the seventh and last king of Rome, reportedly sent a message to his son by dead-heading the tallest poppies in his garden.[173] Lucius Quinctius Cincinnatus, consul in 460 BCE, was forced to sell most of his land and retire to a small farm, where he was subsequently approached by a group of senators while working and asked to serve as dictator in order to defeat the Aequian, Sabine and Volscian tribes.[174] This last case was frequently utilised in later periods as a means of providing an example, or *exemplum*, of old Roman *virtus*.[175]

Literary and documentary evidence attests to the sheer variety of garden space that could be experienced by the Romans, from the *horti* of the imperial, senatorial, equestrian and decurion elite to the *hortus* of the plebeian or peasant, although the terminology utilised to do so is not always precise.[176] Archaeological evidence from the sites around Latium and Campania, and the Bay of Naples in particular, confirms that garden space was not only prevalent but also, like the Roman houses to which it was attached, highly personalised.[177]

From the Classical period onwards, ancient gardens were associated with health and well-being.[178] While the citizens of Classical Greece do not seem to have utilised private gardens to the extent that the citizens of Rome did, we know of a number of prominent public gardens that were used for recreational purposes, and these recreational purposes incorporated care of the body and of the mind.[179] At Athens, the Academy, the Cynosarges and the Lyceum all contained *gymnasia* that contained *stoai* and *xystoi* for walking, *palaistrai* for wrestling practice, *dromoi* for military and athletic training and *exedrai* where students could be educated in philosophy through lectures and seminars. The goals of this philosophical education were *eutaxia*, 'good manners', *euexia*, 'good physical condition', *philoponia*, 'capacity for hard work', and *polymathia*, 'general knowledge'.[180] During the course of the Hellenistic period, Greek architectural features began to be incorporated into the *villae* and *domus* of the Roman senatorial, equestrian and decurion elite; the conceptualisation of the garden as a place for physical and mental stimulation resulted in the institution of the peristyle and the colonnade, and the creation of a designated space for walking, talking and thinking in the Roman garden.[181] Certain architectural features were consciously intended to be the setting for intellectual and philosophical conversations, and were deliberately designed in order to remind visitors who participated in these endeavours of Greek philosophy and its adherents.[182] Thus we see Cicero designating areas of his Tuscan *villa* 'the Academy' and 'the Lyceum' and decorating them accordingly.[183]

The garden has been described as the 'heart and centre' of the ancient Roman home.[184] However, recovering an ancient Roman garden in its entirety, not to mention attempting to reconstruct the myriad ways in which visitors could experience it, is extremely challenging. The necessity of using literary, documentary, architectural, archaeological and bioarchaeological evidence in tandem in order to fully explicate the ancient garden has frequently been noted by scholars.[185] With regard to the ancient Roman garden, to date scholars have approached the subject from a variety of different perspectives, focussing on the garden in literature, art and mythology.[186] It was, however, the pioneering work of Wilhelmina Jashemski that began to fully explore ancient Roman gardens utilising archaeological and bioarchaeological methodologies.[187] A recent attempt to examine the Roman garden using spatial theory has differentiated between the garden as a representational space, as depicted in ancient literature and art, particularly wall painting, and as a physical space.[188] Despite this, the role that ancient Roman gardens played in the acquisition and maintenance of good health and well-being has not yet been thoroughly considered.[189] While the medicinal properties of the wide range of plant material utilised by the ancient Egyptian, Greek, Roman and Byzantine peoples have been acknowledged and examined, these have not necessarily been fully or effectively contextualised.[190]

Gardens are simultaneously 'parts of the real world – actual pieces of land – and also virtual worlds – coherent sets of possible sensory stimuli'.[191] Consequently, a garden can be considered to have two manifestations, the physical and the metaphysical, and meaning is bestowed upon it by the range of human activities that take place within it.[192] The ways in which the ancient Roman garden contributed to the acquisition, maintenance and preservation of good health and well-being are directly related to these manifestations. First, the produce of a garden could be utilised within the home or it could be bartered or sold as a means of providing additional resources. The production and consumption of one's own foodstuffs was a means of aspiring towards the Roman ideal of self-sufficiency, an important feature of Roman self-fashioning, but it was also a practical means of ensuring the household's subsistence and survival.[193] While gardens have been described as being either utilitarian or ornamental, this is somewhat misleading.[194] Ancient Roman gardens were both, albeit in different ways. The Romans did not necessarily appreciate beauty for its own sake, but rather for what that beauty implied and signified, and in the case of the garden, its beauty could simultaneously indicate control over nature and provision of subsistence for the purposes of ensuring the survival and prosperity of the household.[195]

The garden spaces were simultaneously ornamental and utilitarian, and were used not only for ostentatious displays of wealth, but also everyday domestic activities, particularly the preparation and consumption of food.[196] There is considerable potential overlap between the preparation of food and the preparation of medicaments. We have already discussed the ways in which food and drink – whether produced in the home or purchased outside it – could be consumed with health and well-being in mind, as a crucial component in a regimen. It should not be surprising to find that the plants grown in the garden could be utilised in similar ways. There is a considerable amount of overlap with regard to the types of plants that ancient authors tell us were cultivated in household gardens and the types of plants that ancient authors tell us were utilised in certain types of medicaments, and what is notable is the nature and purpose of these types of medicaments. Ancient medicaments were designed to treat symptoms rather than the underlying cause of these symptoms, and so the medicaments we see referred to in ancient literature are all those which it would make sense to keep on hand within the home for the sake of expediency: purgatives, emetics and laxatives, aphrodisiacs and contraception, sedatives, remedies for coughs and sore throats.

The tenth book of Columella's *On Agriculture* is dedicated entirely to horticulture. Columella states that his motivation is the increasing popularity of gardening combined with the fact that there is a dearth of knowledge regarding how to undertake it correctly.[197] However, his work can also be read as meditation on the fruits of Roman imperialism, with his garden containing specimens from all around the Mediterranean and serving as the Roman Empire in microcosm.[198]

While Columella provides practical instructions regarding how to site, lay out and manage a garden, he also advises on what to plant in it and the ways in which these crops can be used. Although the vast majority of plants known in antiquity were considered to have medicinal properties, and the vast majority of medicaments were based on plants, it is worth considering the plants that Columella highlights as being particularly beneficial to health in addition to those he mentions as having other primary purposes.[199] He recommends all-heal and celandine for their general healthy properties.[200] He promotes poppies for their ability to promote sleep and a variety of plants that serve as aphrodisiacs.[201] He advises freedmen and freedwomen to use pepperwort to remove the scars left by branding during their time as slaves.[202] He suggests cress to deal with internal parasites.[203] All of these are fairly mundane health problems that it would behove a household to deal with internally, rather than referring them to an external healthcare practitioner.

The Romans believed that the garden was an intrinsically healthy place in and of its own right. It offered an escape from the hustle and bustle of everyday life, and this was not the sole province of wealthy senators with extensive *peristyles*. Pliny the Elder tells us that the lower classes of the city of Rome 'used to give their eyes a daily view of country scenes by means of imitation gardens in their windows', which has been interpreted to mean that the windowsills of *cenacula* in *insulae* were decorated with window boxes.[204] Martial writes to his benefactor Lupus of the country property that he has bestowed upon him, and compares it unfavourably with the one that he has in his window.[205] While the residents of *insulae* potentially used their window boxes, and perhaps also baskets and pots, to cultivate plants that could be utilised, it is worth considering that these miniature gardens were intended to contribute to health and well-being in a slightly different way, a way that is made explicit in discussions of gardens built on larger scales.

In keeping with the positive connotations of agriculture and horticulture, the maintenance of the garden was thought to be a means of keeping fit preferable to attending the *gymnasium*.[206] Pliny the Elder explicitly links his friend Antonius Castor's cultivation of a garden with his longevity: 'I used to visit his special garden, in which he would rear a great number of specimens even when he passed his hundredth year, having suffered no bodily ailment, and, in spite of his age, no loss of memory or physical vigour'.[207] When exiled to Pontus in 12 CE, Ovid wrote a series of letters to his family members and friends back in Rome. In one addressed to his friend Severus, he writes of how he misses his gardens:

> But, I suppose, the delights of the city have been taken from me in my wretchedness in such fashion that I may have at least what country joys I will! It is not for the fields lost to me that my heart longs, the fair lands in the Paelignian country, nor for those gardens lying on the pine-clad hills which the Clodian and Flaminian roads survey – them I tilled for I know not whom, in them I used in person to guide (nor am I ashamed to say it) the spring water upon the plants; somewhere, if they still live, there are certain trees also planted by my hand, but never is my hand destined to gather their fruit. For all these losses would that it could be my lot even here to have in my exile a plot to till! I would in person, if only I might, pasture the goats as they hang upon the crags, I would pasture the

sheep as I leaned upon my staff; that my breast might not dwell upon its usual cares I would myself lead the plough-oxen beneath the curving yoke, teaching myself the words which the Getic bullocks know, hurling at them the familiar threats. In person would I control the handle of the down-pressed plough and try to scatter seed in the furrowed earth. I would not shrink from clearing away the weeds with the long hoe and supplying the water for the thirsty garden to drink. But whence shall all this come to me between whom and the enemy there is only the breadth of a wall and a closed gate?[208]

Both the *peristyle* and the *viridarium* were utilised for the purposes of maintaining health and well-being. Vitruvius unequivocally states that walking out of doors is extremely beneficial, and that a particularly suitable place to undertake such exercise is through a *porticus* decorated with *viridian* ('green things'):

> The open spaces which are between the colonnades under the open sky, are to be arranged with green plots; because walks in the open are very healthy, first for the eyes, because from the green plantations, the air being subtle and rarefied, flows into the body as it moves, clears the vision, and so by removing the thick humour from the eyes, leaves the glance defined and the image more clearly marked. Moreover, since in walking the body is heated by motion, the air extracts the humours from the limbs, and diminishes repletion, by dissipating what the body has, more than it can carry.[209]

Celsus likewise recommends walking alongside *viridia*.[210] In Gaius Petronius Arbiter's *Satyricon*, runners are depicted training in Trimalchio's *peristyle*, taking the idea of using it as a location for physical exercise to extremes just as so many other aspects of Roman social life are taken to extremes in this section of the novel.[211] For the rationale behind this, we need to consider the Roman opinion of the colour green for, according to Pliny the Elder, 'no colour has a more pleasing appearance', and it serves to sooth the eyes, hence why people enjoy looking at young plants.[212] Plants were not only valued for their pleasing appearances, however. They were also valued for their pleasing scents which could be utilised to augment experiences.[213] We should also consider the role that other features of the garden such as fountains could play: in the course of recommending medicaments that have a soporific effect, Celsus observes that the sound of falling water nearby can promote sleep, too.[214] This can be understood if we consider the ancient conception of the senses, and the ways in which objects were thought to give off particles that were absorbed by the eyes, ears, nose and mouth.

This practice of walking as a leisure activity has been identified as a means of advertising the economic independence of the walker – he is able to use his body for the purpose of doing something other than generating profit – and it has been equated with the water feature as an example of conspicuous consumption.[215] However, that rather misses the point that this activity would be taking place in an economically productive area, as the *peristyles* and colonnades of the wealthy elite were frequently planted with exotic species of tree and flower.[216] Gardens could also be used for relaxation, as a location for reading or being read to, writing or dictating works of literature, and vocal or musical performances. We see plane trees both praised and criticised for their ability to provide shade but little else.[217] They were, however, a prominent feature of just about every garden recorded in Roman literature, and there is archaeobotanical evidence for their presence around the Bay of Naples as well, indicating their popularity.[218]

As we have seen, garden produce could be utilised in a variety of ways for the purposes of benefitting health and well-being. Plants, fruits and vegetables could be utilised as foodstuffs and medicaments either alone or in combination. However, we should also consider more ephemeral qualities such as scent. In addition to recommending that a household grow flowers in the garden in order to sell them, Cato also states that the housekeeper should hang garlands over the hearth on the Kalends, Ides, Nones and any other holy day, and it seems likely that she would have been responsible for making the garlands.[219] The choice of the flowers for garlands was significant in itself. While roses and violets seem to have been consistently popular, certain flowers were associated with particular deities or particular events, and were thus considered more appropriate in specific contexts.

Botanical knowledge was widespread in Graeco-Roman antiquity, and it is possible to reconstruct what people believed the properties of flowers used for garlands to be, and identify some patterns (see Figure 2.4).[220] The rose, the violet

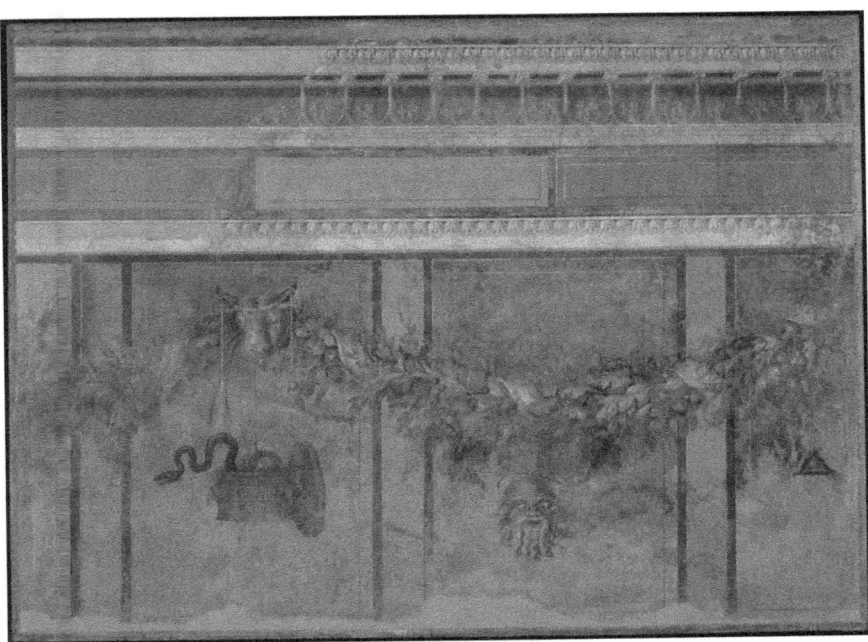

Figure 2.4 A fresco depicting an elaborate garland, Villa of Publius Fannius Synistor, Boscoreale, *circa* 50–40 BCE.

Source: Image courtesy of the Metropolitan Museum of Art Open Access (Metropolitan Museum of Art inv. 03.14.4).

and the myrtle were particularly popular, and we can begin to appreciate why they were considered particularly suitable for use in garlands for *symposia* and *convivia* when we consider their properties: they were believed to have a cooling effect, potentially very useful in a stuffy *triclinium*, and even have a sedative effect, and were also believed to dispel the fumes of wine.[221] Additionally, and potentially more useful still, roses could be prepared in such a way that they took the edge off of perspiration.[222] Conversely, gillyflower and marjoram were not in the habit of being utilised in this way because they were thought to excite the nerves of the head, and stupefy and oppress the head respectively, as well as being warming.[223] Wearing a garland ensured that their flowers and leaves were in proximity to the head, and it was also common practice for petals and leaves to be removed from the arrangement and dipped into wine, ensuring that not only could the scent of the flowers and leaves be tasted and smelled, but also that the plant's additional properties could be utilised, in order to supplement the celebration in a positive way.[224] On certain special occasions the components of garlands were dictated by custom rather than taste or trends – for example, at weddings the bride commonly wore marjoram in her hair not just for its pleasant fragrance, but also because it was sacred to Aphrodite/Venus.[225]

Plants could also be used throughout the home to augment pre-existing spaces, both temporarily and more permanently, and it would appear that certain specimens were considered particularly appropriate to certain spaces, although once again, this was not due to their smell, but the effects that that specific smell was thought to have on those who smelled it.[226] However, it is important to remember that it was not just those plants with pleasant smells that were in demand. Even those that were thought to smell unpleasant could be useful, utilised for fumigation and disinfection, and even as pest control measures.

The agricultural treatises recommend growing flowers in the garden and then selling any surplus to requirements on the estate at the market.[227] Presumably these flowers would be purchased by those who had no garden space of their own, or by professional garland makers, *coronarii*. There is literary and documentary evidence for garland makers, particularly in Rome, which indicates the areas of the ancient city where flowers could be purchased such as the *Via Sacra* and *Portunalia*, the area around the Temple of Portunus in the Forum Boarium, as well as artistic representations of the process proliferating.[228] There is also archaeological and archaeobotanical evidence for the production of flowers on a large scale, such as in the case of the Garden of Hercules (II.viii.6) at Pompeii. This commercial garden was situated next door to a shop selling oils, unguents and perfumes.

Roman domestic religion

One final aspect of the Roman house and garden and the activities that took place within them that it is necessary to consider here is Roman domestic religious belief and practice. The importance of the physical Roman house and garden in respect of the metaphysical Roman domestic religious belief and practice, also known as *sacra privata* or *sacra familiae*, is made explicit in a series of rhetorical questions posed by Cicero in his speech *On His House*:

> What is more sacred, what more inviolably hedged about with every kind of sanctity, than the home of every individual citizen? Within its circle are his altars, his hearths, his household gods, his religion, his observances, his ritual; it is a sanctuary so holy in the eyes of all, that it were sacrilege to tear and owner therefrom.[229]

Horace offers us an insight into what was involved in Roman domestic religious belief and practice in one of his *Odes*:

> If you raise your upturned hands to the sky when the moon is born anew, Phidyle, my country lass; if you placate the gods of your property with incense, with this year's grain, and with a greedy sow, your vine will be fruitful and will not feel the sickening Scirocco, nor will your crops know the blight of mildew, nor your darling nurslings the dangerous season when autumn produces its fruit. The victim marked out for sacrifice, that feeds on snowy Algidus among the oaks and holm oaks or grows fat in Alban pastures, will stain with its neck the pontiffs' axes; but it is not for you to pester the little gods whom you decorate with rosemary and brittle myrtle by slaughtering numerous sheep. If a hand has touched the altar without any gift, not made more persuasive by an expensive victim, it softens the displeasure of the household gods by reverent grain and sputtering salt.[230]

He imagines an act of private worship taking place at a household shrine on a modest country estate, and details the offerings that such a supplicant could make to their household gods – on this occasion, the *Lares* and *Penates* are specified – and the ways in which these household gods could be expected to reciprocate by ensuring protection for that worshipper's household and property.[231] He contrasts the offerings made by his simple supplicant Phidyle – the humble rosemary, myrtle, grain and salt – with those that could be made by her wealthier peers – exotic incense and expensive livestock. Ultimately, if the household gods are satisfied, the outcome is the same.

Concerns over maintaining boundaries, and in turn ensuring the integrity of the house and its household, can be recognised in several household festivals. The first of these is the *Compitalia*, a moveable festival celebrated at the end of December or the beginning of January at the *compitum*, the junction of three or more roads.[232] According to Pliny the Elder, the festival was established by Servius Tullius in order to commemorate his miraculous conception: his mother Ocresia, a slave in the royal household of Tarquinius Priscus, supposedly conceived after seeing a phallus rise up out of the hearth, and Servius was subsequently considered to be the son of the *Lar familiaris*.[233] A broken yoke was hung up to signal the cessation of work.[234] Figures made of wool representing the free members, and balls of wool representing the slave members, of each household were set up at *compita* in the hope that they would serve as adequate substitutes, so preserving the lives of their human counterparts.[235] Both Cato the Elder and Columella describe, in varying levels of detail, how their households celebrated the *Compitalia*.[236] The role that firm boundaries played in ensuring health and well-being is made explicit in Cato the Elder's *On Agriculture*, which gives specific instructions with regard to the warding of a farm against disease and disaster through the *suovetaurilia* ritual, in which a bull, a sheep and a pig were sacrificed.[237] The second of these is the *Terminalia*, celebrated on the 23rd February every year in honour of the god Terminus, who was thought to protect boundary markers, and through this boundaries.[238] As we have seen, according to Varro, Romulus assigned each Roman citizen an inalienable *heredium*, that is, a portion of land to be passed on to their heir, which subsequently became the hereditary family estate.[239] As far as the *Twelve Tables* were concerned, this comprised two *iugera* of land consisting of a *hortus* and an *ager*, land suitable for horticultural and agricultural cultivation respectively.[240] Pliny the Elder stated that one *iugerum* was the area that could be ploughed by an ox over the course of a day – roughly 1.2 acres or half a hectare.[241] While land, not to mention home, ownership changed dramatically from the archaic period, through the middle Republic, and into the late Republic and early Principate, it is important not to disregard the significance of these quantities and their intended purpose – the complete self-sufficiency, in all senses, of a Roman citizen and his family. An individual's land, whether the original *heredium* or a much more extensive estate, requires a boundary in order to define, enclose and protect it. For the Romans, boundaries were physical, whether natural features of the landscape such as rivers, trees or landmarks, or manmade ones such as walls, fences or hedges. Agricultural writers advise their readers to mark out their property very clearly, and land surveyors provide practical and technical information about how exactly this should be done.[242] However, out of necessity boundaries were also metaphysical. When a boundary stone or group of boundary stones were set up, an animal was sacrificed, and its ashes and other offerings placed in a hole dug especially for the purpose.[243] Consequently, interfering with a boundary stone was not only a civic offense but also a religious one.

The relationship between Roman domestic religion and Roman healthcare theory, method and practice seems to have been an extremely close one: concerns over establishing and maintaining the health and well-being of the household and *familia* were deeply embedded in Roman domestic religious belief and practice. However, literary, documentary and archaeological evidence indicates that there was a considerable amount of variety in these not just from household to household, but even within the household itself. Each household worshipped a unique combination of deities.[244] While the standard – if one can call them that – household gods were the *Lares*, the *Penates*, the *Genius* of the *pater familias* and the *Juno* of the *mater familias*, and Vesta, many other deities (and not just Roman ones) were worshipped too. There is even some evidence for Aesculapius being worshipped in a domestic context at Ostia and Pompeii.[245] Private religious behaviour was personal and individual rather than communal, and it is clear from Pompeii, Herculaneum and Ostia that one house might have multiple household shrines, with certain combinations of the members of the household worshipping at each shrine.[246] It is thought that the freeborn and freed members of the household worshipped at the freestanding or niche shrines located in the open areas of the house such as the *atrium* and the *peristyle,* while the slave members of the household worshipped at the shrine paintings in the closed areas of the house such as the kitchen.[247]

The *Lar familiaris* and the *Lares familiares*

The importance of the *Lar* and the *Lares* to the household is made clear by the frequent use of the term as a metonym for the household as a whole.[248] However, it is impossible to establish a definite origin for either the *Lar* or the *Lares*, and it is uncertain as to whether they were originally spirits of the field, and so worshipped at the *compita*, or spirits of the ancestors, and so worshipped at the hearth.[249] There are numerous varieties, although they have in common the role of guarding and protecting their charges, usually in association with a particular physical area.[250] Certainly after the third century BCE one key role was that of the *Lar familiaris*, the guardian spirit and protector of the household.[251] The earliest literary reference to this is found in the prologue to Plautus' *The Pot of Gold*, in which the *Lar familiaris* introduces itself and the other characters, as well as providing some background information:

> For many years already I've been occupying this house and protecting it for the father and grandfather of the man who lives here now. Now this man's grandfather entrusted me, on bended knee, behind everyone's back, with a treasure of gold. He buried it in the middle of the hearth, entreating me to guard it for him. When he died, he didn't even want to make this known to his own son – he was so greedy. He wished to leave him penniless rather than show his treasure to his son. He did leave him a piece of land, not a big one, though, so that he could live on it with great toil and miserably. When the man who'd entrusted the gold to me died, I began to observe whether his son would in any way hold me in greater honour than his father had. He took less and less trouble over me and showed me less respect. I returned the favour: he also died poor. He left a son behind, the one who lives here now, a man of the same character as his father and grandfather. He has one daughter. She worships me every single day with incense or wine or something else and gives me garlands.[252]

Here we see the *Lar familiaris* watching over four generations of the same family and, since the daughter is pregnant, looking forward to the birth of a fifth. It guards not only the household and the *familia* but also property in the form of physical objects.[253] If propitiated, it offers assistance to the propitiator, but if not, it does not. However, the *Lar familiaris*' remit was not restricted to within the house: Albius Tibullus prays to his *Lares* to ensure either that he does not have to go off to war, or, if he does, to protect him while he is away; when one returned from war, one's arms could be set down before them.[254] The importance of the *Lar familiaris* and, later, *Lares*, is underscored by the fact that Cato states that when an estate owner visits his estates, the first thing he should do is greet the *Lar*.[255] Additionally, the

Lar or *Lares* played a role in significant family occasions. When a boy became a man, he would dedicate his *bulla*, his *toga praetexta* and his first beard shavings to it or them, while when a girl was to be married and pass from the guardianship of the *Lares* of her father to that of those of her husband, she took three coins and gave one to her husband, one to his *Lar familiaris* and one to his *Lar compitalis*, and the *Lares* received wedding offerings of frankincense and floral wreaths.[256] *Lares* could be moved to a new residence; when ownership of a house changed hands, the household shrine was frequently repainted to reflect the new owners' *Lares*, while statuettes recovered from various locations in Pompeii and Herculaneum indicate that people fleeing the towns during the eruption of Vesuvius in 79 CE were taking their *Lares* with them. The *Lar* was depicted in the form of a youth either standing or dancing and holding a cornucopia (see Figure 2.5).[257]

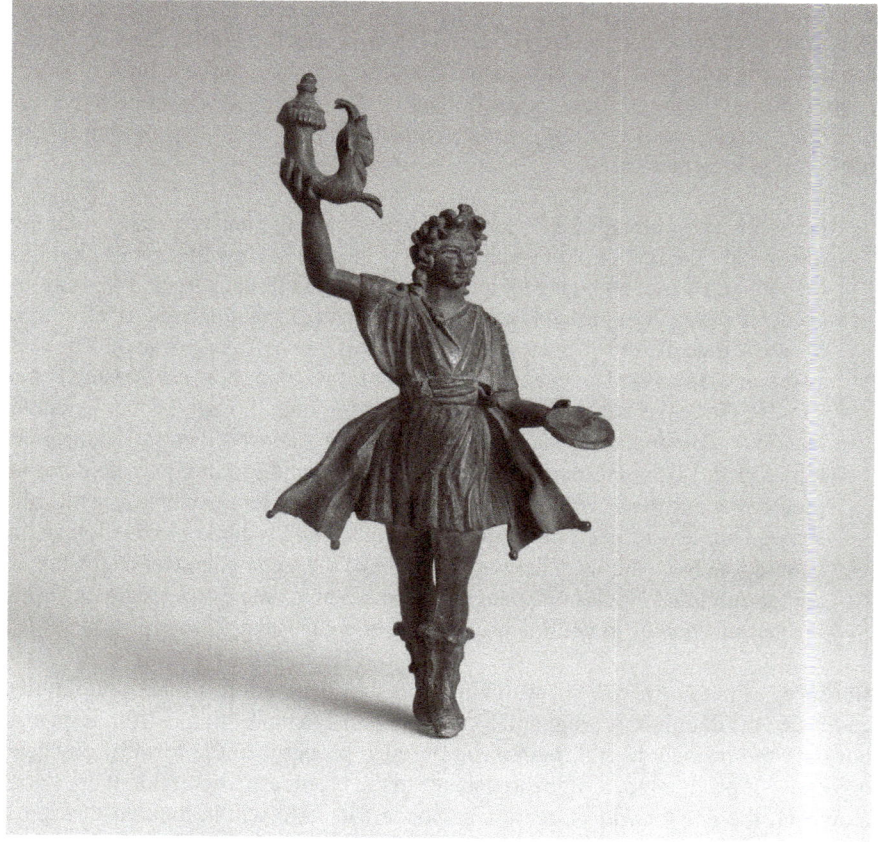

Figure 2.5 A bronze statuette of a *Lar*, dating to the first or second century CE.

Source: Image courtesy of the Metropolitan Museum of Art Open Access (Metropolitan Museum of Art inv. 19.192.3).

The Penates

The origins of the *Penates* are, like those of the *Lares*, obscure.[258] The physical form that they took within the household shrine is likewise unclear.[259] Cicero equates them in importance with the *Lares*, and describes them as the gods of the ancestors and the household.[260] However, they seem to have been particularly associated with the *penus*, the storeroom, and were thought to protect the food supply, thereby ensuring the household's means of subsistence continued, which is relevant to the acquisition and maintenance of health and well-being of the present members of the household.[261] It has been suggested that the choice regarding which deities were included in any given household's *Penates* was driven by personal preference for or attraction to the ideas that they represented.[262] Thus the term *Penates* can be used to refer collectively to all the deities worshipped in a particular household.[263]

The Genius and the Juno

The *Genius* was the guiding numen of the family, the living spirit of the *pater familias* rather than a deity, and was worshipped on his birthday.[264] Consequently, it was a companion for life.[265] Numerous inscriptions dedicated to the *Genii* of specific individuals survive.[266] The *Juno* was the female equivalent.[267] Both of these were associated with generation and procreation, and these are likewise relevant for the health and well-being not just of the present but also of the future members of the household, ensuring the continuity of the family line (see Figure 2.6). According to Isidore, the *Genius* was responsible for the 'life force of all things yet to be born'.[268] Thus the *Genius* had a role to play during the wedding ceremony, when the wedding bed, the *lectus genialis*, was set up in the *atrium*.[269] It is possible that a statuette of the *Genius* was actually placed in the bed to represent the *Genius*' procreative power and ensure the next generation of the household.[270] It has been suggested that the annual celebration of an individual's birthday was akin to the annual celebration of the foundation of a cult since, in essence, an individual's birth was the foundation of the cult of their particular *Genius* or *Juno*.[271] While worship of the *pater familias*' *Genius* is attested during the second century BCE, in the works of Plautus, worship of the *mater familias*' *Juno* is not attested until the late first century BCE, during the Augustan Principate. The *Genius* took the form of a man in a toga and was frequently depicted performing a sacrifice to the *Lares*, presumably on behalf of all the living members of the household that were in his charge (see Figure 2.7).

Vesta

The hearth was the heart of the home and the heart of domestic religious practice. The Latin word used to refer to it, *focus*, emphasises the fostering of the fire on the hearth and stresses the importance not only of starting it but also keeping it alight.[272] The Latin word used to refer to the kitchen, where the fire was generally

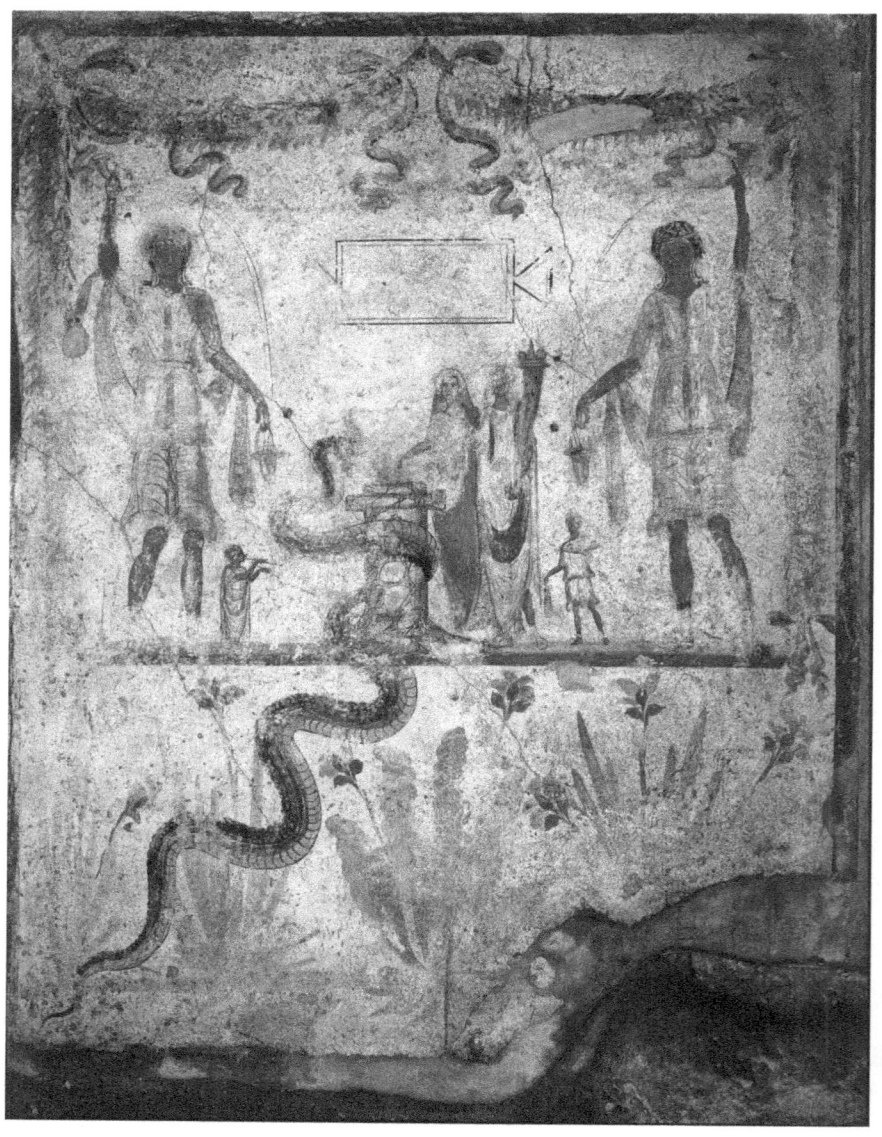

Figure 2.6 A fresco depicting the *Genius* and the *Juno* sacrificing from the House of Julius Polybius in Pompeii (IX.13.1–3), dating from the first century CE.

Source: Image courtesy of Wolfgang Rieger (Licence: CC–PD–Mark).

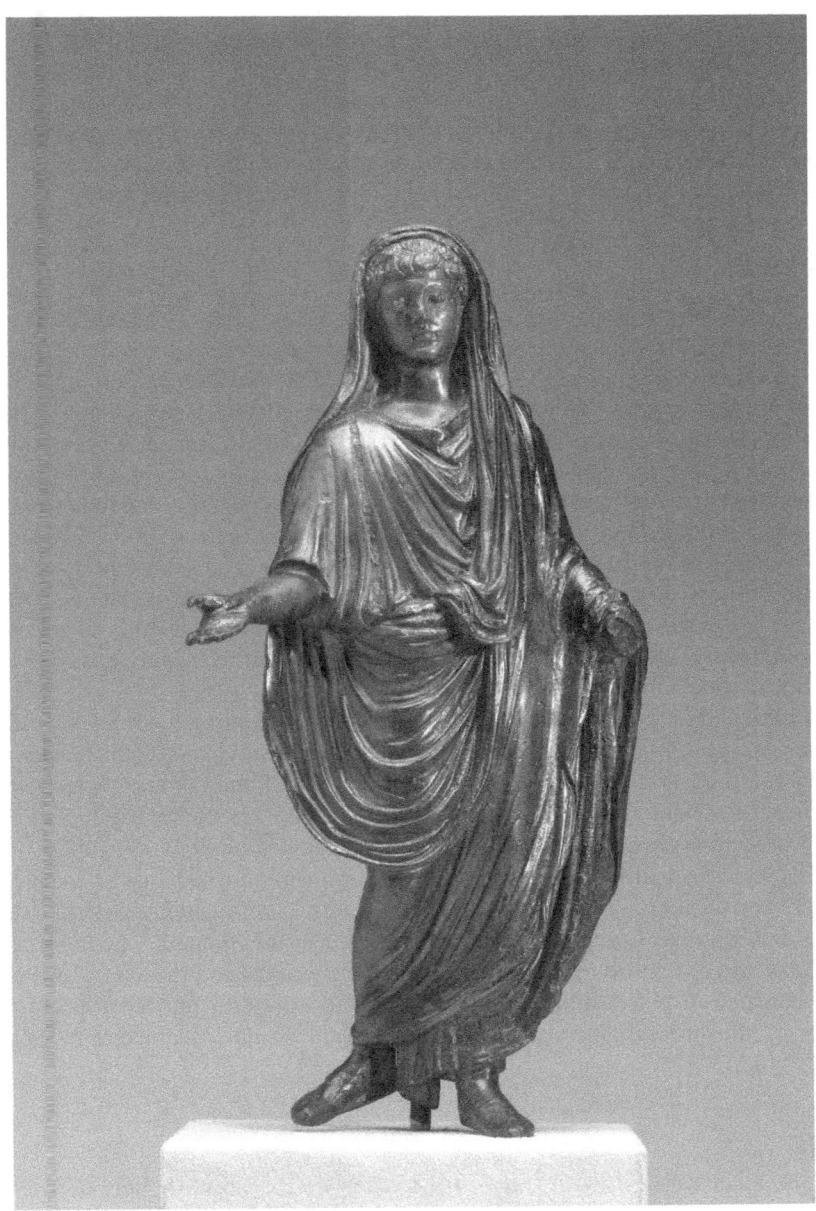

Figure 2.7 A bronze statuette of a *Genius*, dating to the first century CE.

Source: Image courtesy of the Walters Art Museum (Walters Art Museum inv. 54.2329).

located, *culina*, is thought to be derived from *colere*, 'to cultivate', 'to foster', 'to watch over' and also to 'revere in a religious manner'.[273] The presence of a fire in the hearth was used to symbolise the occupation of the house by a living family, and during the *Feralia* on 21st February, part of the *Parentalia* festival, fires were forbidden as the living could not co-exist with the dead.[274] The ability to control fire and by implication heat, light and the ability to cook food was considered a mark of civilisation.[275] The goddess Vesta was particularly associated with the hearth, and was thought to be present there in the form of a living flame.[276]

Conclusion

The Roman house – whether *villa*, *domus*, *insula* or *casa* – was designed and constructed with its potential healthiness in mind and, as such, particular attention was paid to its geographical location; either a healthy site was chosen in the first place, or measures were subsequently taken to ameliorate any problems. There was considerable concern for the natural resources of air, light and water, all of which were fundamental to the experience of occupying and running a house.

The Roman garden had a crucial role to play in the acquisition and maintenance of good health and well-being. The garden space was believed to be beneficial and was utilised as a location for all sorts of activities. The garden produce was utilised not only in food and drink but also in medicaments, and in other ways that were related to ensuring health and well-being such as the production of garlands for ritual activities, or items that could be used to augment a space elsewhere in the house and stimulate the senses.

Additionally, the Roman house and garden were the setting for Roman domestic religious activities, such as the worship of the household gods at the household shrine, on both ordinary and extraordinary occasions, and concerns over establishing and maintaining the health and well-being of the household and *familia* in not just the present but also the future were fundamental to this.

Since the Roman house and its garden were commonly utilised as means of expressing an individual's identity, wealth, status, culture, etc., we should consider the role that health and well-being played in this process. Having examined the ways in which the house and garden were utilised in the acquisition and maintenance of health and well-being, we shall now turn our attention to the actors in this process, and explore the roles played by individual members of the household.

Notes

1　Seneca the Younger, *Moral Epistles* 104.1, 6 (trans. R. M. Gummere): *In nomentanum meum fugi, quid putas? Urbem? Immo febrem et quidem subrepentem. Iam manum mihi iniecerat. Medicus initia esse dicebat motis venis et incertis et naturalem turbantibus modum. Protinus itaque parari vehiculum iussi; Paulina mea retinente exire perseveravi; illud mihi ore erat domini mei Gallionis, qui cum in Achaia febrem habere coepisset, protinus navem ascendit clamitans non corporis esse, sed loci morbum. . . . Quaeris ergo, quomodo mihi consilium profectionis cesserit? Ut primum gravitatem urbis excessi et illum odorem culinarum fumantium, quae motae quicquid pestiferi vaporis obferunt, cum pulvere effundunt, protinus mutatam valitudinem sensi. Quantum deinde adiectum putas viribus, postquam vineas attigi? In pascuum emissus cibum meum invasi. Repeti vi ergo iam me; non permansit marcor ille corporis dubii et male cogitantis. Incipio toto animo studere.*

2 On the city of Rome as an unhealthy place in which to live, see Scobie, 1986; Scheidel, 2003; Davies, 2012.

3 This was not uncommon, particularly during the summer months: for another example of a Roman leaving the city in an attempt to avoid the 'bad air', see Horace going to his Sabine farm, at *Satires* 2.6.18–19.

4 This will be discussed further in Chapter 3, The Roman Household, and Chapter 4, The Transmission of Medical Knowledge.

5 On travel as therapy in antiquity, see Horden, 2005.

6 Pliny the Younger, *Letters* 5.19.6–8 (trans. B. Radice): *Nam ante aliquot annos, dum intente instanterque pronuntiat, sanguinem reiecit atque ob hoc in Aegyptum missus a me post longam peregrinationem confirmatus rediit nuper; deinde dum per continuos dies nimis imperat voci, veteris infirmitatis tussicula admonitus rursus sanguinem reddidit. Qua ex causa destinavi eum mittere in praedia tua, quae Foro Iulii possides. Audivi enim te saepe referentem esse ibi et aera salubrem et lac eiusmodi curationibus accommodatissimum. Rogo ergo scribas tuis, ut illi villa, ut domus pateat, offerant etiam sumptibus eius, si quid opus erit.*

7 See Celsus, *On Medicine* 3.22.8–14 for his recommendations for the treatment of pulmonary tuberculosis, particularly 3.22.10 for the prescription of milk; see Pliny the Elder, *Natural History* 28.33 for a list of possible medicinal uses of milk. See Blake, 2016, p. 96 for Pliny's deliberate presentation of himself in his letters as a kind master who cares about the health and well-being of his slaves.

8 On the street life of ancient Rome, see initially Holleran, 2011 and more comprehensively Hartnett, 2017.

9 Hughes, 1994, pp. 65–66.

10 Hippocrates, *On the Nature of Man* 7; van Tilburg, 2015, pp. 800–802.

11 Hippocrates, *Airs, Waters, Places* 1.1–12 (trans. W. H. S. Jones): Ἰητρικὴν ὅστις βούλεται ὀρθῶς ζητεῖν, τάδε χρὴ ποιεῖν· πρῶτον μὲν ἐνθυμεῖσθαι τὰς ὥρας τοῦ ἔτεος, ὅ τι δύναται ἀπεργάζεσθαι ἑκάστη· οὐ γὰρ ἐοίκασιν ἀλλήλοισιν οὐδέν, ἀλλὰ πολὺ διαφέρουσιν αὐταί τε ἐφ᾽ ἑωυτέων καὶ ἐν τῇσι μεταβολῇσιν· ἔπειτα δὲ τὰ πνεύματα τὰ θερμά τε καὶ τὰ ψυχρά, μάλιστα μὲν τὰ κοινὰ πᾶσιν ἀνθρώποισιν, ἔπειτα δὲ καὶ τὰ ἐν ἑκάστῃ χώρῃ ἐπιχώρια ἐόντα. δεῖ δὲ καὶ τῶν ὑδάτων ἐνθυμεῖσθαι τὰς δυνάμιας· ὥσπερ γὰρ ἐν τῷ στόματι διαφέρουσι καὶ ἐν τῷ σταθμῷ, οὕτω καὶ ἡ δύναμις διαφέρει πολὺ ἑκάστου; similar information is given in Hippocrates, *On the Sacred Disease* 16; see also Lo Presti, 2012.

12 Hippocrates, *Airs, Waters, Places* 2.14–17; 11.11–13; Hulskamp, 2012; Taub, 2004, p. 8.

13 For ancient authors specifying that knowledge of the specific location was crucial and generalising from place to place was problematic, see Geminus, *Introduction to the Phenomena* 17.19 (on astronomy); Ptolemy, *Almagest* 8.6 (on astronomy); Ptolemy, *Four Books* 2.2 (on astrology); see Taub, 2002, pp. 148–149.

14 Hippocrates, *Airs, Waters, Places* 5.21; on the ancient connection between astronomy and agriculture, see Taub, 2002, p. 143.

15 Hippocrates, *Airs, Waters, Places* 1.12–15.

16 Plato, *Laws* 5.747 d – e.

17 *On Architecture* was dedicated to the emperor Augustus, himself a consummate builder, so it is worth speculating on how broadly Vitruvius' recommendations were applied during the early Principate; see Augustus, *Things Done* 19–21 for a list of the buildings that Augustus either built or restored.

18 Taylor, 2003, p. 22.

19 Vitruvius, *On Architecture* 1.1.1.

20 Vitruvius, *On Architecture* 1.1.10; it is of course possible that an architect could collaborate with someone in possession of medical knowledge, or disregard this entirely.

21 Vitruvius, *On Architecture* 1.1.10 (trans. J. Gwilt): *Sine his enim rationibus nulla salubris habitatio fieri potest.*
22 Vitruvius, *On Architecture* 1.1.13, 1.1.15. Bear in mind Quintilian's assessment of Celsus' ability, at *Institutes of Oratory* 12.11.24.
23 For general discussion of Roman attitudes to public health, see Robinson, 1994, pp. 96–112; Koloski-Ostrow, 2015 is far more critical. See van Tilburg, 2015 on the relationship between health and city planning.
24 Vitruvius, *On Architecture* 1.4.1–12, 1.6.1–3.
25 Vitruvius, *On Architecture* 8.6.10; see also Frontinus, *On Aqueducts* 1.11, 2.88, 2.92.
26 Vitruvius, *On Architecture* 1.2.9.
27 Vitruvius, *On Architecture* 1.2.7; see also Plutarch, *Roman Questions* 94.
28 Vitruvius, *On Architecture* 5.3.1 (trans. J. Gwilt): *Corpora propter voluptatem inmota patentes habent venas, in quas insidunt aurarum flatus, qui si a regionibus palustribus aut aliis regionibus vitiosis advenient, nocentes spiritus corporibus infundent.*
29 Vitruvius, *On Architecture* 5.9.5 (trans. J. Gwilt): *Media vero spatia quae erunt subdiu inter porticus, adornanda viridibus videntur, quod hypaethroe ambulationes habent, magnam salubritatem, et primum oculorum quod ex viridibus subtilis et extenuatus aer propter motionem corporis influens perlimat speciem et ita auferens ex oculis umorem crassum, aciem tenuem et acutam speciem relinquit. praeterea cum corpus motionibus in ambulatione calescat, umores ex membris aer exsugendo inminuit plenitates extenuatque dissipando quod plus inest quam corpus potest sustinere.*
30 Vitruvius, *On Architecture* 6.1.1–12. See Nevett, 2015 for discussion of variation in the forms of ancient housing and how to deal with this with regard to theory and methodology.
31 Vitruvius, *On Architecture* 6.5.1–3.
32 Strabo, *Geography* 6.4.1.
33 Strabo, *Geography* 5.7. See Viitanen, 2010, pp. 62–69 for an up-to-date assessment of Campagna's agricultural potential during the Roman period.
34 Strabo, *Geography* 6.1.12, 6.2.4 (trans. H. L. Jones): καὶ τὴν παροιμίαν δὲ ὑγιέστερον Κρότωνος λέγουσαν ἐντεῦθεν εἰρῆσθαί φασιν.
35 Strabo, *Geography* 5.7, 6.1.12.
36 Strabo, *Geography* 5.4.7.
37 Strabo, *Geography* 5.3.7, see also 5.3.2 on the founding of the city. On the disease environment of the city of Rome, see Scheidel, 2003.
38 Vitruvius, *On Architecture* 1.4.11; Strabo, *Geography* 5.3.8; Frontinus, *On Aqueducts* 2.88.
39 Tacitus, *Annals* 15.43 (trans. J. Jackson): *Ceterum un t quae domui supererant non, ut post Gallica incendia, nulla un teaon nec passim erecta, sed dimensis vicorum ordinibus et latis viarum spatiis cohibataque aedificiorum altitudine ac patefactis areis additisque porticibus, quae frontem insularum protegerent . . . ea ex utilitate accepta un tea quoque novae urbi attulere. un te tamen qui crederent veterem illam formam salubritati magis conduxisse, quoniam angustiae itinerum et un tea tectorum non perinde solis vapore perrumperentur: at nunc patulam latitudinem et nulla umbra defensam graviore aestu ardescere.*
40 van Tilburg, 2015, p. 800.
41 Strabo, *Geography* 5.4.8.
42 Viitanen, 2010 argues that archaeological evidence from the vicinity of Rome shows that the majority of *villa*s were built in accordance with the recommendations made in these treatises, indicating that this knowledge was widespread and its tenets widely practiced.
43 For the only modern in-depth study of Cato, see Astin, 1978.
44 Cato the Elder, *Speeches* 128.
45 Varro, *On Agriculture* 1.2.28; Columella, *On Agriculture* 1.1.2; Pliny the Elder, *Natural History* 19.19.57. Greek and Punic treatises were written contemporaneously, but Cato may not have known of these, Dalby, 1998 reissued 2010, p. 16.

46 Cornelius Nepos, *On Great Generals* 2.24.3.1 (trans. J. C. Rolfe): *In omnibus rebus singulari fuit industria; nam et un tea sollers et peritus iuris consultus et magnus imperator et probabilis orator et cupidissimus litterarum fuit*; on Cato as an agricultural writer, see White, 1973, pp. 440–458.
47 Dalby, 1998 reissued 2010, p. 17.
48 White, 1973, p. 447.
49 Dalby, 1998 reissued 2010, pp. 23–24.
50 Cato the Elder, *On Agriculture* 1.1.3 (trans. A. Dalby): *Loco salubri.*
51 Cato the Elder, *On Agriculture* 1.3–4 (trans. A. Dalby): *Uti bonum caelium habeat; ne cclamitosum siet; solo bono, sua uirtute ualeat. Si poteris, sub radice montis siet, in meridiem spectet . . . bonumque aquarium.*
52 Cato the Elder, *On Agriculture* 141. For further discussion of Roman domestic religion and its role in the maintenance of health and well-being, see Chapter 3, The Roman Household.
53 White, 1973, p. 466.
54 Quintillian, *Institutes of Oratory* 10.1.95.
55 Fundania: Varro, *On Agriculture* 1.1.2 Turranius Niger: 2 prologue 6 Quintus Pinnus: 3.1.9.
56 Varro, *On Agriculture* 1.1.8–11.
57 For discussion of the notion that those that live closer to nature are morally superior to those who live in urban centres, see Hughes, 1994, p. 67.
58 Varro, *On Agriculture* 1.2.3 (trans. W. D. Hooper and H. B. Ash): *Vos, qui multas perambulastis terras, ecquam cultiorem Italia vidistis?* On Italy, see also Strabo, *Geography* 6.4.1.
59 Varro, *On Agriculture* 1.2.3–4 (trans. W. D. Hooper and H. B. Ash): *Ego vero, Agrius, nullam arbitror esse quae tam tota sit culta. Primum cum orbis terrae divisus sit in duas partes ab Eratosthene maxume secundum naturam, 4 ad meridiem versus et ad septemtriones, et sine dubio quoniam salubrior pars septemtrionalis est quam un tea, et quae salubriora illa fructuosiora, dicendum utique Italiam magis etiam fuisse opportunam ad colendum quam Asiam.*
60 Varro, *On Agriculture* 1.2.10 (trans. W. D. Hooper and H. B. Ash): *Qui de agri cultura Romanus peritissimus existimatur.*
61 Varro, *On Agriculture* 1.12.1 (trans. W. D. Hooper and H. B. Ash): *Danda opera ut potissimum sub radicibus montis silvestris villam ponat, ubi pastiones sint laxae, item ut contra ventos, qui saluberrimi in agro flabunt. Quae posita est ad exortos aequinocticles, aptissima, quod aestate habet umbram, hieme solem.*
62 Varro, *On Agriculture* 1.12.2; 1.4.4 (trans. W. D. Hooper and H. B. Ash): *Ita enim salubritas, quae ducitur e caelo ac terra, non est in nostra potestate, sed in naturae, ut tamen multum sit in nobis, quo graviora quae un tea diligentia leviora facere possimus. Etenim si propter terram aut aquam odore, quem aliquo loco eructat, pestilentior es fundus, aut propter caeli regionem ager calidior sit, aut ventus non bonus flet, haec vitia emendari solent domini scientia ac sumptu.*
63 For an inscription from Tarentum, see *CIL* IX 235 = *ILS* 2923; see also Martin, 1985, pp. 1960–1962.
64 Columella, *On Agriculture* 7.2.30.
65 Columella, *On Agriculture* 1.1.7–14; 3.9.2; 7.2.3; 2.15.4; 2.10.18.
66 Martin, 1985, pp. 1966–1967.
67 Columella, *On Agriculture* 1.3.2 (trans. H. B. Ash): *Nec rursus pestilenti quamvis feracissimo pinguique agro dominum ad fructus pervenire. Nam ubi sit cum Orco ratio ponenda, ibi non modo perceptionem fructuum, sed et vitam colonorum esse dubiam ve potius mortem quaestu certiorem.* This offers a slightly different perspective on discussions of the use of the house as a means of expressing identity, social status and other desirable qualities, as explored most fully in Wallace-Hadrill, 1994; Hales, 2003.
68 Columella, *On Agriculture* 1.2.3 (trans. H. B. Ash): *Uberi glaeba, parte campestri, parte alia collibus vel ad orientem vel ad meridiem molliter devexis; terrenisque aliis*

atque aliis silvestribus et asperis, nec procul a mari vel navigabili flumine, quo depor-
tari fructus et per quod merces invehi possint.

69 Varro, *On Agriculture* 1.4.4–5 (trans. W. D. Hooper and H. B. Ash): *Quod perma-*
gni interest, ube sint positae villae, quantae sint, quo spectent porticibus, ostiis ac
fenestris. . . . Sed quid ego illum voco ad testimonium? Non hic Varro noster, cum
Corcyrae esset exercitus ac classis et omnes domus repletae essent aegrotis ac funeri-
bus, immisso fenestris novis aquilone et obstructis pestilentibus ianuaque permutata
ceteraque eius generis diligentia suos comites ac familiam incolumes reduxit? Varro's
medical knowledge is discussed in Boscherini, 1993; van Tilburg, 2015 focuses on this
episode specifically.

70 See Wallace-Hadrill, 1994, p. 60 on the reasons why someone might or might not wish
to renovate their house.

71 Cicero, *Letters to Quintus* 21 (3.1).

72 Pliny the Younger, *Letters* 2.7, 5.6.

73 Taylor, 2003, pp. 59–60.

74 Vitruvius, *On Architecture* 6.1.1, 6.5.1–3.

75 Spencer, 2010, p. 62.

76 Edwards, 1993, pp. 1–4, pp. 141–149.

77 See for example Storey, 2004, on the term *insula*.

78 The scholarship on housing in the ancient world is vast and it is impossible to include
it all here. The most important recent works for our purposes here are Wallace-Hadrill,
1994; Hales, 2003.

79 See for example Schmidt, 1990 on Cicero's properties; and Förtsch, 1993 on Pliny the
Younger's.

80 Garnsey, 1979.

81 Edwards, 1993, pp. 29–39.

82 See for example the Auditorium site in Rome, Terrenato, 2001; and the Villa delle
Grotte site at Grottarossa, Becker, 2006.

83 Cato the Elder, *On Agriculture* 1.1–7.

84 Purcell, 1995; Wallace-Hadrill, 1998; Marzano, 2007.

85 Cato the Elder, *On Agriculture* 1.13.6–7.

86 Cato the Elder, *On Agriculture* 1.6.1; see for example the site of Settefinestre, Carandini, 1985.

87 Marzano, 2007, pp. 9–10.

88 Statius, *Silvae* 1.3.6–8. See Myers, 2005 for discussion of Statius' *ekphrasis* and its
relationship with *otium*.

89 Statius, *Silvae* 1.3.92, 108–110.

90 Pliny the Younger, *Letters* 2.17.1 (trans. B. Radice*): Gratiam villae, opportunitatem*
loci, 2 litoris spatium.

91 Pliny the Younger, *Letters* 5.6.1–2 (trans. B. Radice): *Amavi curam et sollicitudinem*
tuam, quod cum audisses me aestate Tuscos meos petiturum, ne facerem suasisti, dum
putas insalubres. Est sane gravis et pestilens ora Tuscorum, quae per litus extendi-
tur; sed hi procul a mari recesserunt, quin etiam Appennino saluberrimo montium
subiacent.

92 Pliny the Younger, *Letters* 5.6.46.

93 Barton, 1996, p. 3.

94 Hales, 2003, p. 99 describes architects as having to 'rework the dream house to fit
irregular plots or downgrade it according to space and resources'.

95 Vitruvius, *On Architecture* 2.8.17, 2.9.16. For the difficulty in identifying rooms in
cenacula in *insulae* with specific reference to the archaeological remains of buildings
in Ostia, see Hermansen, 1982, pp. 17–24.

96 See the advertisements for rented accommodation in these properties at *CIL* IV 138
and *CIL* IV 1136. See Pirson, 1997 for discussion of rented accommodation.

97 Hermansen, 1982, p. 25.

98 According to Jashemski, 1979b, p. 24 gardens and cultivated land occupy 17.7 percent of Pompeii.
99 For the most up-to-date and comprehensive discussion of all aspects of the ancient Roman garden, see the contributions to Jashemski et al., 2018, particularly those found in Part 1, The Main Types of Gardens.
100 Cato the Elder, *On Agriculture* 1.7 (trans. W. D. Hooper and H. B. Ash): *Praedium quod primum siet, si me rogabis, sic dicam: de omnibus agris optimoque loco iugera agri centum, vinea est prima, si vino bono et multo est, secundo loco hortus inriguus, tertio salictum, quarto oletum, quinto pratum, sexto campus frumentarius, septimo silva caedua, octavo arbustum, nono glandaria silva.*
101 Varro, *On Agriculture* 1.23.4; Columella, *On Agriculture* 1.6.24.
102 For general overviews of Roman gardens and gardeners, see Farrar, 1998, 2016. For discussion of the literary evidence for ancient Roman gardens, see Littlewood, 2018; Myers, 2018.
103 For discussion of the technical aspects of creating a Roman garden, see Gleason and Palmer, 2018; for discussion of ancient gardening practices and techniques, see Jashemski, 2018b.
104 Virgil, *Aeneid* 11.318–319; Varro, *On Agriculture* 1.23.5.
105 Pliny the Elder, *Natural History* 19.60; Columella, *On Agriculture* 11.3.8.
106 See for example *Priapea* 2; *Priapea* 3; Martial, *Epigrams* 6.72.
107 On ancient Roman produce gardens, see Jashemski, 2018a; on ancient Roman plants, see Jashemski et al., 2018.
108 See the *menologia rustica Colotianum* and *menologia rustica Vallense* for publicly inscribed farmers' almanacs, *CIL* I² 280–281, *CIL* VI 2305 = *ILS* 8745.
109 Columella, *On Agriculture* 11.3.14–18.
110 Cato the Elder, *On Agriculture* 8.2; Varro, *On Agriculture* 1.23.4.
111 Frayn, 1979, p. 58.
112 Frayn, 1979, p. 64.
113 Seneca the Younger, *On Providence* 3.6.
114 Columella, *On Agriculture* 11.3.37; see also, much later, Palladius, *On Agriculture* 11.4.
115 Cato the Elder, *On Agriculture* 8.2; Varro, *On Agriculture* 1.23.4.
116 Pliny the Elder, *Natural History* 19.52; Columella, *On Agriculture* 10 preface 2.
117 Varro, *On Agriculture* 1.10; Festus, *Latin Glossary* 91.12 L.
118 *Twelve Tables* 7.3; Pliny the Elder, *Natural History* 19.50; von Stackelberg, 2009, p. 10.
119 *Appendix Vergiliana*, *Moretum* 60–84 (trans. H. Rushton Fairclough): *Hortus erat iunctus casulae, quem vimina pauca et calamo rediviva levi munibat harundo, exiguus spatio, variis sed fertilis herbis. nil illi deerat quod pauperis exigit usus; interdum locuples a paupere plura petebat. nec sumptus ullius erat, sed recula curae: siquando vacuum casula pluviaeve tenebant festave lux, si forte labor cessabat aratri, horti opus illud erat. varias disponere plantas norat et occultae committere semina terrae vicinosque apte circa deducere rivos. hic holus, hic late fundentes bracchia betae fecundusque rumex malvaeque inulaeque virebant, hic siser et nomen capiti debentia porra grataque nobilium requies lactuca ciborum, <spinosi asparagi> crescitque in acumina radix, et gravis in latum dimissa cucurbita ventrem. verum hic non domini (quis enim contractior illo?) sed populi proventus erat, nonisque diebus venalis umero fasces portabat in urbem. inde domum cervice levis, gravis aere redibat vix umquam urbani comitatus merce macelli: Cepa rubens sectique famem domat area porri quaeque trahunt acri vultus nasturtia morsu intibaque et Venerem revocans eruca morantem.*
120 Gleason, 2013, p. 16; for elaboration, see Gleason et al., 2018, pp. 482–488.
121 See for example the approach taken by Henderson, 2004; Pagán, 2006, pp. 19–36.
122 For an overwhelmingly literature focussed approach to the study of Roman gardens, see Grimal, 1969; more integrated studies were subsequently inaugurated by Jashemski, 1979b, 1993.

123 See for example Gleason, 1990, 1994 on the Portico of Pompey; Bergmann, 2002 on Oplontis.
124 On archaeological evidence for plant pots, see Macaulay-Lewis, 2006.
125 For Pliny's *villa*, see Pliny the Younger, *Letters* 5.6.
126 See Morvillez, 2018 for a detailed overview of the development of the Roman domestic garden.
127 See for example Cicero, *Letters to Atticus* 23.2 (II.3.2); Vitruvius, *On Architecture* 6.3.10; Pliny the Younger, *Letters* 5.6.38. The *viridarium* is discussed by Purcell, 1987.
128 Purcell, 1996, p. 141.
129 Martial, *Epigrams* 8.14, 8.68; Seneca the Younger, *Moral Epistles* 122.8; Pliny the Elder, *Natural History* 15.47; Macrobius, *Saturnalia* 2.4.14.
130 Vitruvius, *On Architecture* 6.3.1–2.
131 Servius, *Aeneid* 1.7.26; alternatively, Varro, *On the Latin Language* 5.162 attributes it to Atria in Spain.
132 Cicero, *Against Piso* 1.1; Seneca the Younger, *Moral Epistles* 44.5; Juvenal, *Satires* 8.8; on this see Flower, 1996, pp. 185–203.
133 Varro, *On the Latin Language* 5.161.
134 Frontinus, *On Aqueducts* 1.76.2.
135 Wallace-Hadrill, 1994, p. 86, pp. 158–159.
136 Horace, *Epistles* 1.5.31, 2.1.102; for discussion of the role that domestic architecture played in this process, see Wallace-Hadrill 1988, 1994; Hales, 2003.
137 Flohr, 2012.
138 Varro, *On the Latin Language* 5.162.
139 Foss, 1994, p. 69.
140 Ovid, *Fasti* 6.302–306; Virgil, *Eclogues* 7.49–50.
141 Servius, *Aeneid*, 1.726; Allison, 2004, pp. 253–254, p. 259.
142 Varro, *On Agriculture* 1.13.2.
143 Columella, *On Agriculture* 1.6.3. On everyday eating and drinking, see Allison, 2015.
144 Seneca the Younger, *Moral Epistles* 78.23; Juvenal, *Satires* 3.249–253.
145 Vitruvius, *On Architecture* 6.6.1–2, 6.6.4; Columella, *On Agriculture* 8.3.1–2.
146 Columella, *On Agriculture* 1.6.3.
147 See for example the twelve houses with conduit pipes connected to the aqueduct supplying Herculaneum, Jansen, 1991, pp. 154–155.
148 On Roman toilets, see most recently and comprehensively Jansen et al., 2011; on Roman sanitation, see Koloski-Ostrow, 2015.
149 Scobie, 1986, pp. 407–412.
150 Juvenal, *Satires* 3.276–277.
151 Yegül, 2009, p. 45.
152 Cato the Elder, *On Agriculture* 10.2–4, 65, 67; Columella, *On Agriculture* 1.6.
153 Vitruvius, *On Architecture* 6.6; Columella, *On Agriculture* 1.6.
154 Carandini, 1985.
155 Varro cited in Pliny the Elder, *Natural History* 18.73.307–308.
156 Pliny the Elder, *Natural History* 18.127, 19.34.115–116; Columella, *On Agriculture* 12.6.1–2, 12.10, 12.56.
157 Appendix Vergiliana, *Moretum* 13–18.
158 Vitruvius, *On Architecture* 6.5.2 (trans. F. Granger): *Qui autem fructibus rusticis serviunt, in eorum vestibulis stabula, tabernae, in aedibus cryptae, horrea, apothecae ceteraque, quae ad fructus servandos magis quam ad elegantiae decorem possunt esse, ita sunt facienda.*
159 Allison, 2004, p. 121.
160 Cova, 2013, p. 375.
161 Allison, 2004; Kastenmeier, 2007; Basso and Ghedini, 2003; Mols, 1999.
162 Gobbo, 2009, p. 346.
163 Allison, 2004, p. 122.

164 For the *salutatio*, see Polybius, *Roman Histories* 6.53; Vitruvius, *On Architecture* 6.3.4–6; Pliny the Elder, *Natural History* 35.6; Wallace-Hadrill, 1994. On display of the household resources, see Allison, 2004, p. 121, 130.

165 It has been suggested that there was an Italic predisposition towards living in close proximity with nature, see Giesecke, 2007, p. 103.

166 Lucretius, *On the Nature of Things* 5. 925–1025. See Seneca the Younger, *Moral Epistles* 15.15–30 for the view that civilisation and the luxury that accompanies it weakens humans and introduces them to new types of disease.

167 Lucretius, *On the Nature of Things* 2.598–660; Pliny the Elder, *Natural History* 25.1.1, 27.1.1, 27.2.7, 37.77.201.

168 Beagon, 1992, pp. 26–50; French, 1994, pp. 196–206.

169 French, 1994, p. 153. Additionally, natural products such as plants and trees were humanised and used to present entire peoples, dynasties, families and individuals, see Macaulay-Lewis, 2008; Gower, 2011; Totelin, 2012. The Romans sought to conquer, control and utilise the natural world for the benefit of the Roman empire and its people, and Pliny the Elder's *Natural History* and the Flavian Temple of Peace demonstrate this 'botanical imperialism' at its apogee in the late first century CE, see Pollard, 2009.

170 Giesecke, 2007, p. 102.

171 Appian, *Civil War* 1.1.7; Pliny the Elder, *Natural History* 18.5–21.

172 Pliny the Elder, *Natural History* 19.19.49.

173 Ovid, *Fasti* 3.331–348; Plutarch, *Numa* 15.5; Livy, *From the Foundation of the City* 1.54.6; Pliny the Elder, *Natural History* 19.53.169; this story is thought to have been inspired by Herodotus' account of Thrasybulus and Periander, at *Histories* 5.92.6.

174 Livy, *From the Founding of the City* 3.26.1–3, 3.29.4; Dionysius of Halicarnassus, *Roman Antiquities* 10.24.1–10, 25.3.

175 Cicero, *On Ends* 2.12; Perseus, *Satires* 1.73–75; Columella, *On Agriculture* 1 preface 13; Florus, *Epitome* 1.5; Cassius Dio, *fragment* 23.2; Eutropius, *Abridgement of Roman History* 1.17; Vegetius, *Concerning Military Matters* 1.3; Festus, *Latin Glossary* 307.

176 See Landgren, 2004 for consideration of the Latin terminology attested in ancient literary and documentary evidence and its implications.

177 See for example Pompeii; of the estimated two-thirds of the site that has been excavated so far, almost eighteen percent of it was garden space of some sort, with almost six percent of this private/domestic garden space, Jashemski, 1979b, p. 24.

178 This belief survives all the way into the Byzantine period, see Littlewood, 2018, p. 257.

179 On Classical Greek gardens, see Carroll-Spillecke, 1989, 1992; Osborne, 1992. On the Academy and the Lyceum as centres for fostering the health of body and mind, see Giesecke, 2016.

180 Morford, 1987, p. 155.

181 See Nielsen, 2013 for explication of these architectural features; see Simelius, 2015 for discussion of the myriad ways in which the peristyle could be utilised.

182 O'Sullivan, 2011, p. 78.

183 Cicero, *Letters to Atticus* 5.2 (I.9.2), 7.3 (I.11.3), 9.3 (I.4.3); Cicero, *Tusculan Disputations* 2.9; Cicero, *On Divination* 1.8, 2.8. On Cicero's philosophical reading and writing while in exile as both *negotium* and *otium*, see Dewar, 2014.

184 Jashemski, 1996, p. 232.

185 Recently, see Day, 2013; this integrated approach is applied with great success to the Bay of Naples in Jashemski and Meyer, 2002.

186 Literature: Grimal, 1969; Littlewood, 1987, 1992, 2002, 2018; Henderson, 2004; Fagán, 2006; Myers, 2018. Art: Kellum, 1994; Kuttner, 1999; Carroll, 2012. Mythology: Bernhardt, 2008; Giesecke, 2014.

187 Jashemski 1974, 1977, 1979a, 1979b, 1993, 1996; Jashemski and Meyer, 2002.

188 von Stackelberg, 2009, p. 9.

189   See some specific case studies at Ciaraldi, 2000, 2002; Farrar, 1998, pp. 133–134.
190   See generally on ancient uses of herbs for medicinal purposes Jashemski, 1999; Scarborough, 2002; Manniche, 1986, 2006.
191   Ross, 1998, p. 176.
192   Pagán, 2006, p. 1.
193   Virgil, *Georgics* 4.125–133; Horace, *Epodes* 2.47; Columella, *On Agriculture* 11.3.1.
194   Carroll, 2003.
195   Varro, *On Agriculture* 1.2.10.
196   Allison, 2004, pp. 125–126, pp. 131–132.
197   Columella, *On Agriculture* 10 preface 1, 3. Pagán, 2006, pp. 19–36 reads this as a literary rather than a technical work.
198   Pagán, 2006, p. 30.
199   On evidence for the many Roman uses for plants, see Jashemski et al., 2002; Jashemski et al., 2018.
200   Columella, *On Agriculture* 10.103–104. See also Dioscorides, *On Medical Materials* 2.180.
201   Columella, *On Agriculture* 10.104–109. See also Virgil, *Georgics* 1.73–78; Celsus, *On Medicine* 2.32, 3.18.12; Dioscorides, *On Medical Materials* 4.65; Pliny the Elder, *Natural History* 18.61.229.
202   Columella, *On Agriculture* 10.124–126.
203   Columella, *On Agriculture* 10.230–232.
204   Pliny the Elder, *Natural History* 19.59 (trans. H. Rackham): *Iam in fenestris suis plebs urbana imagine hortorum cotidiana oculis rura praebebant*; Linderski, 2001, p. 308.
205   Martial, *Epigrams* 11.18.1–2.
206   Varro, *On Agriculture* 2 preface 2 on the master; see also Martial, *Epigrams* 3.58 on the household slaves.
207   Pliny the Elder, *Natural History* 25.5.9 (trans. H. Rackham): *Visendo hortulo eius in quo plurimas alebat centesimum annum aetatis excedens, nullum corporis malum expertus, ac ne aetate quidem memoria aut vigore concussis.*
208   Ovid, *Letters from Pontus* 1.8.39–62 (trans. A. L. Wheeler): *At, puto, sic urbis misero est erepta voluptas, quolibet ut saltem rure frui liceat! non meus amissos animus desiderat agros, ruraque Paeligno conspicienda solo, nec quos piniferis positos in collibus hortos spectat Flaminiae Clodia iuncta viae. quos ego nescio cui colui, quibus ipse solebam ad sata fontanas, nec pudet, addere aquas: sunt ubi, si vivunt, nostra quoque consita quaedam, sed non et nostra poma legenda manu. pro quibus amissis utinam contingere possit hic saltem profugo glaeba colenda mihi! ipse ego pendentis, liceat modo, rupe capellas, ipse velim baculo pascere nixus oves; ipse ego, ne solitis insistant pectora curis, ducam ruricolas sub iuga curva boves, et discam Getici quae norunt verba iuvenci, adsuetas illis adiciamque minas. ipse manu capulum pressi moderatus aratri experiar mota spargere semen humo. nec dubitem longis purgare ligonibus herbas, et dare iam sitiens quas bibat hortus aquas. unde sed hoc nobis, minimum quos inter et hostem discrimen murus clausaque porta facit?*
209   Vitruvius, *On Architecture* 5.9.5 (trans. F. Granger): *Media vero spatia quae erunt subdiu inter porticus, adornanda viridibus videntur, quod hypaethroe ambulationes habent, magnam salubritatem, et primum oculorum quod ex viridibus subtilis et extenuatus aer propter motionem corporis influens perlimat speciem et ita auferens ex oculis umorem crassum, aciem tenuem et acutam speciem relinquit. praeterea cum corpus motionibus in ambulatione calescat, umores ex membris aer exsugendo inminuit plenitates extenuatque dissipando quod plus inest quam corpus potest sustinere.*
210   Celsus, *On Medicine* 1.2.6.
211   Petronius, *Satyricon* 28.
212   Pliny the Elder, *Natural History* 37.62–63 (trans. H. Rackham): *Quippe nullius coloris aspectus iucundior est*; observed by Landgren, 2004, p. 157; on garden paintings in antiquity, see Bergmann, 2008; on concepts of colour in antiquity, see Bradley, 2009.

213 See for example mint, thought to lift people's spirits; Pliny the Elder, *Natural History* 23.147; see also Draycott, 2015, pp. 71–72.

214 Celsus, *On Medicine* 3.18.15.

215 O'Sullivan, 2011, p. 79.

216 Columella, *On Agriculture* 3.8.4.

217 Cicero, *On Divination* 2.30.63; Ovid, *Metamorphoses* 10; Virgil, *Georgics* 4.146.13–14; Horace, *Odes* 2.11.13. Plane trees did, however, have medicinal uses: Pliny the Elder, *Natural History* 12.13; Dioscorides, *On Medical Materials* 1.107.

218 Meiggs, 1982, pp. 276–278; Jashemski et al., 2002, pp. 145–146.

219 Cato, *On Agriculture* 143.

220 Hardy and Totelin, 2016.

221 Pliny the Elder, *Natural History* 21.10.14, 21.18.35; Dioscorides, *On Medical Materials* 1.99.1, 4.121; Athenaeus, *Dinner Sophists* 15.675 E.

222 Dioscorides, *On Medical Materials* 1.99.3.

223 Athenaeus, *Dinner Sophists* 15.675 E; Dioscorides, *On Medical Materials* 3.39.1.

224 Draycott, 2015.

225 Catullus 61.6–7.

226 Draycott, 2015, pp. 71–72.

227 Cato the Elder, *On Agriculture* 8.2; Varro, *On Agriculture* 1.23.4; Columella, *On Agriculture* 1.6.24.

228 Via Sacra: Ovid, *Fasti* 6.791–792; Portunalia: Fronto, *Epistles* 1.7; *CIL* VI 9227, 9282, 9283.

229 Cicero, *On His House* 109 (trans. N. H. Watts): *Hic arae sunt, hic foci, hic di penates, hic sacra, religiones, caerimoniae continentur: hoc perfugium est ita sanctum omnibus, ut inde abripi neminem fas sit. Quo magis est istius furor ab auribus vestris repellendus, qui quae maiores nostri religionibus tuta nobis et sancta esse voluerunt, ea iste non solum contra religionem labefactavit, sed etiam ipsius religionis nomine evertit.* According to Festus, *sacra publica* were performed on behalf of the entire Roman people or large sections of the Roman people at public expense, while *sacra privata* were performed on behalf of individuals, households or *gentes* at private expense, see *Latin Glossary* 245. This firm separation between public and private religious belief and practice has recently been questioned by Bendlin, 2000, p. 135; he has argued in favour of religious pluralism and a religious marketplace. For the most comprehensive discussions of the so-called *sacra privata*, see Marquardt, 1886; de Marchi, 1896–1903; Samter, 1901; more recently, see Orr, 1978; Harmon, 1978; Bassani and Ghedini, 2011; Maiuri, 2013; most recently, see Flower, 2017.

230 Horace, *Odes* 3.23 (trans. N. Rudd): *Caelo supinas si tuleris manus nascente Luna, rustica Phidyle, si ture placaris et horna fruge Lares avidaque porca, nec pestilentem sentiet Africum fecunda vitis nec sterilem seges robiginem aut dulces alumni pomifero grave tempus anno. nam quae nivali pascitur Algido devota quercus inter et ilices aut crescit Albanis in herbis victima pontificum securis cervice tinguet: te nihil attinet temptare multa caede bidentium parvos coronantem marino rore deos fragilique myrto. immunis aram si tetigit manus, non sumptuosa blandior hostia mollivit aversos Penatis farre pio et saliente mica.*

231 For a new study that focuses on Roman domestic religious belief and practice and the *Lares* in particular, see Flower, 2017.

232 For a general overview, see Scullard, 1981, pp. 58–60; Holland, 1937; Sartorio, 1988. For detailed discussion, see Flower, 2017, pp. 162–174.

233 Pliny the Elder, *Natural History* 36.204; see also Dionysius of Halicarnassus, *Roman Antiquities* 4.2.1; Plutarch, *On the Fortune of the Romans* 10.

234 Persius, *Satires* 4.26–32.

235 Dionysius of Halicarnassus, *Roman Antiquities* 4.14; Macrobius, *Saturnalia*, 1.7.34–35; Paul ex Festus, *Latin Glossary* 239 L, 272–273 L.

236 Cato the Elder, *On Agriculture* 5.3, 57.1; Columella, *On Agriculture* 1.8.6–20, 11.1.22–23.

237 Cato the Elder, *On Agriculture* 141.
238 Ovid, *Fasti* 2.639–684.
239 Varro, *On Agriculture*, 1.10.2.
240 *Twelve Tables* 7.3; see also Paul ex Festus, *Latin Glossary* 91.12 L.
241 Pliny the Elder, *Natural History* 18.2.7, 18.3.9.
242 Varro, *On Agriculture* 1.14, 1.15; Columella, *On Agriculture* 5.10.1. Dilke, 1971; Campbell, 2000.
243 Siculus Flaccus, *On Agreements About Lands* 11.
244 Bodel, 2008, p. 248. See Peterson, 2012, p. 331 for the suggestion that after the earthquake in 62 CE households incorporated a multiplicity of gods into their shrines as a means of enlisting extra protection.
245 Renberg, 2007, p. 135.
246 See Cato the Elder's opinion that the *dominus* should dictate the worship of the entire household, *On Agriculture* 143. Boyce, 1937; Orr, 1973, 1978; Fröhlich, 1991; Bakker, 1994; Bodel, 2008, pp. 265–266.
247 Foss, 1997.
248 Catullus 31.9; Horace, *Satires* 1.2.56; Virgil, *Georgics* 3.44; Lucan, *Civil War* 2.331, 2.729, 5.537, 7.346; Martial, *Epigrams* 10.61.5. See also *Digest* 25.3.1.2 for the law stating that a man's home was where his *Lar* was located in the event that he owned multiple residences.
249 For the former position, see Wissowa, 1902, pp. 166–174; for the latter, see Samter, 1901, pp. 105–108; see also Waites, 1920; Holland, 1937; Scheid, 1990, pp. 587–598. However, see now Flower, 2017.
250 Cicero, *Timaeus* 68.
251 Bettini, 2013.
252 Plautus, *The Pot of Gold* 3–25 (trans. W. De Melo): *Hanc domum iam multos annos est quom possideo et colo patri auoque iam huius qui nunc hic habet. sed mihi auos huius opsecrans concredidit auri thesaurum clam omnis: in medio foco defode, uenerans me ut id seruarem sibi. is quoniam moritur (ita auido ingenio fuit), numquam indicare id filio uoluit suo, inopemque optauit potius eum relinquere quam eum thesaurum commonstraret filio; agri reliquit ei non magnum modum, quo cum labore magno et misere uiueret. ubi is obiit mortem qui mi id aurum credidit, coepi conseruare, ecqui maiorem filius mihi honorem haberet quam eius habuisset pater. atque ille uero minus minusque impendio curare minusque me impertire honoribus. item a me contra factum est, nam item obiit diem. is ex se hunc reliquit qui hic nunc habitat filium, pariter moratum ut pater auosque huius fuit. huic filia una est. ea mihi cottidie aut ture aut uino aut aliqui semper supplicat, dat mihi coronas.* For discussion of this passage, see Flower, 2017, pp. 31–35.
253 See also Ovid, *Fasti* 5.133–142.
254 Tibullus, *Elegies* 1.10.15–32; Ovid, *Tristia* 4.8.22.
255 Cato the Elder, *On Agriculture* 2.1.
256 Persius, *Satires* 5. 30–31; Propertius, *Elegies* 4.1.131–132; Ovid, *Fasti* 3.77 –790; Pliny the Younger, *Letters* 10.116; Petronius, *Satyricon* 29.8; Suetonius, *Nero* 12; Varro, *De Vita Populi Romani* 1, cited by Nonius Marcellus; Plautus, *The Pot of Gold* 385–386. Clarke, 1991, pp. 7–12; Dixon, 1992, pp. 133–159; Johansson, 2010.
257 Boyce, 1937, pp. 108–109; Pollini, 2008 on the two types.
258 Dubourdieu, 1989.
259 Pollini, 2008, p. 393.
260 Cicero, *Republic* 5.5; Cicero, *On the Responses of the Haruspices* 37.
261 Servius, *Aeneid* 3.12.
262 Bodel, 2008, p. 262.
263 Servius, *Aeneid* 2.514; Flower, 2017, pp. 48–50.
264 Tibullus, *Elegies* 1.7.49–54, 2.2.1–10, 3.11.8–9; Censorinus, *On the Birthday* 2.2. Künckel, 1974; Mattero, 1992; Flower, 2017, p. 6.

265 Horace, *Epistles* 2.2.187–189.
266 See for example *CIL* X 861, an inscription found on the household shrine of Marcus Epidius Rufus at Pompeii and dedicated to his *Genius* and *Lares* by two of his freedmen; *CIL* X 860, an inscription found on a herm in the house of Caecilius Iucundus and dedicated to the *Genius* of Lucius by one of his freedmen.
267 Tibullus, *Elegies* 4.6.1; Petronius, *Satyricon* 25; Pliny the Elder, *Natural History* 2.16.
268 Isidore, *Origins* 8.11.88f; Apuleius, *On the God of Socrates* 15.151f; Festus, *Latin Glossary* 84.3–7; Martianus Capella, *On the Seven Disciplines* 2.152.
269 Johansson, 2010, pp. 140–142.
270 Johansson, 2010, p. 142.
271 Argetsinger, 1992, p. 176.
272 Varro quoted in Servius, *Aeneid* 12.118 and Isidore, *Origins* 20.10.
273 Tibullus, *Elegies* 1.1.5–6; Ovid, *Tristia* 1.3.40–45; Servius, *Aeneid* 3.134.
274 Ovid, *Fasti* 2.563–66. For a general overview, see Scullard, 1981, pp. 74–76; Dolansky, 2011, p. 127 describes the *Parentalia* as being 'fundamental' to Roman society and of 'paramount importance' to the Roman family.
275 Orr, 1973, pp. 34–37, 1978, pp. 1560–1561.
276 Ovid, *Fasti* 6.301–308; Virgil, *Aeneid* 9.258–259; Servius, *Aeneid* 1.292.

3   The Roman household

Introduction

Gaius Castricius Calvus Agricola, son of Titus, of the Stellatine tribe, the well-wishing patron of good [either farmers or freedmen] – especially of those who [worked hard and] well to cultivate their fields, and [who looked after] their own bodies carefully (the most important requirement [for farmers]); who fed themselves, and [who looked after] whatever possessions they had. Let anyone who wishes [to live] in a truly good and free fashion [hold these] precepts for true: The first is that you should want to be loyal [to your lord], respect [your parents and keep] your promises [. . . not win a bad] reputation. A man who does no [harm and keeps his promises] will have a pleasant [and trouble-free life], happily and with a clear conscience. Agricola teaches you to remember these precepts, which [he did not learn from philosophers, but from] nature and experience.

To Lucius Castricius, freedman of Gaius. I mourned his death because he deserved it, and [arranged his burial and provided a place;] and I had this memorial made to him so that [all freedmen should have an] incentive to be loyal to their patrons.

Also to Castricia Helena, freedwoman of Gaius, because [she too was loyal].[1]

An inscription from Forum Livi (modern Forli in Tuscany) offers an insight into the workings of the household of Gaius Castricius Calvus Agricola, or at least the way in which Agricola wanted his household to work, and be seen to be working, during the early years of the Augustan Principate. Agricola's priorities, it seems, reflected the name by which he preferred to be known (*agricola* = 'husbandman, agriculturist, ploughman, farmer, peasant'), and consequently the inscription serves two purposes. The first is a didactic one, it espouses a specific course of action regarding the way to live a productive life; the second is honorific, as it highlights specific members, both male and female, of Agricola's household who chose to do as he recommended. Agricola makes an explicit link between the health and well-being of the individual and the success that they can expect to have in life. He foregrounds the necessity of self-care and goes as far as to state that he did not learn this from others, but rather from himself. This is despite the fact that it accords with the general consensus regarding health and well-being found in a variety of ancient literary genres.[2] He does, however, aim to share this knowledge, not only with the members of his own household, but also with anyone else who might happen to see and read the inscription.[3] Thus, he is offering himself and his household as *exempla*.

Over the last thirty years interest in the Roman household and family has increased significantly but studies have until recently been dominated by social historians who utilise ancient literary evidence and, to a lesser extent, ancient documentary evidence for the information these can provide.[4] Attempting to reconstruct the composition of the Roman family and household and the roles played by their members based solely on literary and documentary evidence is, unfortunately, problematic. Ancient Roman literary evidence, no matter what the genre or content, was written in most cases by elite citizen males. To understand how the Roman household and family were composed and what the roles played in them by men, women and children, freeborn, freed or slave, it is necessary to attempt to distinguish the writer's views of the thoughts and deeds of other members of ancient Roman society from what those other members actually thought and did.[5] Additionally, there was no standard, typical, normal Roman household or family despite the tendency to generalise about family life. The Roman household could contain any number or combination of family members, slaves, freedmen and freedwomen, other clients, close and distant relatives and potentially even tenants or lodgers.

The 'best' literary evidence for the Roman household and family comprise Roman legal writings pertaining to the household and literary discussions of family life. These elucidate certain aspects not only of how people behaved but also of how they were expected to behave towards members of their household and family, which in turn helps us reconstruct social mores and values.[6] The institution of the household and family was of fundamental importance to the Romans and, particularly from the Augustan Principate onwards, was thought to be intrinsically linked to and representative of the institution of the Roman state. Roman commentators directly linked the fall of the Republic and the subsequent civil wars to moral decline, a significant component of which was associated with household and family life, and which Augustus' so-called moral legislation was an attempt to address.[7] Thus accounts of ancient Roman family life of the Regal period and the early and middle Republic are presented as having been infinitely superior to those of the late Republic and early Principate, although these should be read as idealising legend rather than historical description and treated accordingly.[8] Stereotypes such as the tyrannical *pater familias*, the virtuous *mater familias* and the wicked and scheming step-parent, while not necessarily reflecting actual practices, do at least help us reconstruct moral positions and ideologies.[9]

Yet study of the Roman world has long been dominated by concern for the representation of masculine power.[10] This concern has extended beyond studies of ancient literary and documentary evidence to those of archaeological evidence, particularly material culture, approaching the latter with entrenched assumptions regarding its implicit masculinity.[11] If the ancient literary and documentary evidence regarding the roles of members of the household in the acquisition and maintenance of health and well-being is somewhat problematic, is it possible to clarify the situation by focussing on archaeological and bioarchaeological evidence and material culture? *Instrumentum domesticum*, household objects that attest the myriad different activities that took place within the domestic environment on a daily basis, provide us with the opportunity to study ancient domestic life and better understand household organisation, consumption and production, social status and aspiration.[12] Pompeii and, to a lesser extent, Herculaneum offer us just such an opportunity. Household objects work in conjunction with household architecture to define a space and imbue it with meaning not only for the inhabitants of the house but also for the visitors to the house.[13] Yet studies of assemblages have shown that the distribution of artefacts in domestic contexts does not necessarily conform to the information contained in the ancient literary evidence and that there is not necessarily any correlation between the size, decoration and artefact assemblage of a room.[14] Also, areas of the house were multifunctional and activities were organised on a temporal rather than a spatial basis; they were both domestic and economic.[15]

As we saw in the previous chapters, concerns over the acquisition and maintenance of good health and well-being were widespread in ancient Greece and Rome. From this starting point, this chapter will examine the roles played in domestic healthcare theory, method and practice by the members, both free and slave, of the Roman household. It will explore the legal responsibilities that the members of the household had towards each other regarding healthcare, the ideal of the household regarding healthcare and the reality of the household regarding healthcare utilising literary, documentary, archaeological and bioarchaeological evidence. It will also consider the ramifications of domestic healthcare for relationships within the household.

Terminology

It is impossible to speak of the Roman household and family in the sense of there being only one type or even one typical type of either in any place at any period, let alone in Italy from the beginning of the first century BCE to the end of the first century CE.[16] Even the Latin terminology associated with the subject is problematic and imprecise.[17]

Yet if we are to examine, analyse and discuss the role (or roles) that the members of the Roman household and family played in the acquisition and maintenance of health and well-being during the late Republic and early Principate, it is first necessary to address and to clarify who, exactly, is meant when English terms such as 'household' and 'family' are used. The Latin words *domus* and *familia* had a wide range of meanings that do not correspond precisely with the English words often utilised to stand in for them.[18] *Domus* can be used to refer to the physical house or, in fact, the home, no matter what architectural form that place of residence might take.[19] It can also be used to refer to the household, covering both family members and freed slaves or slaves, or even to the broader kinship group. Finally, it can be used to refer to the patrimony. *Familia* is considered to have at least six definitions, and these definitions cover both people and property with a significant overlap between the two.[20] The first encompasses all people subject to the control of the *pater familias*, whether they are relations, freed slaves or slaves, and this comprises a household, while the second is restricted to the slaves of a household. The third is extended to all the servants (so presumably both freed slaves and slaves) resident in one place. The fourth is a group of people closely associated by blood or affinity, and this comprises a family. The fifth is a school. The sixth is a legal one and refers to one's estate which consists of the household and the household property. It is worth noting that these definitions do not remain static. Rather, the emphasis placed upon the Roman household and family changed over the course of the Late Republic and into the Augustan Principate, expanding from the agnatic *familia* to the wider kinship *domus*, with the latter becoming something of a status symbol, a visual sign of the current level of wealth and power of the owner.[21]

Additionally, these terms are utilised most frequently in legal contexts, although they also feature in rhetorical ones, focusing on the ideal of the Roman household and family rather than the reality. While the types of households and families highlighted in ancient Roman literature tend towards the idealised, with emphasis placed upon what we would refer to as the 'nuclear' family, consisting of the triad of the father, mother and children, other types of evidence indicate that Roman households and families were much more complicated than that.[22] As a result, although it is certainly possible to speak of the Roman nuclear family consisting of father, mother and children, it is clear that when considering the family in relation to the household, it is also necessary to factor in additional kin and non-kin individuals, and their proximity to the nuclear family.[23] Since this nuclear family was by no means static due to a combination of mortality, divorce and remarriage, much-needed stability could have been provided by non-kin within the household and kin without it.[24] Roman families were particularly subject to constant alteration and adaptation according to changes in circumstance.[25] This occurred whether the family was imperial, senatorial, lower class, military or slave.[26] Consequently the precise composition of the Roman household could vary considerably. Elite households were large and composed of potentially considerable numbers of specialised slaves and freed slaves, while those further down the social scale were smaller and composed of fewer slaves and freed slaves with overlapping duties.[27] There is substantially more evidence for elite families in urban areas than there is for any other type of family in urban areas, or even rural areas, despite the fact that peasant families played an important part in the Romans' self-conceptualisation.[28] So, since Roman households and families came in all shapes and sizes, and comprised a wide range of members, for the duration of this discussion, I shall utilise the term 'household' as a means of casting a wide net and including all the individuals within a specific place of residence, whether freeborn, freed slaves or slaves, related by blood or marriage, or formally employed or simply engaged.

The *pater familias*

A case in point regarding the considerable flexibility of the Roman household can be found if we examine the term *pater familias*. It is found most frequently in

Roman legal texts and is used to denote either the head of a family or the owner of an estate.[29] A male Roman citizen, provided he had been released from the control of his own father, whether through his father's death or emancipation prior to his father's death, was in possession of *patria potestas* and *dominium* over his children, his wife if their marriage had been accompanied by *manus*, his slaves and his property.[30] Thus in the eyes of the law a young child would be a *pater familias* if he had no living father, while a grown man would not be if his father were still living and he had not been emancipated, provided that some sort of property was possessed.[31] In theory, *patria potestas* granted the *pater familias* absolute power over those subject to his authority for the duration of his lifetime.[32] There is thus a tendency to assume that the *pater familias* was an autocratic and all-powerful figure, and that *patria potestas* embodied arbitrary tyrannical power.[33] While this may have been the case in the eyes of the law, it may not have been the case in everyday life.[34]

Theoretically, the *pater familias'* power over his offspring began prior to a child's birth, as an unborn child conceived within marriage was considered to be its father's property, with Roman resistance to the practice of abortion resulting from its being perceived as interfering with paternal rights.[35] The *Twelve Tables* state that not only does a father have the power of life and death over a son born within a lawful marriage, but also that a father should immediately put to death a son recently born 'who is a monster or has a form different from that of members of the human race'.[36] This power was exercised upon the birth of a child, as it was the *pater familias'* decision whether to acknowledge and accept it into the family.[37] It is perhaps this responsibility for monitoring unborn children and accepting newborn children into the household, combined with the ongoing power of life and death over the household's members, that has led to the assumption that the *pater familias* was directly responsible for the household's health and well-being. That this was the case is frequently asserted in discussions of Roman medicine, but is there any real evidence to support it?[38]

Cato the Elder is often presented as the archetypal example of a *pater familias* taking charge of his household's health and well-being, and while Cato's surviving literary works indicate that he did, in fact, do so, we have to wonder how typical such behaviour was.[39] After all, Plutarch's *Cato the Elder* also includes details regarding Cato's very involved approach to parenting his son, which involved being present when his wife bathed the child, and later teaching him to read, tutoring him in law and training him in athletics, martial skills and sport, none of which seems to have been typical behaviour of a father at this time, as these duties would normally have devolved onto slave members of the household.[40] Is what we are seeing here from Plutarch and, to a lesser extent, Pliny the Elder, an attempt to present Cato as a highly idealised *pater familias* and a suitable example for others to attempt to live up to? The agricultural treatises of Cato, Varro and Columella certainly highlight the role of the *pater familias* in caring for the health and well-being of the members of his household, not to mention his livestock, but we should not assume that this was always, in fact, the case. In fact, other sources place responsibility for the health and well-being of the members of the household squarely in the hands of the *domina*, a logical extension of her role in relation to household management and the provision of food and drink.[41]

Under what circumstances might a *pater familias* have been in a position to be directly responsible for the mental and physical health and well-being of his entire household? He needed to have a combination of authority and opportunity. In the early and middle Republic, most women seem to have transferred to the husband's *manus* upon marriage, but this practice seems to have gradually ceased, until in the first century BCE it was extremely unusual. It has been suggested that this system reflected the conditions of Roman society during this time, with women moving physically from their fathers' holdings to their husbands' and remaining there for life, with their own property becoming subsumed into that of their new families.[42] Considering the time at which Cato was living and his preference for tradition, it is likely that his marriages included *manus*, meaning that both of his wives and any slaves that they brought into the household with them became subject to his authority. Under circumstances such as these, it would have been considered appropriate for him to dictate regimen. Additionally, it would appear that his son and his son's wife and child lived with him, even after the son's mother died and he remarried.[43] Therefore Cato was in possession of both authority and opportunity. However, the *pater familias* was not always in the enviable position of being able to combine authority with opportunity. If a marriage was undertaken without *manus*, a wife and any slaves she brought into the household with her did not become subject to her husband's authority, but rather remained subject to that of her father, or, if *sui iuris*, herself or her guardian, which meant that it was not necessarily appropriate for the *pater familias* to dictate regimen to them as he did with his own dependents. Who, then, would have been responsible for them? Would a wife married without *manus* have needed to return to her family home, or send any ailing slaves back to her family home, to seek medical treatment there if she were still within the power of a father or a guardian? Or would she, if *sui iuris*, treat any ailments she or her slaves suffered herself, without recourse to her husband?

Even if the *pater familias* was inclined to manage the health and well-being of his household, he was not necessarily always present, but would have been frequently absent from the household, whether on secondment to a province, away on business or simply out of the house. Thus, his responsibilities must have devolved onto someone else, whether formally or informally, and it is likely that someone was appointed to make decisions regarding the healthcare of the members of the household in his absence. Investigations into Roman demography have suggested that a high number of Roman households did not, in fact, have a living *pater familias*, and that by the time most Romans were aged thirty they did not have a living father, let alone a grandfather or great grandfather.[44] In the case of Cato the Elder, although he lived to the age of eighty-five and oversaw the lives of his firstborn son (who actually predeceased him) and grandson, his second son was born when he was eighty years old, and so was left without a father when he was five years old. It is difficult to image a five-year-old, although technically a *pater familias*, or even a fourteen-year-old, not only technically a *pater familias* but also an adult, managing the health and well-being of the members of his household. Would his mother or perhaps his guardian taken charge of his household staff?

The *pater familias* of the family was not necessarily the *dominus* of a particular residence or the household. The *pater familias* might become incapacitated through illness or insanity and be put in the charge of his relatives for as long as was necessary.[45] Upon the death of their father, siblings might continue to live together in the family home, pooling their resources as a means of preserving the family property and fortune, particularly if there was not much of either to start with.[46] While the eldest sibling might nominally be in charge (as in the case of Appius Claudius Pulcher, aged twenty or twenty-one when his father died in 76 BCE and left him responsible for two younger brothers and three younger sisters), this would likely be subject to continuous negotiation. In either of these scenarios, if a specific issue related to health and well-being arose, a domestic council, a *consilium*, could be formed in order to discuss how to deal with it.[47] Additionally, young men of the senatorial and equestrian classes often set up independent households prior to marriage, but these households would likely be funded by their *pater familias*, with the young man perhaps being in receipt of an allowance or *peculium* to cover day-to-day living expenses.[48]

Finally, it is important to note that, while the term *pater familias* is gendered male, it does not necessarily follow that a woman could not fulfil the role of head of a family or of owner of an estate.[49] There is both literary and documentary evidence not only for estates owned by women, but also for women not only owning slaves but also freeing slaves and subsequently acting as their patron, and for families in which only the woman was actually freeborn or a freed slave, so the only one in a legal position to own anything.[50]

Marriage and the *mater familias*

Whatever the size of the household, one fundamental determinant as to how, precisely, it operated was the type of marriage ceremony that was performed, as the result dictated whether marriage was accompanied by *manus*.[51] In the early days of the Roman Republic, marriage seems to have generally been accompanied by *manus*, which meant that a woman was under the control of her husband, and this occurred through one of three methods: by *usus*, by *confarreatio* or by *coemptio*. *Usus* and *confarreatio* seem to have been the methods available to the freeborn, whatever their class, while *coemptio* was restricted to patricians. Under Roman law, uninterrupted possession of a moveable object for one year, or an unmoveable object for two years, conferred legal ownership of that object on to the individual in possession of it.[52] Thus a woman came under the control of her husband by *usus*, 'usage', if she remained under his roof for one full year without a break, although she could prevent this if she spent three nights away from it.[53] This type of marriage seems to have become obsolete by the second century CE, perhaps abolished by Augustus, or perhaps, due to the decline of marriage by *manus*, simply ceasing to be necessary.[54] A woman came under the control of her husband by *confarreatio*, 'emmer-wheat', if a particular offering was made to

Jupiter Farreus during the wedding ceremony by the Pontifex Maximus and the Flamen Dialis, with the *manus* created by the grain which went into the sacrificial loaf that comprised the offering.[55] This type of marriage was highly unusual, probably unpopular due to the complicated requirements of the ceremony in addition to the restrictions that came with it, but it does seem to have survived for longer than marriage by *usus*, perhaps due to the fact that certain priesthoods were only open to those whose parents had been married in that way. A woman could be brought under the control of her husband by *coemptio*, 'formal purchase', at any time during the marriage, and this formal purchase included her property.[56]

A man who had been released from the paternal authority, *patria potestas*, of his *pater familias*, which usually but not always occurred as a result of the death of the *pater familias*, was himself a *pater familias*.[57] Thus his children, whether sons, *filii familias*, or daughters, *filiae familias*, were subject to his paternal authority. His wife, however, would only be subject to his authority if their marriage had been accompanied by *manus*. If this was the case, she was released from the paternal authority of her own *pater familias*, and transferred to that of her husband, becoming a *mater familias* in the process. If their marriage had been done without *manus*, she remained a *filia familias* until the death of her own *pater familias*.[58] It is also worth considering the consequences of the Roman tendency towards asymmetric marriage, and how a large disparity in age between a husband and wife might have affected the power dynamics of their marriage in relation to the health and well-being not only of the husband and the wife, but also their dependents.[59]

As discussed previously, whether a household had a *mater familias* or not depended upon whether the marriage had taken place with or without *manus*. If the female head of the household was a *mater familias*, she would have been subject to the will of the *pater familias*, just as the other members of the household were. If she was not, she would have been in nominal charge of her household within the household. In either case, we might expect a considerable amount of negotiation to have taken place between husband and wife regarding how the health and well-being of all of the members of their household were to be dealt with. It would seem to have been the case that the female head of the household, whether *mater familias* or not, was responsible for certain aspects of the running of that household.

The belief that division of labour between husband and wife was the key to a successful household was an ancient one, expressed most fully by Xenophon in his discussion of estate management in general and that of Ischomachus in particular.[60] According to Ischomachus, he delegated all the indoor work to his wife, which left him free to concentrate on the outdoor work. While the precepts of the treatise are not specifically mentioned in surviving Roman works, the treatise is known to have circulated in Rome in the first centuries BCE and CE, as Cicero translated it and Philodemus critiqued it.

A key component of the Roman wedding was the bride smearing pig or wolf fat on the doorposts of her new husband's home, supposedly as a means of keeping anyone doing harm to members of the family with potions.[61] However, there are indications that practices changed over time and women became less willing to perform duties that they considered menial. While Titus Maccius Plautus (*circa* 254–184 BCE) explicitly links the female head of the household with the garden, Columella tells us that by his time, 'the ancient practice of the Sabine and Roman mistresses of households has not only become out of fashion but has absolutely died out', leading to these duties devolving onto the female head of the slave household.[62] Book 12 of Columella's *On Agriculture*, which focuses on the house-keeper, gives us a good idea of what the duties of the female head of the household had been but had come to be devolved onto the housekeeper. Likewise, while Titus Livius Patavinus (59 BCE–17 CE) presents Tanaquil gathering supplies to treat her husband's wounds and Pliny the Younger describes the care that Gnaeus Domitius Tullus' wife lavished upon him, Lucius Apuleius Madaurensis (*circa* 124–*circa* 170 CE) has Psyche's sister complain about having to administer to her husband:[63]

> The other chipped in: 'As for [my husband], he's bent and bowed with arthritis, and scarcely ever pays homage to my charms. I'm forever massaging his twisted and frozen fingers, and soiling these delicate hands of mine with his odious fomentations, sordid bandages, and fetid poultices. Instead of playing the role of a normal wife, I'm burdened with playing his doctor'.[64]

In the *Cupid and Psyche* interlude of Apuleius' novel *The Golden Ass*, Psyche's nameless sisters are aggrieved to find that, while their husbands are old, bald and ill, their younger sister's husband is young and handsome in addition to being exorbitantly wealthy. Psyche's sisters explicitly compare their circumstances to Psyche's, not only their husbands but also the ramifications of being married to such men. One of Psyche's sisters gives a detailed description of the duties she performs for her husband, and she is clearly not happy about these; she goes so far as to complain that performing them renders her abnormal. While it is undeniable that this is a work of fiction and, more significantly, Apuleius has deliberately constructed the characters as a means of setting Psyche and her sisters up in opposition to each other, making the sisters particularly unsympathetic in the process, it is worth considering why he chose domestic medical practice as a means of doing this, to the extent of having one of them utilise technical language in the process.[65] We have to wonder, is this a realistic portrayal of an elite Roman woman in the middle of the second century CE? Were elite Roman women of this period not only undertaking domestic medical practice but also entirely comfortable with medical theory and method as well? And was this considered normal or abnormal, something that they were happy to do or something that they were not? Psyche is a princess and her sisters are queens, and women occupying such high positions might well be expected to consider such menial duties beneath their dignity, particularly when equipped with large complements of slaves; certainly it is a common refrain in ancient literature of the late first and early second centuries CE that elite women are refusing to fulfil the roles required of them, in contrast to their venerable ancestors, and these roles are devolving onto their slaves.[66]

Cassius Dio has Augustus justify his moral legislation by asking the rhetorical question:

> is there anything better than a wife who is chaste, domestic, a good house-keeper, a rearer of children; one to gladden you in health, to tend you in sickness; to be your partner in good fortune, to console you in misfortune; to restrain the mad passion of youth and to temper the unseasonable harshness of old age?[67]

The Romans regarded marriage as an institution designed for the production and rearing of legitimate children as a means of ensuring the continuance of the family line.[68] Thus we might expect particular attention to be paid to the health and well-being of women of child-bearing age and children.[69] As we have seen, particular regimens were recommended for pregnancy, infants, children and adolescents.[70]

Dominus, Domina and devolution

The Roman household was often compared to the Roman state. Seneca declared that '[our ancestors] held that a household was a miniature commonwealth', while Pliny the Younger went further, stating that 'the house provides a slave with a country and a sort of citizenship'.[71] Just as in the Roman state, in the Roman household each member had a role to play and that role was, to a degree, determined by particular factors. The roles of family members were broadly divided according to gender, with the male members of the household (primarily the *pater familias, dominus* or *vilicus*) undertaking certain tasks in relation to mental and physical health and well-being and the female members of the household (primarily the *mater familias, domina* or *vilica*) undertaking others. Depending on the nature and composition of the individual family, these roles might devolve onto alternative family members, for example the *pater familias* or *mater familias* might delegate some of their duties to freed or slave members of the household if they possessed them, or they might undertake these duties themselves if not.[72] However, it is clear that there was considerable asymmetry in male and female participation in the labour force, whether that labour took place in an urban or rural context.[73]

In households where the *pater familias* or *mater familias*, or *dominus* or *domina*, are absent, their responsibilities nominally appear to have devolved onto the *vilicus* or *vilica*.[74] However, many other members of the household possessed varying levels of skill and expertise in relation to domestic medical practice. While these would certainly include the physician or the midwife, if the household was large enough or affluent enough or possess one or other of these specialists, we should also include the nurse of any infants or young children, the pedagogue of any older children, personal attendants with responsibility for massage, oils, perfumes, cosmetics or bathing and those responsible for the acquisition, provision and preparation of food and drink. One household could potentially include a variety of potential practitioners of domestic medical practice, with adjacent, overlapping or independent sets of medical knowledge.[75] Consequently, the Roman household could be considered a medical marketplace in miniature.

Over the course of the first century BCE, the gradual erosion and finally complete cessation of traditional republican avenues of power and glory caused elite Romans to search for alternative ways of differentiating and distinguishing themselves from their peers.[76] One means of doing this was through their private residences, particularly those residences located outside of the city of Rome, and the households that resided in them. There is a noticeable increase in slave numbers over the course of the first century BCE, and in conjunction with this increase in numbers comes an increase in slave occupations and specialisations.[77] For legal purposes, the Roman *familia* was considered to comprise two parts, the *familia urbana* and the *familia rustica*. This distinction was partly down to residence, the assumption being that a Roman citizen possessed both an urban and a rural residence, but mainly down to duties. However, both categories contained potentially limitless occupations and potential duties, and they expanded through the first century BCE. In a well-ordered household (and a well-ordered household was considered desirable and something to aspire to), there was a distinct hierarchy resulting in a clear chain of command. Slave labour could be either functional (*officia*) or skilled (*artificia*), and promotion and demotion were both possible.[78] The necessity of the members of a household knowing their role and playing it effectively if a household is to be well-run and well-ordered is highlighted in Roman literature. Only a well-run and well-ordered household can be a successful household. There is a performative aspect to this. The Roman household was viewed as a representation and reflection of its owner. Petronius deliberately presents Trimalchio's household as not conforming to the proper order, with his slaves performing tasks inappropriate to their assigned duties.[79]

This begs the question; how did this impact the running of the household? Was a household full of individuals armed with medical knowledge a positive thing or a negative thing?

Rationale

Recent scholarship on the ancient Roman household and family has described the institution as 'the primary site of production, reproduction, consumption and the intergenerational transmission of property and knowledge undergirding production in the Roman world'.[80] When viewing the Roman household and family as not just a social unit but also an economic one, considering the role that health and well-being played is crucial. As we have seen, concerns over the acquisition and maintenance of good health and well-being were widespread in ancient Greece and Rome, with regimen seen as the way to achieve the best possible state of it. And, as we have seen, there was also a substantial moral component to this. As a result, it is not surprising that the health and well-being of individual household members was seen as being fundamental to the health and well-being of the household as a whole. There was a substantial moral component to this too, as a well-ordered household had not only a functional but also a moral dimension and represented an ideal to strive for.[81] If the household was to maximise its social and economic potential and be as productive as possible, and the head of that household was to be taken seriously and accorded respect and recognition, they needed to take health and well-being seriously.

The head of the household, whether male or female, not only needed to be physically and mentally healthy themselves in order to set the tone, but they also had to bear in mind the health of their dependents.[82] Female members of the household needed to undertake not only the productive labour of domestic activities such as spinning and weaving, but also the reproductive labour of pregnancy, childbirth and childrearing.[83] Slaves, freedmen and freedwomen needed to perform their assigned duties effectively. Yet reconstructing the precise contributions made by individual members of the household can be tricky, particularly when we take into consideration the fact that households were highly individualised. The literary evidence that is the most systematically and methodically informative about domestic activities – the agricultural treatises of Cato the Elder, Varro and Columella – first focuses primarily upon agricultural estates and the *familia rustica* that inhabits and operates them, and second addresses itself to the estate owner and what he (or potentially she) either does or should do. Cato, for example, uses the passive voice and second-person singular throughout his treatise, which results in the occlusion of the slave labour and the absorption of it into the agency of the estate owner, and Varro and Columella write in similar ways.[84] Other types of evidence can be useful here. Documentary evidence such as epitaphs can provide names and occupations, and sometimes, particularly in relation to female members of the household, descriptions of duties that they performed particularly well, although we do have to take into account the prevailing ideology behind these.[85] Archaeological evidence for daily life such as household objects can indicate not only what domestic activities were taking place, but also where they were taking place and who was undertaking them.[86] However, it must be borne in mind that activities relating to health and well-being are difficult to reconstruct precisely because, being centred upon the physical body of the individual, they are entirely ephemeral (the consumption of food and drink, the process of bathing and anointing, undertaking physical or mental exercise, etc.).

So, how best to ensure the health and well-being of all of the members of the household? The head of the household was legally obliged to provide food, clothing and shelter to their dependents.[87] Beyond this, they might choose to purchase a slave healthcare practitioner or, if that was not feasible, engage a freeborn or freed one. In the Republic, many prominent Romans had personal physicians. These include Gaius Julius Caesar, Marcus Licinius Crassus, Gaius Verres, Marcus Antonius, Gaius Octavius (later Augustus), Calpurnius Piso and Marcus Porcius Cato Uticensis.[88] In the early Empire, the household of Livia boasted at least physician (*medicus*), but the fact that a supervisor of physicians (*supra medicos*) is also attested implies that there were more, while the presence of an infirmary orderly (*ad valetudinarium*) implies that there was, in fact, an infirmary where those physicians, amongst others, plied their trade. There was also a midwife (*obstetrix*) and a wet nurse (*nutrix*) to tend to pregnant and postpartum women and their infants. Additionally, individuals such as the caterer (*opsonator*), the baker (*pistor*), the masseuse (*unctrix*) and the person in charge of the perfumed oils (*ad unguenta*) also had roles to play in regimen (see Figure 3.1).[89] While the possession of such highly specialised staff could be viewed as Livia's household conforming to the discourse of *luxus* and *luxuria*, it is also possible to argue that such staff were necessary if the household were to fully engage with the theories, methods and practices surrounding regimen.[90]

Identifying the physical locations in which any sort of medical practice was undertaken is difficult, as the only architectural requirements for such a location were space and light, and these were not necessarily always met. Additionally, the equipment utilised for medical practice could range from vast *instrumentaria* to a single multifunctional instrument, from comprehensive pharmacopeia to a single multipurpose ointment. Such items were portable, so could easily be transported from one area of a building to another, and perishable, particularly the organic components. It is difficult to identify instruments used specifically and exclusively for medical practice in the absence of supportive contextual information. While some medical instruments are indicative of a high level of specialisation and are consequently rare in the archaeological record, others are more generic and were commonly used outside of medical situations (see Figure 3.2).

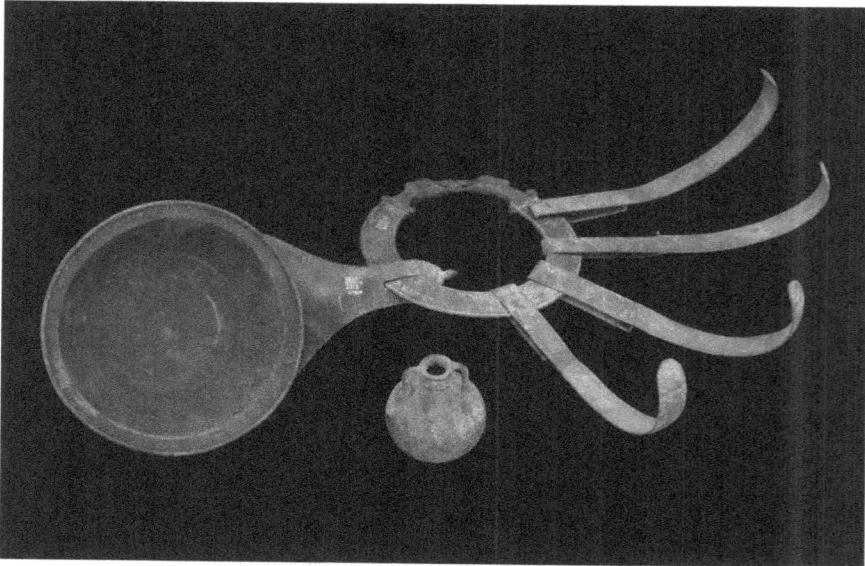

Figure 3.1 A bronze strigil set; a copy of an item supposedly recovered from Pompeii and currently housed in the Naples National Archaeological Museum and dating from *circa* 199 BCE–79 CE.

Source: Image courtesy of the Wellcome Library (Wellcome Collection/Science Museum inv. A128412).

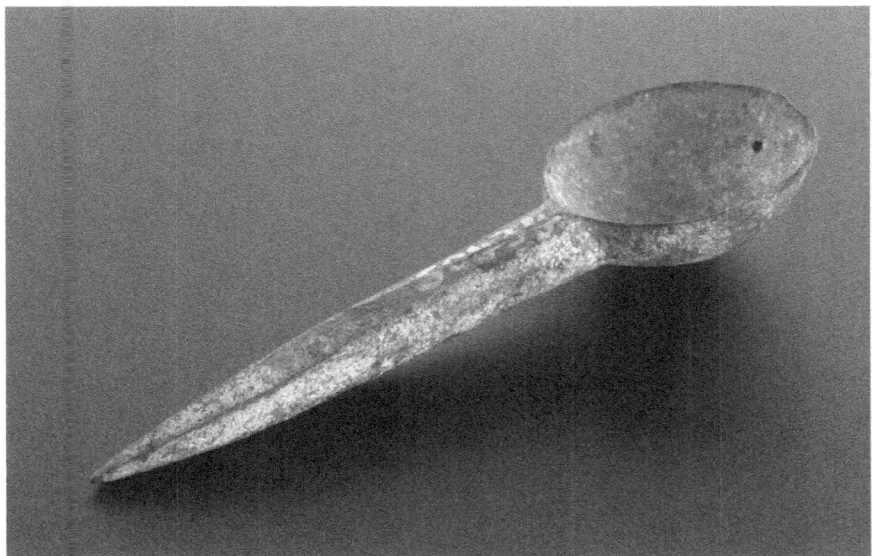

Figure 3.2 A bronze spoon and pick combined, *circa* 199 BCE–500 CE.
Source: Image courtesy of the Wellcome Library (Wellcome Collection/Science Museum inv. A113622).

While there have been occasional archaeological discoveries of surgeries, there have also been discoveries of houses containing medical instruments whose purpose is less clear. At Pompeii, medical instruments have been found at over twenty locations, indicating that some sort of medical activity was taking place on a variety of premises.[91] The practitioners could have been homeowners, they could have been freedmen or freedwomen or slaves.[92] In professional terms, there is also a significant amount of overlap between physicians, pharmacists and ointment makers and sellers (see Figure 3.3).[93] Thus if a household did possess a medical practitioner, there is a range of potential responsibilities relating to health and well-being that they could have held.

However, Varro suggests initiating a standing agreement with a local physician just as one might with a fuller or other type of artisan whose expertise was not necessarily required.[94] The household of Cicero does not seem to have included a permanent, full-time physician. Rather he seems to have been in the habit of engaging them as and when their services were required, and he did so upon the recommendations of friends.[95] There are indications that physicians were engaged to treat not just family members, but also slaves and freedmen and freedwomen.[96] However, one of the central tenets of Roman household management was not spending money on anything that you could produce yourself.[97] As we have seen, Cato took responsibility for all the members of his household, and Varro divided

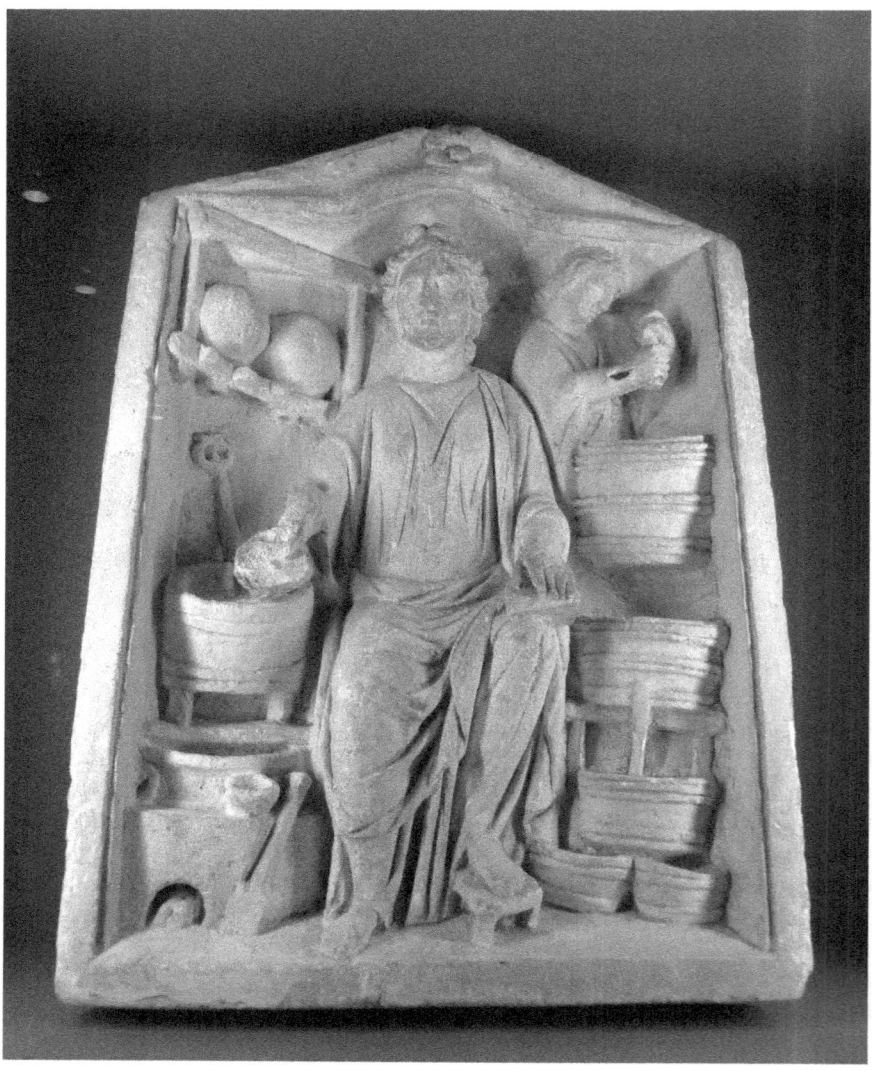

Figure 3.3 A stone funerary relief depicting a woman who has been variously identified as a doctor, a pharmacist and a soap-maker, dating from the second century CE.

Source: Image courtesy of Carole Raddato (Licence: CC–BY–SA–2.0).

health problems into those that could be dealt with by anyone, and those that should be dealt with by a physician.[98] Thus it would make sense from an economic standpoint to minimise the number of occasions upon which a physician was consulted, as in addition to paying for the physician, it would also be necessary to pay for the treatment that they recommended.[99] Considering that there was a long tra-ditional of hostility to professional medical practitioners amongst the Romans, it is hardly surprising that people might choose not to consult them at all, preferring instead to monitor and manage their own health and well-being, and there is no reason to assume that it was only the owners of agricultural estates that did so.[100] Frugality, whether as a result of ideology or necessity, was likely widespread.

So the health and well-being of all members of the household were monitored because all members of a household, no matter how young or old, were expected, if not required, to be productive, and an individual's ability to be productive was dependent upon their state of health and well-being. It was in the best interests of the head of the household that all the members of their household were as physically and mentally healthy as possible. Cato notes the importance of the household being in good condition, its members neither sick nor hungry, and that the estate manager in particular needs to be healthy and well-rested.[101] He sets out how much and what sort of food and drink different types of slaves should be allocated.[102] He suggests reducing the rations of slaves that are sickly.[103] Varro criticises Hortensius for caring less for the health and well-being of his slaves than for his fish.[104] He offers advice on how to treat slaves, recommending scold-ing rather than beating, and the provision of incentives and rewards such as larger rations of food and clothing, occasional exemption from work and permission to work for themselves.[105] Columella offers guidance for maintaining the slaves whether they be in good health or poor health, recommending that they be well looked after so as to foster loyalty and obedience.[106] If slaves become sickly, it might become necessary for the owner to cut their losses and sell them or, if no one was prepared to buy them, simply abandon them, although those who did so could suffer opprobrium from their peers.[107] Alternative courses of action included taking care of them, even in cases of terminal decline, perhaps assign-ing them less labour intensive duties.[108] After all, as both Varro and Horace point out, assigning the right person to the right task is crucial.[109] As is clear from the epitaphs found in *columbaria*, members of elite households had clearly defined and rather specialised duties. Elite households in which slaves had multiple duties were looked down upon, although modest households probably had fewer slaves with more general duties as a matter of course.[110] Columella highlights the ten-dency for estate owners to appoint the wrong estate manager through sheer igno-rance, and the problems that result.[111] Ultimately, as Martial makes clear, a happy estate like his friend Faustinus' *villa* at Baiae is a productive estate.[112] The good health of slaves is a matter of economic self-interest rather than philanthropy, although philanthropy had its place.[113]

Acquisition, preparation and provision

There are several specific areas of household activity that it is necessary to con-sider when exploring the roles played by members of the household in relation to health and well-being. The first is the acquisition of the items necessary for the maintenance of health and well-being, whether in the form of raw materials or ready-made. The second is the preparation of the items necessary for the maintenance of health and well-being. The third is the provision of care and attention. The agricultural treatises of Cato, Varro and Columella provide a significant amount of information regarding the running of a rural household and up to a point this information can be applied to the running of an urban household as well.

Acquisition

The process of acquiring items for the household varied considerably depending on whether the household was located in a rural or an urban context. As we have seen, the writers of the agricultural treatises promoted self-sufficiency as highly desirable, and it features as an ideal in numerous other works of literature. However, it has been suggested that the emphasis placed upon self-sufficiency and the boasting undertaken by those who claim to have achieved it indicates that it was far from usual.[114] Certainly people seem to have cheated as a means of making a point.[115] Self-sufficiency was likely more achievable in rural contexts, at least as far as agricultural estates were concerned as, depending upon its size and situation, an agricultural estate could comprise land for the cultivation of crops, vineyards, olive groves, gardens, orchards, grazing and pasture.[116] Thus it could produce not just the Mediterranean triad of grain, grapes and olives, but also fruit, vegetables, flowers, herbs, meat and dairy products. It might also produce specialist and luxury products through ventures such as apiculture, aviculture and pisciculture.[117] Additional produce could be gathered in the wild, and game could be hunted.[118]

As far as rural residences were concerned, ideally as much as possible was produced on the estate and processed within the household.[119] These products were subsequently utilised by members of the household and any surplus to requirements were sold in order to raise the money necessary to buy items that could not be produced on the estate.[120] Cato recommends suitable places to purchase particular products.[121] Some of this would be utilised by the members of the household while that which was surplus to requirements would be sold at nearby settlements in order to raise the money necessary to buy the items that could not be produced within the household.[122] This could be the case with both standard items such as the products of agriculture and horticulture, potentially sold at *nundinae*, and with more specialist ones such as the products of apiculture, aviculture and pisciculture, potentially sold at *macellae*.[123]

As far as urban residences were concerned, those with ties to agricultural estates or market-gardens in the *suburbium* could receive produce directly and regularly.[124] It is possible that a high percentage of Romans were fed directly from estates, whether their own or those of family members, friends or acquaintances. Consequently, those who resorted to purchasing staples that their estates should have provided for them were publicly excoriated.[125] Those occupying urban residences that were themselves in possession of land were able to grow some or perhaps most of what they needed. Those who were lacking land or connections to those in possession of it had to purchase what they needed, although the extent of their purchasing power could vary considerably.[126] Foodstuffs and other items could be purchased from a variety of locations ranging from wholesalers in *fora* to hawkers on the street, with some sellers even visiting homes directly. Visual evidence such as wall paintings, reliefs and mosaics frequently depict such transactions, while epigraphic evidence attests to the sheer variety of manufacturers, dealers and sellers operating (see Figure 3.4). Depending upon the storage space available in urban residences, consumers might be in a position to buy in bulk and store items until such as time as they were needed, or they might need to buy in small quantities on a daily basis, or they might even buy an item as and when it was required for immediate consumption.[127]

As stated at the outset of this monograph, one of my aims is to emphasise just how one-sided previous work undertaken on ancient Roman medicine has been and establish just how inter-related many aspects of daily life were with medical theories and practices, as well as situating them squarely in the home. One of the ways of doing this is to examine the consumer landscape of the ancient city or town, as there is a significant amount of evidence for the production and distribution of items that consumers would then have had the opportunity to purchase and utilise in domestic medical practice.

Iron from Noricum was particularly prized, and it was made into tools and instruments near Comum and Sulmo that were then sold at Rome.[128] Copper

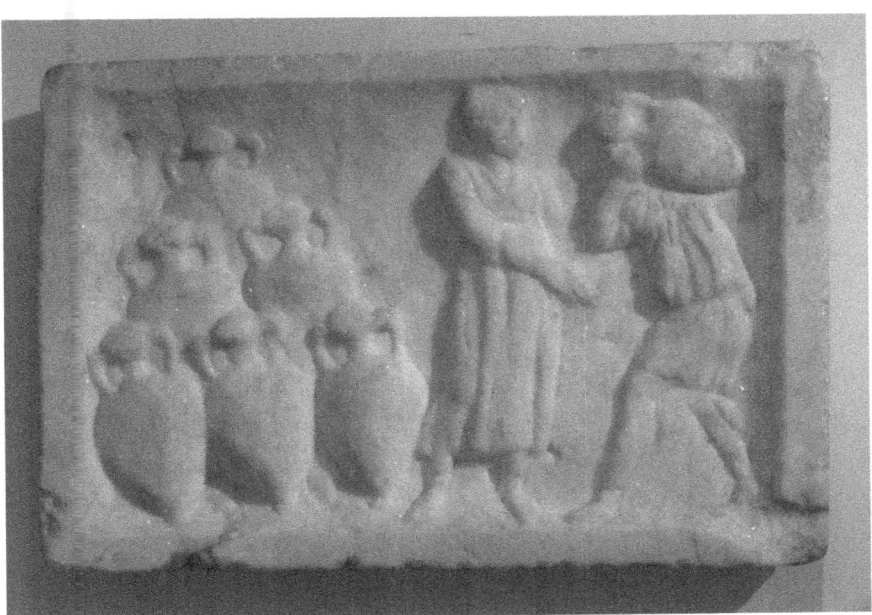

Figure 3.4 A relief of workers transporting *amphorae*, dating from the second century CE.

Source: Image courtesy of the Metropolitan Museum of Art Open Access (Metropolitan Museum of Art inv. 25.78.63).

and bronze were likewise processed in Capua and then sold at Rome and other locations in Italy.[129] Instruments such as probes, spatulas, spoons, tweezers and even scalpels would have been readily accessible to consumers (see for example the terracotta tomb reliefs of metal-workers that display their shops and wares) (see Figure 3.5), and have frequently been found in domestic contexts.[130] Pottery

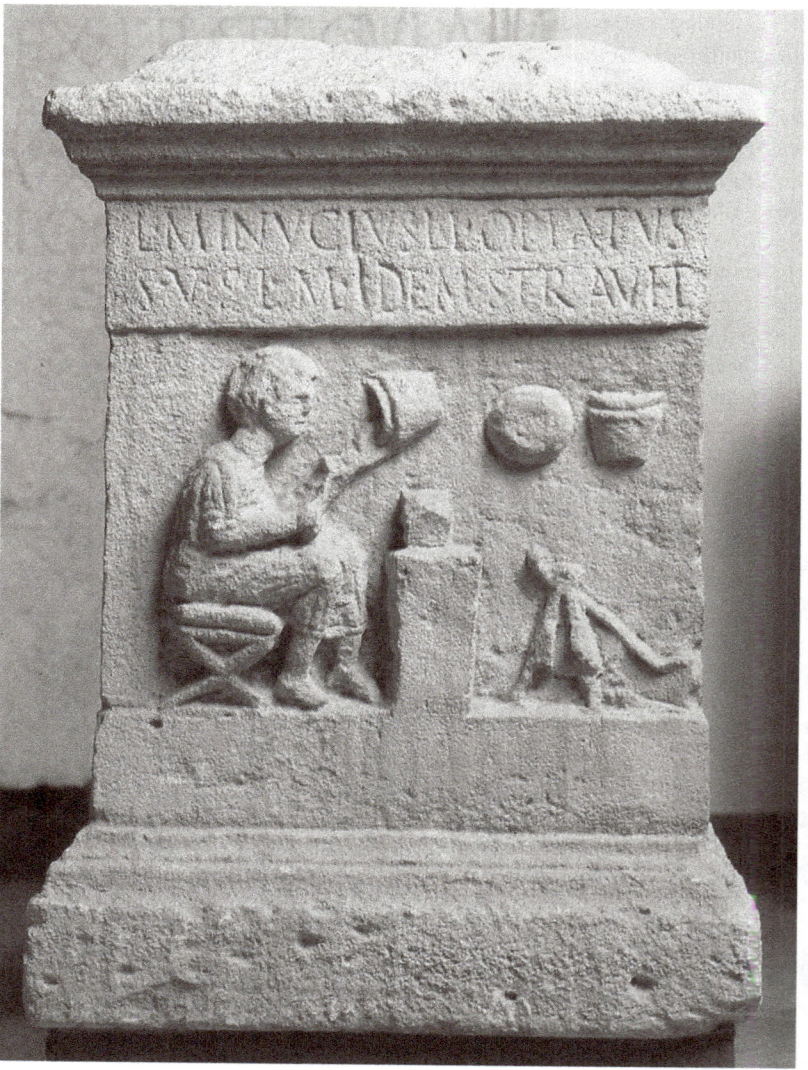

Figure 3.5 A scene from the altar of Lucius Minucius Optatus, dating from the first century CE.

Source: Image courtesy of the Museo Nazionale Atestino di Este, with the permission of the Ministero per i beni e le attività culturali – Polo museale del Veneto.

came from Arretium.[131] While it is questionable whether glass was manufactured at Rome, it was certainly sold there.[132] Inscriptions and reliefs attest numerous individuals employed in these industries, not only as metal-workers, potters, and glass-blowers, but also as sellers and distributors. Excavations have revealed a metal-worker's shop with evidence of medical instrument production at Pompeii.[133] Consumers were in a position to exercise choice over their purchases.[134]

There was also a thriving trade in the vast array of organic materials required for domestic medical practice. While specialists provided certain types of raw materials (literary and documentary evidence attests the existence of seed sellers, resin sellers, cinnamon sellers, frankincense sellers, root cutters, garland sellers, etc.), other individuals working in the medicament industry produced and sold spices, drugs, ointments, unguents, oils, perfumes and incense (see Figure 3.6).[135] Unsurprisingly, Rome's industry is the best attested. During the latter part of the first century CE, the *Horrea Piperataria* was constructed to provide a location for the storage and sale of pepper and spices from Egypt and Arabia, but prior to that there were many smaller sites doing much the same thing.[136] During the late Republic and early Principate, the *Via Sacra* and the *Vicus Tuscus* (subsequently renamed the *Vicus Tuarius*) were where dealers and sellers of these items

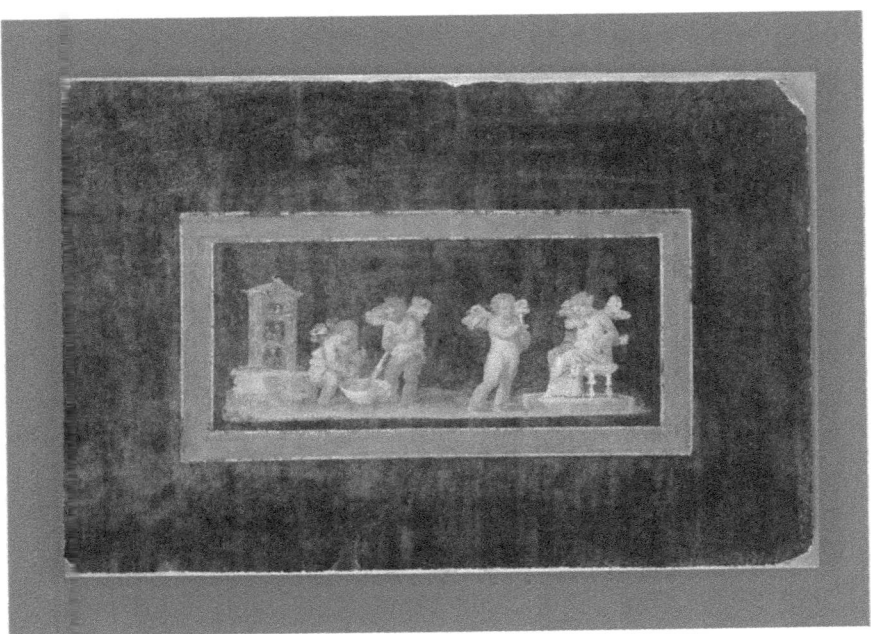

Figure 3.6 A fresco depicting cupids and Psyche making perfume, dating from the first century CE.

Source: Image courtesy of the J. Paul Getty Museum, Open Content Program (J. Paul Getty Museum inv. 72.AG.81).

congregated.[137] Capua was also an influential centre of production and distribution, with the name of the street upon which the trade was centred there giving its name to similar locations in other cities and towns, and the activities of the Faenii attested in Rome, Puteoli, Ischia and as far afield as Lugdunum.[138] Excavations at Pompeii have revealed a commercial nursery with an aromatics shop located next door (see Figure 3.7).[139] Excavations at a site outside Pompeii have revealed what has been interpreted as evidence of the manufacture of Mithridatium on an industrial scale.[140] On occasion, both full and empty containers inscribed with the name of the druggist or the drug have been found, indicating that consumers had the option of seeking out particular 'brands' of medicament.[141]

Who in the household was responsible for the acquisition of foodstuffs, medicaments and other medical paraphernalia such as *instrumentaria*? Depending upon the nature of the household, either the master or the mistress, or the bailiff or the housekeeper, filled these roles, presumably with some level of oversight over necessary expenditure. However, in larger households, slaves, freedmen and freedwomen had particular responsibilities relating to the acquisition of items necessary for the maintenance of health and well-being. Thus, the head herdsman had oversight of the livestock and the related produce, although there might also

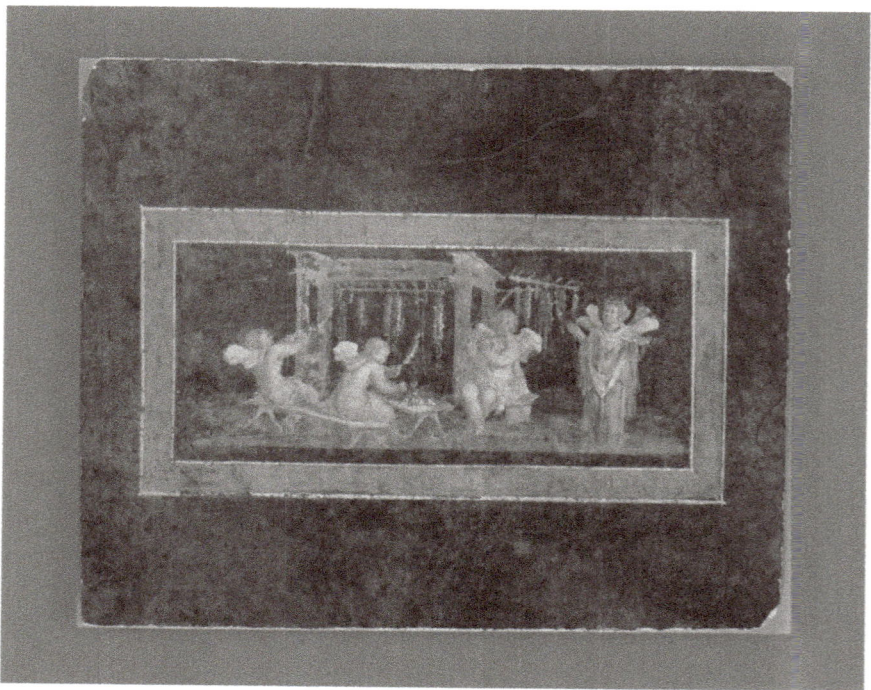

Figure 3.7 A fresco depicting cupids hanging garlands, dating from the first century CE.

Source: Image courtesy of the J. Paul Getty Museum, Open Content Program (J. Paul Getty Museum inv. 72.AG.82).

be shepherds, goat herders and grooms, and so provided the household with meat, dairy products, leather and wool. The gardener maintained the kitchen garden and provided the household with herbs, fruit and vegetables.[142] Other slaves might be responsible for individual purchases, and Plautus offers an insight into this process, presenting a street trader hawking his wares: 'I'm selling Greek sudorific ointments, or other, emollient ones against hangover'.[143] Such items could have been acquired for either communal or individual usage.

Preparation

Once the items necessary for the maintenance of health and well-being had been acquired, it was necessary to prepare them for consumption and usage by the members of the household. A considerable amount of effort went into the preparation of food and drink on a daily basis, even before considerations such as the role that foodstuffs had to play in health and well-being were concerned (see Figure 3.8).[144] Seneca iterates how much work could go in to managing a household's dietary regimen and the necessity of filling a range of sensory and gustatory requirements:

> Think also of the poor purveyors of food, who note their masters' tastes with delicate skill, who know what special flavours will sharpen their appetite, what will please their eyes, what new combinations will rouse their cloyed stomachs, what food will excite their loathing through sheer satiety, and what will stir them to hunger on that particular day.[145]

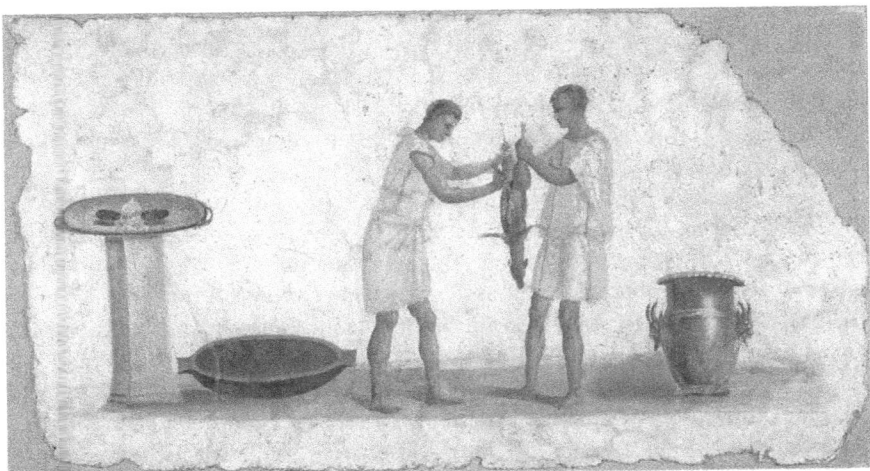

Figure 3.8 A fresco depicting two slaves preparing a meal, dating from the early second century CE.

Source: Image courtesy of the J. Paul Getty Museum, Open Content Program (J. Paul Getty Museum inv. 72.AG.112).

The management of the household's inventory seems to have been the responsibility of the mistress of the house or, in her absence, the housekeeper. Columella describes the responsibilities of the housekeeper in relation to the preparation of food, drink and medicaments in considerable detail.[146] However, in larger households these responsibilities could devolve onto specific individuals. The storekeeper (*cellarius*) maintained the stores of dried goods, relish, oil and wine.[147] The cook (*cocus* or *coquus*) prepared the daily meals. According to Livy, the first cooks arrived in Rome in 189 BCE, either as war booty or luxury purchases, in the wake of Gnaeus Manlius Vulso's campaign in Galatia.[148] Although kitchens were undesirable places and cooks had low reputations, it is likely that they were knowledgeable about the healthy properties of foodstuffs, and that they applied this knowledge as a matter of course either at the instigation of their master or mistress, or on their own initiative.[149] The cook in Plautus' *Pseudolus* describes the beneficial effects of his food in comparison to his peers':

> I don't season dinner the same way as other cooks, who serve up seasoned meadows in their pans, who turn the guests into oxen and present them with herbs and then continue to season those herbs with other herbs: they add sorrel, cabbage, beet, spinach; they put in coriander, fennel, garlic, horse parsley; they pour in a pound of silphium; and they grate wretched mustard, which makes the eyes of those who grate it cry before they've grated it. When these people cook dinners and season them, they don't season them with seasonings but with screech owls to eat up gustes' intestines while they're still alive. That's why people live such short lives here, because they stuff herbs of this type into their bellies, frightening to mention, let alone to eat. Humans eat herbs which farm animals don't eat. . . . You can say so boldly; people who eat the dainties I season can live for even two hundred years each.[150]

While this can be read as Plautus utilising the comic stereotype of the boastful cook, it does offer an example of someone tasked with food preparation passing judgement on the healthful qualities of what they prepare.[151] Trimalchio is extremely appreciative of his cook's skills.[152]

While there is a considerable amount of literary evidence for the enjoyment of food and drink for its own sake, foodstuffs were also prepared with their perceived healthful properties in mind. This was true not only for staples such as grain, wine and oil, but also fruit and vegetables, and even more unusual items such as meat, fish and dairy products. So although the vast majority of foodstuffs were considered to have healthful properties in and of themselves, they could also be prepared in such as way or consumed in such a way as to harness and maximise these healthful properties, either as a means of prevention or one of therapy.

Thus the majority of the recipes that Cato provides for wine have some sort of medicinal purpose, but he does specifically differentiate between what is required to produce wine simply for drinking and what is required to produce a wine for therapy.[153] His hellebore wines can be used as laxatives, his capers or juniper berries wine as a diuretic, his juniper wood wine for gout, his myrtle wine for indigestion, his pomegranate wine for colic and diarrhoea and his fennel and pomegranate wine for indigestion, retention of urine and tapeworms. Horace recommends spikenard in wine as a remedy for depression.[154] Columella states that many people consider wine suitable for the treatment of internal complaints, but that squill wine is particularly good for promoting digestion, invigorating the body and dealing with a troublesome cough, while pennyroyal wine is also good for dealing with coughs, and myrtle wine is good for colic.[155] Must, produced as part of the wine-making process, also had medicinal uses.[156] Columella includes the preservation of fruit and the production of fruit syrup in the duties of the housekeeper.[157] Marcus Gavius Apicius (*circa* early first century CE) recommends a way of keeping grapes fresh and advises that once the grapes are needed the water in which they were stored can be given to the sick as a type of honey water, a recipe for a substitute for salted fish that is recommended for sick stomachs and as an aid to digestion and a recipe for mild aromatic salts that can be used to aid digestion and move the bowels, but also as a preventative measure against a range of illnesses.[158]

The medicaments produced within the household seem to have been primarily concerned with certain aspects of health and well-being, notably digestion and reproduction. Thus, we see a wide range of evidence for the production of remedies for indigestion, as well as assistance to the digestive tract such as purgatives, emetics, laxatives and diuretics. We also see evidence for the regulation of the reproductive capabilities of the members of the household that range from aphrodisiacs for both male and female members of the household, to aids for conception, to treatment for a variety of prenatal and postnatal conditions, as well as aids for contraception and even the procurement of abortions.[159]

The fact that Roman domestic medical practice seems to have been primarily concerned with certain health issues should not come as a surprise if we consider these health issues from a practical point of view. As far as the issues surrounding digestion are concerned, not only was the digestive process a fundamental feature of the maintenance of good health and well-being, but it was also an area where expediency was a factor. It was simply not feasible for an individual to summon a physician every single time that they suffered an attack of indigestion, constipation or diarrhoea. As far as issues surrounding reproduction are concerned, expediency could also be a factor here, particularly in relation to the use of aphrodisiacs and contraceptives.

Members of the household performed roles specifically concerned with the use of medicaments such as oils, unguents and perfumes, and it is probable that these roles required them to undertake a certain amount of preparation of these items.

Provision

As we have seen, there was an expectation that members of the elite should bear a certain amount of responsibility for their own health and well-being. According to Seneca the Younger,

> each man knows best the defects of his own body. And so one relieves his stomach by vomiting, another props it up by frequent eating, another drains and purges his body by periodic fasting. Those whose feet are visited by pain

abstain either from wine or from the bath. In general, men who are careless in other respects go out of their way to relieve the disease which frequently afflicts them.[160]

The master or mistress of the household was ultimately responsible for the health and well-being of its members. Thus, we see the master dealing with his slaves' health problems, such as Charinus recommending Acanthio swallow Egyptian resin dipped in honey for his lungs.[161] While some slave owners seem to have sold or abandoned ailing or elderly slaves, others seem to have maintained them, albeit reluctantly.[162] In larger households there appears to have been a significant amount of infrastructure dedicated to monitoring and maintaining the health and well-being of slaves. Columella states that the bailiff should deal with minor injuries, but that in the case of more serious conditions he should take the sufferer to the infirmary and advise on a course of treatment.[163] The provision of this treatment and the day-to-day running of the infirmary is the responsibility of the housekeeper.[164] There is also evidence for the assault or corporal punishment of slaves, and it is probable that slaves treated thus received some level of care, if only to facilitate their return to their duties.[165]

A range of slaves contributed to the personal care of the free members of the household in relation to their bodies. If a household possessed a bathhouse, it might also possess bath staff or attendants (*balneator, faber balneator*). A barber (*tonsor, tonsatrix*) would cut and style the hair of the male members of the household, while a lady's maid (*ornatrix*) would not only style the hair of the female members of the household but also prepare and apply cosmetics.[166] A number of slaves provided head and body massage using oils (*tractator, tractatrix, unctor, unctrix*), and this could be done with therapeutic benefits in mind (*iatralipte*).[167] Some slaves were tasked with taking care of the oils specifically (*unguentarius, unguentaria*).

A range of slaves contributed to the personal care of the free members of the household in relation to their minds. A reader (*anagnastes*) would read aloud, and a poet (*poeta*) would compose and potentially also read their work, both of which would be particularly appreciated as a distraction from pain or discomfort. Singers and musicians of various types (*cantor, cantrix, citharoedus, musicarius, musicus, symphoniacus*) would sing and play (see Figure 3.9). A philosopher (*philosophus*) could offer an opportunity for education and debate, and Plutarch is particularly effusive regarding the healing powers of philosophical enquiry.[168]

The nurse's responsibilities could extend well beyond maintaining a child while it was young.[169] For nurses that remained with their charges into adulthood, such as those who accompanied their mistresses into a new household upon their marriage, they could serve as a repository of knowledge regarding subjects such as contraception, conception, abortifacients, pregnancy and childbirth. Ovid presents Canace's nurse as being the only person privy to her pregnancy and actively seeking to terminate it:

What herbs and what medicines did my nurse not bring to me, applying them with bold hand to drive forth entirely from my bosom – this was the only

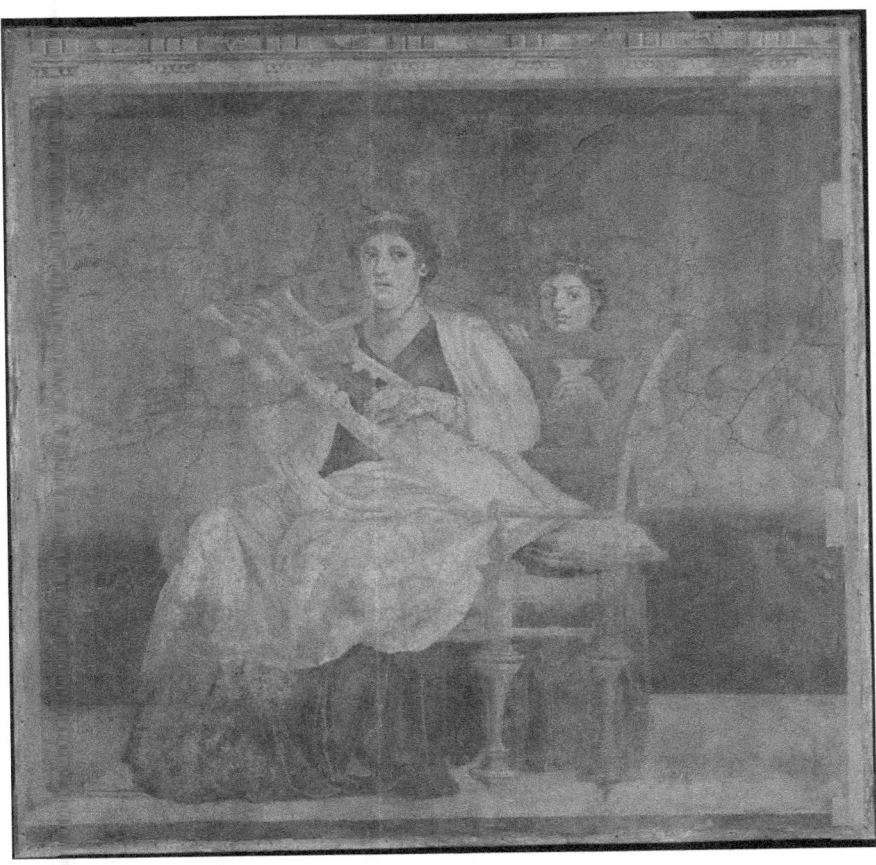

Figure 3.9 A fresco depicting a woman playing a kithara, Villa of Publius Fannius Synistor, Boscoreale, *circa* 50–40 BCE.

Source: Image courtesy of the Metropolitan Museum of Art Open Access (Metropolitan Museum of
Art inv. 03.14.5).

secret we kept from you – the burden that was increasing there? Ah, too full
of life, the little thing withstood the arts employed against it, and was kept
safe from its hidden foe![170]

There is also a significant amount of overlap between the provision of veterinary medicine to the household's livestock and the provision of medicine to the
household's human members.[171]

All servile members of the household had general duties relating to the maintenance of health and well-being as the need arose, and the fact that these are
difficult to separate out from general duties of the Roman slave indicates how

integrated healthcare theory and practice were in the ancient Roman household. Plautus offers a number of examples of slaves simultaneously performing menial domestic tasks and providing a basic level of mental and physical healthcare, such as taking care of someone feeling faint by fetching a chair and some water, recommending medical treatment for grief, and holding someone's head to either prevent them from vomiting or assist them while they do it.[172] In Petronius' *Satyricon*, a slave bandages his master Trimalchio's arm, albeit not to his master's taste by using white wool instead of purple, while Giton administers to Eumolpus by binding the cut on his forehead with cobwebs soaked in oil.[173] Celsus recommends using children or women for massage and rubbing due to their softer touch.[174]

Household resources and Roman domestic religion

The members of the household – freeborn, freed and slave – and their labour were resources that could be utilised in the service of domestic religious belief and practice. While numerous ancient writers state that either the master of the household or his proxy should be the one to lead domestic worship, other members of the household clearly had important roles to play.[175] It was the responsibility of the mistress of the household or her proxy to maintain the hearth and the household shrine, sweeping the hearth every evening in preparation for the following day, and making garlands to hang around it on the *Kalends, Nones, Ides* and other feast days.[176]

There was no single equivalent to the Greek *miasma*, (that is defilement, the impairment of a thing's form or integrity) in the Latin language.[177] There were, however, numerous ways of referring to the act of soiling, staining, fouling, defiling and thus polluting something (*polluere, inquinare, foedare, funestare, scelerare, maculare*, etc.).[178] There were also a variety of ways of referring to dirt itself. These could be both descriptive and thus not necessarily pejorative, such as *lutum* (not only mud and mire, but also the dust sprinkled on wrestlers, or the clay used by potters), *caenum* (dirt, filth, mud, mire) or *spurcitia* (dirt, filth, smut, dung). However, they could also be more loaded, such as *sordes* (not just dirt and filth, but also uncleanness, squalor) or *illuvies* (dirt, filth, uncleanness of the body). What of cleanliness and being clean, both physically and metaphysically? *Lotus* referred to the process of washing or bathing and the state of physical cleanliness that resulted from it, while *mundus* signified cleanliness in the sense of niceness, neatness and elegance.[179] Purity, however, was another matter. *Purus* signalled that someone was free from dirt in the sense of being clean and pure, while *castus* indicated that someone was morally pure, unpolluted and guiltless, particularly with regard to matters of sexual propriety and impropriety. Yet Romans prioritised looking and feeling clean and tidy.[180] Consequently, a particularly elegant or distinguished Roman would often be labelled *lautus* (well-washed), his toga *candidus* (shining white, clear, bright).[181] This carefully cultivated image, the result of *cultus* (labour, care, cultivation and, above all, culture) would ideally only be deviated from at certain times on specific occasions where the contrast would be most apparent, such as during the mourning period.

It was not just the personal cleanliness and tidiness of the individual that was considered a priority, but also that of their home. The agricultural treatises of Cato, Varro and Columella advise that for an estate to be successful it needs to be organised, orderly and above all clean.[182] Cicero's invective against Piso incorporates criticism of the state of his household: 'The table piled not with shellfish or fish, but with huge joints of tainted meat; slatternly slaves do the waiting, some even old men; cook and hall-porter are one; neither breadmaker nor wine-cellar on the premises; the bread from a bakehouse, the wine from a tavern'.[183] Slovenly housekeeping was considered inexcusable, leading Horace to exclaim 'Common brooms, napkins, and sawdust, how little do they cost! But if neglected, how shocking is the scandal! To think of your sweeping mosaic pavements with a dirty palm-broom, or putting unwashed coverlets over Tyrian tapestries'.[184] Just as there was a moral dimension to keeping your person clean and tidy, so there was to keeping your home clean and tidy. Juvenal's fourteenth satire, the subject of which is the bad example that parents can set their children, devotes a lengthy section to the importance of having a clean and tidy home at all times:

When a guest is expected, none of your household will get a break. 'Sweep the marble floor! Polish the columns till they shine! Get that dried-up spider along with all her web. One of you wipe the plain silver, and you, the embossed vases!' The master's voice rages as he stands over them, holding the rod. You get terribly anxious in case your friend, when he comes, is offended by the sight of your reception room fouled with dog turds or the colonnade splashed with mud, when one little slave boy equipped with just a half bucket of sawdust can put this right; and yet you don't make any effort to ensure that your son sees a home that's pure and completely flawless, and without reproach?[185]

Both Horace and Juvenal emphasise how simple a clean and tidy home is to accomplish, making a failure to do so all the more reprehensible. They also indicate that there is more at stake than just neatness. Horace is concerned that expensive, luxurious possessions be treated with the appropriate care, going so far as to call it *flagitium* (a shameful act or disgraceful thing) if they are not, while Juvenal is keen to ensure that the home is *sancio* (made sacred, rendered inviolable) and *sine labe* (not only without blemish, but also without stigma, or without disgrace). This relationship between cleanliness and sanctity is particularly significant when the ubiquity of domestic religious practice is taken into account.

Different members of the household played complementary roles in domestic religious activity.[186] Even children contributed, at least in part, to prepare them for the time when they would be adults and responsible for their own domestic religious activity.[187] Garlands were hung, incense was burned, a variety of different types of food and drink such as spelt, grain, fruit and wine were offered and on occasion animals such as cows, sheep and pigs were sacrificed. When first excavated a number of household shrines from Pompeii and Herculaneum were found to have the remnants of offerings still on them. Literary evidence suggests that particularly devout individuals worshipped their household gods daily; in Plautus' *The Pot of Gold*, the *Lar* makes a point of commenting on the daughter of the household's daily devotions, comparing and contrasting her favourably with her neglectful father, although the circumstances are such (she is unmarried, pregnant and desperate) that this could be an aberration.[188] Pliny the Elder comments on the practice of offering any food that is dropped on the floor during dinner to the household gods, and depending upon the skill or care with which food was served and consumed, this could have occurred infrequently or frequently.[189]

Foodstuffs

One final thing to consider regarding the relationship between Roman domestic religious belief and practice and Roman domestic healthcare theory, method and practice is the use of the household's resources to worship the household gods, thus using the household resources of the present, those same resources that were utilised in household healthcare practice, to perpetuate the household's prosperity and ensure the household resources of the future. While the household gods all seem to have been associated and concerned with the family's health and well-being in very particular ways, a focus on the acquisition, storage and preparation of food is a recurring theme.[190] Consider the connection between food and drink and health and well-being, and the concept and importance of regimen for both healthy and unhealthy individuals, at all stages of their lives. The Roman agricultural treatises tell us exactly what was supposed to be produced on the estate and kept in the storeroom and the purposes to which these items were supposed to be put by specific members of the household, such as the housekeeper, which included use in a range of medicaments. There are clear connections being made between domestic religious practice, food and drink, and health and well-being within ancient Roman households.

Cato includes instructions on how to undertake a range of domestic festivals utilising items produced onsite. In order to make a dedication to ensure the health of oxen, one must offer emmer, fat, lean meat and wine to Mars and Silvanus.[191] On another feast day dedicated to oxen, one must offer wine and roast meat from either a herd or a flock to Jupiter and Vesta.[192] Prior to harvesting, one must offer a female piglet to Ceres, incense and wine to Janus, Jupiter and Juno.[193] He provides recipes for a number of different sacred cakes, and it is a logical assumption that the ingredients required were sourced from the agricultural estate and the cakes were baked by a member of the household, in all probability the housekeeper.[194] Poems written in honour of the god Priapus suggest that household produce was utilised for the purposes of making offerings to him, and these offerings changed according to the time of year. Flowers grown in the garden were used to create garlands, which were probably made by the female members of the household.[195] Although painted garlands are found on many household shrines, some also include hooks indicating where the real garlands were hung.

In Pompeii and Herculaneum, more household shrines have been found to be located in kitchens than in any other room, and consequently domestic religious practice seems to have been related more closely to the storage and preparation of food than to the eating of it.[196] In a handful of houses, these connections are made explicit in the form of the wall paintings that accompany the household shrines located in kitchens.[197] The House of Aufidius Primus (I.x.18), the House of Sutoria Primigenia (I.xiii.2), the House of Pansa (VI.vi.1), the House of Octavius Primus (VII.xv.12), the House of the Pork (IX.ix.3) and Villa 6 at Terzigno all include depictions of foodstuffs, particularly pork and fish, in prominent positions around the household shrine. What is the significance of all these animal products, and why were they included alongside the more standard images of the household deities? Considering that the paintings are thought to have served religious purposes, providing a place of worship for the slave members of the households in which they appear, it is possible that the reason for including these particular products was likewise religious.

Alternatively, we could interpret these paintings as having some sort of economic symbolism, as there are certainly examples of Pompeian household shrines referring to the business interests of the household and *familia*, such as that in the House of the Sarno Lararium (I. xiv.7) which depicts scenes of work taking place on the River Sarno.[198] If we consider the contents of the paintings in this light it becomes appropriate to consider the position of these foodstuffs, particularly pork and fish, in the Roman diet, whether consumed during the course of a religious ritual, or otherwise. Pork was the most common sort of meat consumed in Roman Italy, eaten by the rich and the poor alike, and while fish is harder to pin down as far as levels of consumption are concerned, since Campania was a significant centre for the production of pigs and pork products, and Pompeii in particular was an important centre for the production of salt-fish products, it is likely that both foodstuffs were readily available to the residents of these six houses, whether fresh or processed and preserved.[199] While some pork and fish products could be consumed fresh, for the most part they were preserved and stored, ensuring provisions for the future.

Conclusion

Concerns over the maintenance of health and well-being were integral to the Roman household and each member of the household had a specific part to play. It would appear that there were duties regarding domestic healthcare and depending upon the nature of the individual household these were undertaken by specific members. In order to be successful, a household needed to be in possession of the resources necessary in order to undertake extensive healthcare practice, and this included not only purchased or produced medicaments, but also equipment such as medical instruments, containers, cloth, food and drink. Collectively, the Roman household contained the resources necessary to provide a high level of expertise regarding the maintenance of health and well-being.

Having examined the members of the household who were responsible for domestic medical practice, and the means by which they did so, now we shall turn to exploring their knowledge, skills and expertise, and the ways in which these were acquired.

Notes

1   *CIL* XI 600 (trans J. F. Gardner and T. Wiedemann): *C. Castricius T. f Calvus trib(unus) [mil(itum) leg(ionis) . . .] Stellatina [Agr]icola, bonoru[m libertorum] benevolus [patronus] maxsimeque eorum, qui agros bene [et strenue coolant, qui] corporis cultus, quod maxime opus est [agricolis, curam gerant], qui se alant, cetera quaequomque habe[nt tueantur]. Praecepta vera, qui volt ver[e] bene et libere v[ivere], haec habeto:] Primum est pium esse: [domino bene] cupias, ver[ere parentes, . . . f]idem bonam [praestes, . . . noli maledicere ne male] audias. Inn[ocens et fidus qui erit,] suavem vitam [et offense carentum] hon[este l]ae[teque] peraget. Haec non a d[octeis vireis institutus, sed n]atura sua e[t us]u Agricola meminisse docet vos. L. Castricio L(uci) C(ai) l(iberto) . . . ob merita quod eius mortem dolui et fu[nus feci et locum dedi, ide]mque monumentum hoc ei feci, ut cu[rent omnes liberti fidem pr]aestare patroneis; item Ca]striciae C(ai) l(ibertae) Helenae, quod et [ipsa pia fuit].*
2   For discussion, see Chapter 1, Health and Well-being in the Roman Republic and Principate.
3   For further discussion of this, see Chapter 4, The Transmission of Medical Knowledge.
4   The bibliography is vast, but for key works see Rawson, 1986, 1991; Bradley, 1991; Kertzer and Saller, 1991; Dixon, 1992; Rawson, 1992; Rawson and Weaver, 1997; Saller, 1994; Dixon, 2001; George, 2005; Dasen and Späth, 2010; Rawson, 2011; Laurence and Strömberg, 2012.
5   Allison, 2007, p. 345.
6   Gardner, 1998, p. 268.
7   See for example Sallust, *Civil War* 10–13, 25; Horace, *Odes* 3.6, 24; Appian, *Civil War* 4.13. Aspects of this are discussed in Severy, 2003; Milnor, 2005.
8   See for example Livy, *From the Founding of the City* preface 8–9; Dionysius of Halicarnassus, *Roman Antiquities* 2.24–26.1; Valerius Maximus, *Memorable Deeds and Sayings* 4.4.8–9; Seneca the Younger, *Moral Epistles* 87.41; Juvenal, *Satires* 6.286–351. See Dixon, 1991 for discussion of the creation of a sentimental ideal of the Roman family.
9   Dixon, 1991, 1997, p. 152.
10 Lefebvre, 1991, p. 49; McDonnell, 2006 on masculine *virtus*; Olson, 2017 on masculine dress.
11 Allison, 2015, p. 117.
12 Berry, 1997, p. 183; Allison, 2013.
13 Berry, 1997, p. 183; Allison, 2004.
14 Berry, 1997, p. 185.
15 Berry, 1997, p. 194; Dickmann, 2011.
16 Gardner, 1998, p. 1 notes the contrast between the universal and unchanging legal construct of the *familia* and actual family groups.
17 Saller, 1984, p. 337, 1994, p. 74.
18 *OLD* s.v. *domus*; *OLD* s.v. *familia*.
19 For further discussion of the different types of Roman residence and their role in the acquisition and maintenance of health and well-being, see Chapter 2, The Roman House and Garden.
20 *Digest* 50.16.195.1–4.
21 Saller, 1984, p. 337, p. 351; see also Cooper, 2007 for discussion of this change of emphasis over a longer period of time into Late Antiquity.
22 For discussion of the evidence for the ancient Roman nuclear family, see Saller and Shaw, 1984.
23 Bradley, 1991, p. 143.
24 Treggiari, 1991, p. 412.
25 Dixon, 1992, p. 160; for reservations about the ability to identify changes to the family over time see Saller, 1994, p. 4.

26 Imperial: Treggiari, 1975b; senatorial elite: Bradley, 1991; lower classes: Rawson, 1966; military: Allison, 2011; slaves: Treggiari, 1975a.
27 See for example Treggiari, 1975a, 1975b.
28 See for example Livy, *From the Founding of the City* preface 8–9; Valerius Maximus, *Memorable Deeds and Sayings* 4.4.8–9; Juvenal, *Satires* 6.286–351; Seneca the Younger, *Moral Epistles* 87.41. For discussion see Dixon, 1992, p. 13.
29 Saller, 1999, p. 184.
30 On *Patria Potestas*, see Crook, 1967.
31 *Digest* 1.6.4, 32.50.1.
32 Dionysius of Halicarnassus, *Roman Antiquities* 2.26–27; *Sextus Empiricus* 3.211; Aulus Gellius, *Attic Nights* 5.19; *Digest* 82.2.11.
33 Saller, 1994, p. 2, p. 102.
34 Saller, 1987, 1994.
35 See for example Cicero, *In Defence of Cluentius* 32; Quintilian, *Institutes of Oratory* 8.4.11; *Digest* 48.19.39.
36 Cicero, *Laws* 3.8.19; Gardner, 1998, pp. 121–123.
37 Harris, 1986; Shaw, 2001 for discussion of the *tollere liberos* ritual.
38 Albutt, 1921, p. 24.
39 Pliny the Elder, *Natural History* 29.8.15; Plutarch, *Cato the Elder* 23.4; Bradley, 2005, pp. 71–72; Draycott, 2016.
40 Plutarch, *Cato the Elder* 20.2–4.
41 This will be discussed further later in this chapter; see also Chapter 4, The Transmission of Medical Knowledge.
42 Dixon, 1992, pp. 41–42, p. 76.
43 Plutarch, *Cato the Elder* 24.1–2.
44 Perkin, 1997, p. 144; Huebner and Ratzan, 2009.
45 See for example Valerius Maximus, *Memorable Deeds and Sayings* 8.6.1.
46 See for example the Aelii Tuberones: Valerius Maximus, *Memorable Deeds and Sayings* 4.4.8 and Plutarch, *Aemilius Paullus* 5.6, 22.9; the Licinii Crassi: Plutarch, *Crassus* 1; the Claudii Pulchri: Varro, *On Agriculture* 3.16.2. Are these simply stories of 'virtuous poverty'? See Gardner, 1998, p. 70.
47 On the role of the *pater familias* and the *consilium* in regulating the behaviour of family members, see Perry, 2015.
48 See for example Marcus Caelius Rufus: Cicero, *In Defence of Caelius* 7.17–18; Seneca the Younger, *On Clemency* 1.15.2–7.
49 Gardner, 1995, p. 378; Saller, 1999, p. 187.
50 For female estate owners, see for example Varro's wife Fundania: Varro, *On Agriculture* 1.2; Valeria Maxima *CIL* VI 3484 = *ILS* 7459. For female heads of household, see Carlsen, 2011. For freeborn or freed slave females in family groups with slave males, see Flory, 1984.
51 On Roman marriage, see Treggiari, 1991; Dixon, 2011; on the Roman wedding, see Hersch, 2010; Larsson Lovén and Strömberg, 2009.
52 Cicero, *In Defence of Flaccus* 84.
53 *Twelve Tables* 6.2; Gaius 1.111; Aulus Gellius, *Attic Nights* 3.2.12–13; Macrobius, *Saturnalia* 1.3.9.
54 Treggiari, 1991, p. 21.
55 *Digest* 1.112; Pliny the Elder, *Natural History* 18.10; Festus, *Latin Glossary* 78 L.
56 *Digest* 1.113–114.
57 *Digest* 50.16.195.2.
58 Cicero, *Topica* 14; Aulus Gellius, *Attic Nights* 18.6.8–9.
59 See Saller, 1987 on male age at marriage; see Shaw, 1987 on female age at marriage; see Harlow and Laurence, 2002, pp. 79–103 on marriage and the life course; see Shelton, 1990 for a case study of Pliny the Younger and Calpurnia's asymmetric marriage. See Dixon, 1988 on the Roman mother.

60 Xenophon, *On Estate Management* 7.3.
61 Pliny the Elder, *Natural History* 28.135, 142; Hersch, 2010, pp. 177–180.
62 Plautus, *The Braggart Soldier* 193–194; Columella, *On Agriculture* 12 preface 10.
63 Livy, *From the Founding of Rome* 1.41.1; Pliny the Younger, *Letters* 8.18; Apuleius, *Metamorphosis* 5.10.
64 Apuleius, *Metamorphosis* 5.10 (trans. A. S. Kline): *Suscipta alia: 'Ego vero maritum articulari etiam morbo complicatum curvatumque ac per hoc rarissimo Venerem meam recolentum sustineo, plerumque detortos et duratos in lapidem digitos eius perfricans, fomentis olidis et pannis sordidis et foetidis cataplasmatibus manus tam delicatas istas adurens, nec uxoris officiosam faciem, sed medicae laboriosam personam sustinens'.*
65 McCreight, 2006; Langslow, 2000.
66 See for example Columella, *On Agriculture* 12 preface 9. However, see also Suetonius, *Divine Augustus* 73.1 for claims that the women of Augustus' household made his clothes.
67 Cassius Dio, *Roman History* 56.3.3–5 (trans. E. Cary): πῶς μὲν γὰρ οὐκ ἄριστον γυνὴ σώφρων οἰκουρὸς οἰκονόμος παιδοτρόφος ὑγιαίνοντά τε εὐφρᾶναι καὶ ἀσθενοῦντα θεραπεῦσαι, εὐτυχοῦντί τε συγγενέσθαι καὶ δυστυχοῦντα παραμυθήσασθαι, τοῦ τε νέου τὴν ἐμμανῆ φύσιν καθεῖρξαι καὶ τοῦ πρεσβυτέρου τὴν ἔξωρον 4αὐστηρότητα κεράσαι;
68 See for example Plautus, *Captives* 889; Suetonius, *Divine Julius Caesar* 52.3; Aulus Gellius, *Attic Nights* 17.21.44.
69 Israelowich, 2015, pp. 71–86. On the health of infants and children, see for example Garnsey, 1991; Bradley, 2005; Gourevitch, 2010; Graham and Carroll, 2012.
70 On pregnancy and childbirth, see Israelowich, 2015. On infants and children, see Dasen, 2004.
71 Seneca the Younger, *Moral Epistles* 47.14 (trans. R. M. Gumere): *Domum pusillam rem publicam esse iudicaverunt*; Pliny the Younger, *Letters* 8.16.2 (trans. B. Radice): *nam servis res publica quaedam et quasi civitas domus est.*
72 See for example the case of Baucis and Philemon in Ovid, *Metamorphoses* 8.630.
73 Saller, 2011, p. 120.
74 On the *Vilicus*, see Carlsen, 1995; on the *Vilica*, see Carlsen, 1993; Roth, 2004.
75 For further discussion of this, see Chapter 4, The Transmission of Medical Knowledge.
76 Roller, 2001, p. 6.
77 Bradley, 1994, p. 66.
78 *Digest* 50.15.4.5, 32.65.1.
79 Petronius, *Satyricon* 28.8, 34.3.
80 Saller, 2011, p. 116; see previously, 2003.
81 Cooper, 2007.
82 See for example Seneca the Younger, *Moral Epistles* 96 for one household's downward spiral.
83 See for example the case of Pliny the Younger's wife who miscarried due to ignorance, Pliny the Younger, *Letters* 8.10 and 8.11.
84 Reay, 2005, p. 335; Blake, 2012 goes as far as referring to slaves as 'prosthetics'; Joshel and Peterson, 2014, pp. 164–165.
85 Treggiari, 1975b, 1976; Joshel, 1992.
86 Allison, 1997, 2004; Berry, 1997, 2007
87 Cato the Elder, *On Agriculture* 56–58; Varro, *On Agriculture* 1.63; Columella, *On Agriculture* 2.9.16, 12.52.18, 12.52.21; Pliny the Elder, *Natural History* 14.35–36, 18.87, 18.90; Suetonius, *Galba* 7.2; Apuleius, *Metamorphosis* 6.11, 6.20; *Digest* 15.3.3.1, 15.3.3.7, 33.7.12 preface, 33.7.18.3.
88 Caesar's physician: Suetonius, *Divine Julius Caesar* 42; Crassus' physician: Cicero, *On Oratory* 1.62; Verres' physician: Cicero, *Verrine Orations* 3.83; Octavian: Suetonius, *Divine Augustus* 59 and Cassius Dio, *Roman History* 53.30; Piso's physician: Cicero, *On the Responses of the Haruspices* 35, *Against Piso* 83; Cato the Younger's physician: Plutarch, *Cato the Younger* 70.2.

89 Treggiari, 1975b; Hasegawa, 2005.
90 On Livia's interest in health and well-being, see Barrett, 2002, pp. 108–112.
91 Baiquez, 1994, pp. 78–96.
92 See for example the probable freedman Aulus Pumponius Magonianus at VIII. ii.10–12.
93 See for example Apuleius, *Metamorphosis* 10.8–11 in which a physician is commissioned to prepare a medicament.
94 Varro, *On Agriculture* 1.16.4.
95 Alexio: Cicero, *Letters to Atticus* 377.1 (XV.1.1); Metrodorus: Cicero, *Letters to Atticus* 378.2 (XV.1a.2); Unnamed at Cumae: Cicero, *Letters to Friends* 41.2 (XVI.14.2); Asclapo: Cicero, *Letters to Friends* 123 (XVI.4), 124 (XVI.5), 127 (XVI.9), 286 (XIII.20).
96 See for example the case of Cicero engaging Marcus Curius in conjunction with Asclapo to treat his slave Tiro, Cicero, *Letters to Atticus* 125.3 (VII.2.3), 126.12 (VII.3.12), 186.2 (IX.17.2).
97 Varro, *On Agriculture* 1.22.1.
98 On Cato: Pliny the Elder, *Natural History* 29.8.15 and Plutarch, *Cato the Elder* 23.4. Varro, *On Agriculture* 2.1.21–23. See also Varro's inclusion of the example of a stabbing requiring the treatment of a physician, *On Agriculture* 1.69.3.
99 For female physicians in the Roman Republic and Empire, see Flemming, 2000, pp. 383–392; Parker, 1997.
100 Criticism of physicians in historical treatises: Livy, *From the Founding of the City* 40.56.11, 42.47.6; Tacitus, *Annals* 12.67.2; Tacitus, *Agricola* 43.2; SHA *The Three Gordians* 28.5. Criticism of physicians in scientific treatises: Pliny the Elder, *Natural History* 29; Aulus Gellius, *Attic Nights* 18.10. For discussion, see Amundsen, 1974, p. 320.
101 Cato the Elder, *On Agriculture* 5.2; 5.5.
102 Cato the Elder, *On Agriculture* 56; 57; 58.
103 Cato the Elder, *On Agriculture* 2. While this could be interpreted as an example of parsimoniousness, it could also be the result of Cato's belief in altering regimen as a therapeutic strategy, see Plutarch, *Cato the Elder* 23.4.
104 Varro, *On Agriculture* 3.17.8.
105 Varro, *On Agriculture* 1.17. On treating slaves well as 'slave manipulation', see Bradley, 1987, p. 21. On 'slave manipulation' as a means of maintaining social and economic order, see Bradley, 1987, p. 51.
106 Columella, *On Agriculture* 11.1.18; 12.1.6.
107 Selling old or sick slaves: Cato the Elder, *On Agriculture* 2.7. Abandoning old or sick slaves: Suetonius, *Divine Claudius* 25.2. Opprobrium: Plutarch, *Cato the Elder* 4.5; 5.1.
108 Caring: see for example the case of Seneca's wife's blind clown, Harpaste, Seneca the Younger, *Moral Epistles* 1.50. Assigning other duties: see for example the case of Seneca's former playmate, Felicio, reassigned as a door porter, Seneca the Younger, *Moral Epistles* 12.3.
109 Varro, *On Agriculture* 2.10; Horace, *Epistles* 1.14.
110 Joshel, 1992, p. 87.
111 Columella, *On Agriculture* 1 preface 13–18.
112 Martial, *Epigrams* 3.58.
113 See Blake, 2016, p. 96 for discussion of Pliny the Younger's presentation of himself as a caring master who considers the health and well-being of his slaves, simultaneously connecting himself with and separating himself from certain of his peers.
114 Holleran, 2012, p. 248.
115 Ovid, *Art of Love* 2.263–266; Martial, *Epigrams* 7.31.
116 Cato the Elder, *On Agriculture* 1.7.
117 Varro, *On Agriculture* 3.
118 On gathering wild plants, see Frayn, 1979. On Roman hunting, see Grattius, *The Chase*; Appian, *On Hunting*.

119 Varro, *On Agriculture* 1.22.1.
120 Cato the Elder, *On Agriculture* 8.2; Varro, *On Agriculture* 1.23.4.
121 Cato the Elder, *On Agriculture* 135.
122 Cato the Elder, *On Agriculture* 8.2; Varro, *On Agriculture* 1.23.4.
123 Holleran, 2012; Frayn, 1993.
124 See for example Martial, *Epigrams* 7.30, 7.49 for bailiffs and tenants sending produce to their owners and landlords.
125 Cicero, *Against Piso* 67.
126 Holleran, 2012.
127 Cova, 2013.
128 Pliny the Elder, *Natural History* 34.41; see Petronius, *Satyricon* 70 for Trimalchio gifting his cook with a set of knives made from Noricum steel; sales depot in Rome: *CIL* VI 250.
129 Pliny the Elder, *Natural History* 34.20; see inscriptions found on copper and bronze utensils attesting origins: *CIL* XV 7074–7105.
130 Bliquez, 1994.
131 Martial, *Epigrams* 14.98; Pliny the Elder, *Natural History* 35.46; see inscriptions found on pottery attesting origins: *CIL* XV 4925–6063.
132 Strabo, *Geography* 16.2.25.
133 Bliquez, 1994, pp. 83–84; for an overview of the design and manufacture of medical instruments, see Bliquez, 2015, pp. 14–20.
134 Holleran, 2012.
135 On drugs and the drug trade in antiquity, see Nutton, 1985. On occupations within the drug industry, see Totelin, 2016; Korpela, 1995.
136 Cassius Dio, *Roman History* 72.24 claims that Domitian was responsible, although it is possible that Vespasian constructed the *Horrea* and Domitian simply dedicated it.
137 See *CIL* VI 1974 for Marcus Poblicius Nicanor; Horace, *Epodes* 2.1.269–270.
138 Pliny the Elder, *Natural History* 21.16–17; on the Faenii, see *CIL* VI 5680, 9932, 9998 and X 1962, 6802.
139 Jashemski, 1979a.
140 Ciaraldi, 2000.
141 See for example an anti-aging preparation marketed as 'bloom of youth', at Smith, 1992.
142 Plautus, *Three Coin Day* 2.4.7, *The Braggart Soldier* 2.2.38; Varro, *On the Latin Language* 6; Cicero, *Letters to Friends* 16.18.2; Horace, *Epodes* 1.18.36; Columella, *On Agriculture* 10.229, 11.1.2.
143 Plautus, *Stichus* 226–227 (trans. W. De Melo): *Uel unctiones Graecas sudatorias uendo uel alias malacas, crapularias*; see also *Three Coin Day* 406–410 for an indication of how ruinously expensive such items could be.
144 Roth, 2007 on the sheer labour intensiveness of providing food in a pre-industrial society.
145 Seneca the Younger, *Moral Epistles* 47.8 (trans. R. M. Gummere): *Adice obsonatores, quibus dominici palate notitia subtilis est, qui sciunt, cuius illum rei sapor excitet, cuius delectet aspectus, cuius novitiate nauseabundus erigi posit, quid iam ipsa satietate fastidiat, quid illo die esuriat.*
146 Columella, *On Agriculture* 2.2.1. See also Martial, *Epigrams* 1.55, 10.48
147 Plautus, *The Braggart Soldier* 3.2.31 and *The Captives* 4.2.115; Columella, *On Agriculture* 11.1.19, 12.39 and 12.4.2; Pliny the Elder, *Natural History* 19.12.62, 188.
148 Livy, *From the Founding of the City* 38.27, 39.6.
149 See Cicero, *On Duties* 1.150–151. For possible reasons as to why cooks were undesirable, see for example Martial, *Epigrams* 10.66 for a wine-pourer promoted to cook who now has a face blackened with soot and hair that smells of grease; Green, 2015 discusses the physical toll that cooking could take on a slave's body.
150 Plautus, *Pseudolus* 811–830 (trans. W. De Melo): *Non ego item cenam condio ut alii coqui, qui mihi condita prata in patinis proferunt, boues qui conuiuas faciunt herbasque oggerunt, eas herbas herbis aliis porro condiunt: Apponunt rumicem,*

brassicam, betam, blitum, indunt coriandrum, feniculum, alium, atrum holus, eo laserpici libram pondo diluont, teritur sinapis scelera, quae illis qui terunt prius quam triuerunt oculi ut exstillent facit. ei homines cenas ubi coquont, quom condiunt, non condimentis condiunt, sed strigibus, uiuis conuiuis intestina quae exedint. hoc hic quidem homines tam breuem uitam colunt, quom hasce herbas huius modi in suom aluom congerunt, formidolosas dictu, non esu modo. quas herbas pecudes non edunt, homines edunt . . . audacter dicito; nam uel ducenos annos poterunt uiuere meas qui esitabunt escas quas condiuero.

151 See Wilkins, 2000 on the boastful cook of Greek comedy; see also Lowe, 1985 on cooks in Plautine comedy.
152 Petronius, *Satyricon* 2.70.12.
153 Cato the Elder, *On Agriculture* 114, 115, 122, 123, 126, 127.
154 Horace, *Odes* 4.12.16–20.
155 Columella, *On Agriculture* 12.32, 33, 35, 38.
156 Columella, *On Agriculture* 12.36; Dioscorides, *On Medical Materials* 5.5; Pliny the Elder, *Natural History* 12.131, 23.7.
157 Columella, *On Agriculture* 12.10.5, 12.42.1.
158 Apicius, *The Art of Cooking* 1.12.1, see also his recipes for oxygarum to promote digestion at 1.20; Apicius, *The Art of Cooking* 9.13.3, and on the medicinal uses of salted fish, see Curtis, 1991; Apicius, *The Art of Cooking* 1.13.
159 Riddle, 1992.
160 Seneca the Younger, *Moral Epistles* 1.68 (trans. R. M. Gummere): *Nota habet sui quisque corporis vitia. Itaque alius vomitu levat stomachum, alius frequenti cibo fulcit, alius interposito ieiunio corpus exhaurit et purgat. Ii, quorum pedes dolor repetit, aut vino aut balineo abstinent. In cetera neglegentes huic, a quo saepe infestantur, occurrunt.*
161 Plautus, *Merchant* 138–139, 144–146. See also Pliny the Elder and Plutarch on Cato the Elder.
162 Seneca the Younger, *Moral Epistles* 1.50.
163 Columella, *On Agriculture* 11.1.8.
164 Columella, *On Agriculture* 12.1.6, 12.3.7–8.
165 See for example Ovid, *Art of Love* 3.235–244; Ovid, *Amores* 1.14.12–18; Martial, *Epigrams* 8.23; Juvenal, *Satires* 6.487–495; Seneca the Younger, Moral *Epistles* 47.2–5. On the laws pertaining to the punishment of slaves, see Watson, 1987, pp. 115–133.
166 See Olson 2008, 2009 on Roman female adornment, but 2012 on Roman male adornment.
167 Seneca the Younger, *Moral Epistles* 66.52; Martial, *Epigrams* 3.82.13.
168 Plutarch, *The Education of Children* 10.
169 Bradley, 1986.
170 Ovid, *Heroides* 11.39–44: *Quas mihi non herbas, quae non medicamina nutrix attulit audaci supposuitque manu, ut penitus nostris – hoc te celavimus unum – visceribus crescens excuteretur onus? A, nimium vivax admotis restitit infans artibus et tecto tutus ab hoste fuit!* See also Juvenal, *Satires* 6.594–597.
171 Cato the Elder, *On Agriculture* 70, 71, 73, 96, 102, 103; Varro, *On Agriculture* 2 1.21–23, 2.2.20, 2.3.8, 2.5.18, 2.7.16, 2.10.10; Columella, *On Agriculture* 6 (on oxen), 7 (on sheep, goats, pigs and dogs); Grattius, *The Chase* 344–346, 354–358, 351–365, 392–395, 413–419, 473–476.
172 Plautus, *Weevil* 312–313, *Merchant* 140, *Rope* 510.
173 Petronius, *Satyricon* 15.54, 98.
174 Celsus, *On Medicine* 3.21.11.
175 Cato the Elder, *On Agriculture* 143.1, 5.3; Columella, *On Agriculture* 1.8.5.
176 Cato the Elder, *On Agriculture* 143.2; Flower, 2017, pp. 40–45.
177 On *miasma* in ancient Greek religion, see Parker, 1983; on pollution and purity in ancient Greek religion, see Bendlin, 2007; on pollution in Roman religion, see Lennon, 2014.

178 Lennon, 2014; on pollution in ancient Rome, see also Bradley and Stow, 2012; Bradley, 2012; Lennon, 2012; on pollution more generally, and the argument that dirt is simply matter out of place, see Douglas, 1966.
179 See Yegül, 1992; Fagan, 1999a on baths and bathing; see Bradley, 2002 on *fullonica* and laundry.
180 DeLaine, 1999, p. 13.
181 According to Seneca the Younger, *The Pumpkinification of Claudius* 13.2, a freshly bathed man both looked and felt radiant; see Bradley, 2002, p. 23 for discussion of the important role that clean clothes played in this presentation.
182 See for example Cato the Elder, *On Agriculture* 2.3–4, 39.1, 39.2, 141, 143.2; Varro, *On Agriculture* 3.5.2; Columella, *On Agriculture* 11.2.27, 11.2.82–83, 12.P. 4, 12.3.8–9, 12.18.3.
183 Cicero, *Against Piso* 67 (trans. N. H. Watts): *Exstructa mensa non conchyliis aut piscibus, sed multa carne subrancida; servi sordidati ministrant, non nulli etiam senes; idem coquus, idem atriensis; pistor domi nullus, nulla cella; panis et vinum a propola atque de cupa.*
184 Horace, *Satires* 2.4.81–84 (trans. H. R. Fairclough): *Vilibus in scopis, in mappis, in scobe quantus consistit sumptus? neglectis, flagitium ingens. ten lapides varios lutulenta radere palma et Tyrias dare circum illuta toralia vestis.*
185 Juvenal, *Satires* 14.59–69 (trans. S. M. Braund): *Hospite venturo cessabit nemo tuorum. 'verre pavimentum, nitidas ostende columnas, arida cum tota descendat aranea tela, hic leve argentum, vasa aspera tergeat alter'. vox domini furit instantis virgamque tenentis. ergo miser trepidas, ne stercore foeda canino atria displiceant oculis venientis amici, ne perfusa luto sit porticus, et tamen uno semodio scobis haec emendat servulus unus: illud non agitas, ut sanctam filius omni aspiciat sine labe domum vitioque carentem?*
186 Hänninen, 2013, p. 46.
187 Mantle, 2002, pp. 100–102; Prescendi, 2010.
188 Plautus, *The Pot of Gold* 25.
189 Pliny the Elder, *Natural History* 28.5.26; the popular *asarotos oikos* mosaic design offers an indication of what the floor of a triclinium might look like after a banquet, with plenty of potential offerings available – for an example see Musei Vaticani inv. 10132, made by Heraclitus and dating from the second century CE, found in a *villa* on the Aventine Hill.
190 Foss, 1997, p. 199.
191 Cato the Elder, *On Agriculture* 83.
192 Cato the Elder, *On Agriculture* 132.
193 Cato the Elder, *On Agriculture* 134; Ovid, *Fasti* 1.171–174, 349–354.
194 Cato the Elder, *On Agriculture* 75–82; Glinister, 2014 on sacred cakes.
195 Cato the Elder, *On Agriculture* 8.2.
196 Boyce, 1937, pp. 105–06; Orr, 1973, pp. 98–99; Foss, 1997, p. 217.
197 For more extensive discussion of this set of household shrines, see Draycott, 2017; Flower, 2017, p. 170, observing this, notes that '*lares* were associated both with a special feast but also with a supply of pork in every season'.
198 Clarke, 2003, pp. 78–81.
199 On pigs in Roman Italy, see King, 1999; MacKinnon, 2001. On fish, see Curtis, 1991, pp. 148–158.

4 The transmission of
medical knowledge

Introduction

> Not even the woods and the wilder face of Nature are without medicines, for there
> is no place where that holy Mother of all things did not distribute remedies for the
> healing of mankind, so that even the very desert was made a drug store. . . . Such
> things alone had Nature decreed should be our remedies, provided everywhere,
> easy to discover and costing nothing – the things in fact that support our life.
> Later on the deceit of men and cunning profiteering led to the invention of the
> quack laboratories, in which each customer is promised a new lease of his own
> life at a price. At once compound prescriptions and mysterious mixtures are glibly
> repeated, Arabia and India are judged to be storehouses of remedies, and a small
> sore is charged with the cost of a medicine from the Red Sea, although the genuine
> remedies form the daily dinner of even the very poorest. But if remedies were to be
> sought in the kitchen-garden or a plant or a shrub were to be procured thence, none
> of the arts would become cheaper than medicine. It is perfectly true that owing to
> their greatness the Roman people have lost their usages, and through conquering
> we have been conquered. We are the subjects of foreigners, and in one of the arts
> they have mastered even their masters.[1]

In this passage, Pliny the Elder, having already established that Nature is a nurturer and provider akin to a maternal figure, highlights the role that the natural
world plays in therapeutics, and states that Nature provides simple remedies in
comparison to the compound and complex ones developed by mankind. He promotes the household garden as a more cost-effective alternative to purchasing
ready-made medicaments. As we saw in the previous chapter, the members of the
ancient Roman household played significant roles in the maintenance of health
and well-being, and the household garden was indispensable in these endeavours
during the middle and late Republic and the early Principate both through its presence within the home, and through the way in which the plants grown in it were
utilised by members of the household. How did people acquire this knowledge?

In the previous chapters I argued against the prevailing view that the *pater
familias*, or *dominus*, acted as the family physician, and proposed an alternative
scenario: that every member of the household, whether male or female, whether
freeborn, freed slave or slave, possessed some degree of medical knowledge, skill

and experience, and that they utilised these in the service of the household on a regular basis. It is easy to see why the subject of ancient Roman domestic medical practice has not, to date, garnered much attention or interest from scholars of either medical or social history: it is not overtly attested in the literary, documentary or archaeological records, and where it does appear, an argument can be made that it does so precisely because either the individuals or the occasions concerned are atypical.[2] I, however, argued against this, too, and suggested that the reason that Roman domestic medical practice does not enjoy sustained and detailed discussion by ancient authors is because it was an integral and fundamental part of the successful running of the household; many aspects of daily life do not feature in literary sources for precisely this reason, although documentary and archaeological evidence can be more informative about them.[3] Roman domestic medical practice was not *meant* to be obvious: unlike professional medical practitioners from outside the household, the professional and/or amateur medical practitioners from inside the household were not in open competition with each other for patients, payment, public recognition or prestige, or at least no more open competition than they would have been under any other circumstances. Their activities were subordinated to the status of the *dominus* or *domina* and their prosperous and successful household management.[4] On the contrary, when some aspect of Roman domestic medical practice does become obvious and makes its way into the historical record, it is because something has gone horribly wrong. Members of the household are subjected to accusations of deliberately or inadvertently misusing their medical knowledge, and this opens the inner workings of the household up to scrutiny.

William Fitzgerald has observed that it is a paradox of domestic slavery that for a slave to serve their master or mistress properly, it was necessary for them to not only be in possession of knowledge, skills and experience that their master or mistress was not, but to also show a certain amount of initiative regarding when it was appropriate to use them.[5] While the master or mistress might want their slaves to be as automata, acting as extensions of their will, they simultaneously needed their slaves to be individuals, and to think and act independently in order to serve them effectively.[6] Sarah Blake has proposed that we view the master (or even the mistress) as a hybrid self, a person composed of both the individual and their servile apparatus, with slavery an 'enabling infrastructure'.[7] She notes that when slaves function as they are meant to, they are unremarkable and, due to their proximity and their ubiquity, are entirely integrated with and so cannot be separated out from their master (or mistress).[8]

In Kate Cooper's analysis of 'the calculated performance of domestic virtue by Roman men', she considers the means by which the *pater familias* made his *domus* available to the scrutiny of his peers and rivals.[9] For a man to achieve success (whether political, economic or social), a well-ordered household was a virtual necessity. Whether the household was actually well-ordered, or whether it simply appeared to be, was entirely negotiable. A key feature of a well-ordered household was the *pater familias*' ability to elicit recognition of his authority from his subordinates within the household.[10] The possibility that a master or a mistress might become dependent upon their slave or slaves preyed on the minds of ancient authors.[11] Such an inversion of the natural order of the superiority of the master/mistress and inferiority of the slave was cautioned against by Cato the Elder.[12] Some slave owners were less concerned, however, and openly presented their slaves' labour as external to and separate from themselves, albeit to approbation from certain of their peers. How was medical knowledge conceptualised within this schema? On the one hand, as we have seen, an educated Roman citizen was expected to have a degree of medical knowledge. On the other, medicine as a profession was inherently degrading, and in the Rome and Italy of the late Republic and early Principate, primarily undertaken by immigrants, whether freeborn, freed slaves or slaves.[13]

The period with which this study is primarily concerned saw not only the transmission of diverse knowledge from the Greek world to the Roman, but also the transformation of this knowledge from Greek to Roman.[14] There is a clear connection between the acquisition of territory and the acquisition of knowledge.[15] Territories, along with their natural resources, peoples and bodies of knowledge were appropriated for the benefit of the Roman people. Yet it is unlikely that any single individual was in possession of all of this knowledge and in a position to transmit all of it; even encyclopaedists such as Varro, Celsus and Pliny the Elder had not read everything that they might have done, however much they might try and indicate otherwise.[16] Rather, these authors 'represent themselves as heroic explorers of the bookworld, bringing back precious nuggets of information and organising them in a rational fashion for the benefit of fellow Romans'.[17] The most visible demonstration of this process is in the works of literature that survive. However, books were not the only means of transmitting knowledge.

The first chapter of this study examined the concept of health in the city of Rome and central Italy during the late Roman Republic and early Principate, and argued that concerns regarding the acquisition, maintenance and preservation of health and well-being were not only prevalent throughout Roman society but also heavily influenced Roman behaviour. The second chapter examined the house and garden of sites where domestic healthcare took place and argued that concerns about health and well-being were literally built into the house and garden. The third chapter surveyed the roles played in domestic healthcare by the members of the household, and it is evident that a considerable number and wide variety of people were in possession of some degree or form of medical knowledge. In this chapter, I shall examine the myriad ways in which the transmission of medical knowledge from outside the Roman household to inside it could occur, who was responsible for this transmission, and how they ensured that it occurred, and offer a thorough consideration of all aspects of domestic medical knowledge, both professional and popular, leading to an acknowledgement of the significance of all members of the household and their contributions to healthcare.

Roman technical knowledge

There seems to have been a general agreement that ancient medicine comprised three areas: diet, drugs and surgery.[18] However, there was no recognised canon of medical knowledge or curriculum for medical training; indeed, each medical sect had wildly different theories, methods and practices. There was no formal process of accreditation or regulation of medical practitioners and, as we have seen, there was considerable overlap between their practices, so a physician, a trainer and a masseuse could all be doing very similar things, as could a physician, a pharmacist and a perfumer.[19] It was in the practitioners' interest to promote him or herself at the expense of his or her peers, to disseminate their knowledge whilst denigrating that of others.

In antiquity, all types of technical knowledge, including medicine, could be transmitted in one of three ways: through reading, through listening and through personal experience.[20] However, there were complex interactions between written and oral traditions, and between the elements of formal education or training and informal socialisation that comprised personal experience, and notions of expertise and authority were fluid. Therefore, while one might read a treatise or listen to one being read, this could result in a conversation about its contents during which one or more of the participants proffers information based on their own experiences, deepening and enriching both the knowledge and the experience. The conversation between Varro and his friends at the Temple of Tellus in the first book of his *On Agriculture* provides a good example.[21] They discuss the work of the father and son team Saserna the Elder and Younger, the first Latin treatise on agriculture to have been written since Cato the Elder's, published at some point between 146 BCE and 57 BCE.[22] The character Varro suggests that they discuss the Sasernae's remedy for foot trouble, since one of his companions is actually suffering from it.[23] The character of Stolo proceeds to relate the charm:

> 'I will tell you', said Stolo, with a smile, 'in the very words in which he wrote it (at least I have heard Tarquenna say that when a man's feet begin to hurt he may be cured if he will think of you): "I am thinking of you, cure my feet. The pain go in the ground, and may my feet be sound". He bids you chant this thrice nine times, touch the ground, spit on it, and be fasting while you chant'.[24]

While the character Varro agrees that the charm is a marvel, since he does not consider it relevant to the subject of agriculture, the group agrees to discard it.[25] While fictitious, or at the very least fictionalised, it demonstrates how this process could work.

Literary transmission

When considering literary transmission, it is not so simple as to differentiate between technical and non-technical literature, the former written by specialists for their peers and the latter written by non-specialists for their peers, despite claims to the contrary.[26] What we might call technical language, the language used to write and speak about a given activity by a group of people who share expertise in or knowledge of this activity, is evident in Latin literature from the third century BCE.[27] Its usage was not confined to specialists but was part of the public domain and the vernacular.[28] Thus we see various types and levels of medical knowledge expressed not only in medical literature but in works from all literary genres.[29] The last two centuries BCE saw considerable development in Roman intellectual life.[30] With regard to medicine specifically, Greek technical works on subjects related to healthcare such as anatomy, surgery, botany, minerology and pharmacology arrived in Rome and were either read in the original Greek or translated into Latin (see Figure 4.1).[31]

A work of literature containing medical information (and, as we have seen, this does not necessarily have to be a work of medical literature) that a Roman might

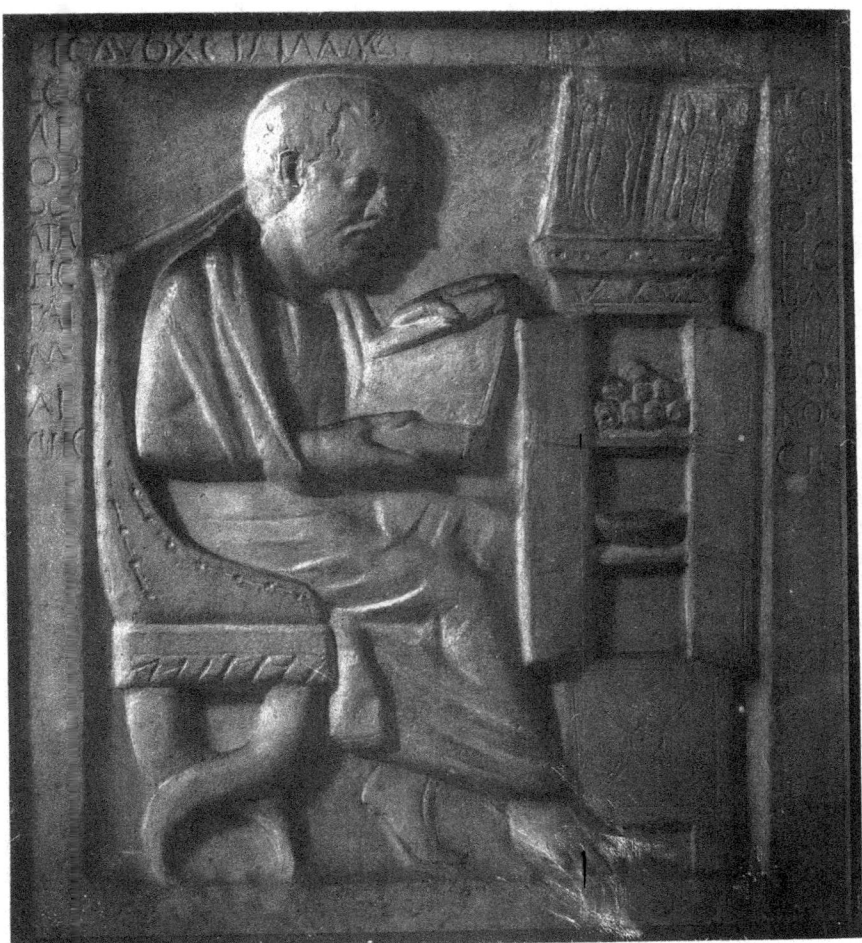

Figure 4.1 A relief of a doctor in his study; a copy.

Source: Image courtesy of the Wellcome Library (Wellcome Collection inv. M0001579).

read or have read to them could take one of a number of forms. The first of these is the highly technical theoretical work, conceived in its entirety as a means of covering one or more subjects, such as Scribonius Largus' *Compositions* (*circa* 47–48 CE), Dioscorides' *On Medical Materials* or Soranus' *Gynaecology*. Such treatises would, in all likelihood, be written by physicians and other specialist practitioners, disseminated by and circulated amongst them and potentially educated and interested laymen. We see one example of this in the case of Cicero's reading of Nicon of Acragas' treatise on dietetics borrowed from his physician acquaintance, and Nicon's pupil, Sextus Fadius:

> I have taken away a book, from Nico's pupil Sextus Fadius: *Nico on Heavy Eating*. What a charming physician, and how docile a patient he would find me! But our friend Bassus told me nothing about that book – though he seems to have told you![32]

However, there are also indications that some treatises on medical subjects were written by specialists specifically for laymen, such as the works by Pseudo-Dioscorides and Galen entitled *euporista* ('easy to procure').[33]

The second type is likewise a highly technical theoretical work, but conceived of as a means of covering a medical subject as only one part of a much larger work, such as Varro's no longer extant encyclopaedia *Disciplines*, Celsus' encyclopaedia *Arts*, of which only the eight books focusing on medicine out of a total of twenty-six have survived, or Pliny the Elder's encyclopaedia *Natural History*, of which thirteen of the thirty-six books are devoted to medicine. Such treatises were not generally written by physicians or other specialist practitioners but rather educated and interested laymen, expressions not only of their own liberal arts educations, but also the subjects that it was desirable for a member of the senatorial, equestrian or decurion elite to be conversant with. Medical knowledge was one crucial part of the liberal arts, of *enkyklios paideia* or *artes liberales*, although the extent to which people immersed themselves in it has been heavily debated.[34] Such treatises would, in all likelihood, have had a wider circulation, but would also have been more likely to suffer editing and epitomisation, and it is questionable how useful they were in a moment of crisis.

The third type is a more informal treatise, a compilation of material accrued over a period of time, such as the recipes for prescriptions included in Cato the Elder's *On Agriculture* or *To His Son*.[35] Relatively few households were likely to have been in possession of substantial libraries comprising specialist treatises or comprehensive encyclopaedia, and even those that were might have found such works difficult to utilise in case of an emergency.[36] Much more accessible, in several respects, was a notebook containing a small selection of useful recipes for prescriptions and instructions for basic procedures. Use of such a notebook, a *commentarius*, is attested in a variety of cases. The Latin word indicates notes or memoranda written down without care and is used particularly in relation to historiography.[37] In one sense, this seems particularly appropriate as such notebooks were used to record a household's medical history, each generation adding their own theories, methods and practices for posterity, as Cato seems to have done for his sons and as his readers were potentially inspired to do, presuming they were not in the habit of doing so already, so there is an element of historiography. Certainly, Varro refers to this practice on several occasions.[38] He states that one should read the works of authorities such as Mago the Carthaginian, make notes to refer to later and add their own writings, too.[39] Pliny the Elder likewise refers to the notebooks of Mithridates VI of Pontus in which he recorded his research into poisons and antidotes.[40] In another sense, the very fact that people were making such notes or memoranda on these subjects shows that they were taking care.

How could people access works of literature that they did not own themselves? Prior to the late first century BCE, there were no public libraries in the city of Rome. Rather, private libraries could be found in the homes of the wealthy elite in Rome, and their alternative residences in Latium and Campania.[41] A significant portion of these collections arrived in Rome as the spoils of conquests of Hellenistic kingdoms. Particularly famous acquisitions were the library of the Macedonian kings, acquired by Lucius Aemilius Paullus Macedonicus in 168 BCE, the library of Apellicon of Teos, acquired by Lucius Cornelius Sulla Felix in 86 BCE, and the libraries of Mithridates, one acquired by Lucius Licinius Lucullus in 70 BCE, another by Pompey in 65 BCE.[42] Caesar planned a public library and went so far as to commission Varro to begin work on it, but was assassinated before he could realise this ambition.[43] Gaius Asinius Pollio set up Rome's first public library in the Temple of Liberty in 39 BCE, which comprised Greek and Latin sections, and Augustus set up two more on the Palatine and in the Temple of Peace, likewise comprising Greek and Latin sections.[44] Apellicon of Teos' library is known to have contained the works of Aristotle and Theophrastus, while Mithridates' library is known to have contained works on botany and pharmacology.

There is a considerable amount of evidence for the transmission of medical knowledge from Mithridates' library to Rome and central Italy in the late Republic and early Principate. In the wake of his victory, Pompey commissioned one of his freedmen, the *grammaticus* Lenaeus, to translate Mithridates' works into Latin.[45] In the late first century CE, Pliny the Elder was able to consult Mithridates' handwritten notes, and slightly later Plutarch was able to do the same.[46] Mithridates' poison antidote, *Mithridatium*, was of particular interest to the Romans.[47] It has been suggested that Lucius Lutatius Paccius, an incense seller who claimed to be a member of Mithridates' family in his epitaph, and another Paccius, possibly his son, who bequeathed a special remedy to the emperor Tiberius in 14 CE, were in fact producing and selling *Mithridatium* in Rome.[48] The physician Andromachus prescribed a version of the antidote to the emperor Nero. Archaeological excavation of a villa near Pompeii uncovered a vat of a substance, the ingredients of which correspond with ancient references to those of *Mithridatium*, so it is possible that the antidote was being manufactured on an industrial scale and so was more readily accessible by 79 CE.[49]

The extent to which individuals could access private collections is debateable. Access was probably reliant on the possession of sufficient contacts through the patronage system, and physical proximity was also a factor, whether the collection was located in Rome or easily accessible areas of Latium and Campania. Lucullus, for example, is known to have permitted Cicero and Marcus Porcius Cato Uticensis (Cato the Younger) to work in his library.[50] Consequently access to these works might depend on patronage and connections.[51] Once access was gained, it might be possible to make personal copies of works consulted, although the process of making copies could be problematic, whether due to the poor quality of the original manuscripts, or the lack of skill on the part of the copyists.[52] This was frequently found to be the case with technical literature: Strabo complains about the copies made of Aristotle's and Theophrastus' works in the library of Apellicon of Teos, Varro notes that copyists could struggle with technical language and Pliny the Elder observes that copyists often failed to reproduce botanical illustrations in herbals accurately, rendering the plants unrecognisable.[53] Educated Romans were well aware of the drawbacks of relying solely on written information. This perhaps explains why some Roman citizens preferred to copy treatises themselves, rather than relying on others to do it for them.[54]

It might have been possible to purchase medical literature through bookshops.[55] The book trade expanded over the course of the first century CE, which meant that access to literature was partially removed from the bonds of friendship.[56] Booksellers and the secondhand market could serve as a means of making technical literature more accessible, although there were likely limitations about what was available at any one time. More informal literary works, copied piecemeal, might include notes taken during public or private lectures.[57]

Additionally, we should not forget that, in order for these works to circulate among members of the elite, their highly educated slaves and freedmen and freedwomen had to read and copy them, and it is likely that they absorbed a considerable amount of technical information in the process. They would subsequently be in a position to disseminate that knowledge among other members of their household, and perhaps even utilise it if the occasion called for it and the need arose.

Oral transmission

Ancient Roman culture has been described as an 'active oral culture'.[58] Consequently, illiteracy or a low level of literacy was not necessarily a barrier to the acquisition of medical knowledge, or any other type of knowledge, for that matter. Technical information was frequently transmitted verbally in antiquity, and the process of this verbal transmission could take several forms.[59]

First, oral transmission could occur formally through a public lecture or a demonstration. These sorts of displays were common in the Hellenistic period, occurring in Rome as early as the second century BCE, and involved individuals presenting their theories, methods and practices to an audience.[60] Asclepiades of Bithynia is known to have done this in Rome, and it is likely that itinerant physicians like Lucius Clodius did likewise whenever they arrived at a sizeable settlement.[61] Such events were recognised as being part of the cultural life of a city.[62] While some lectures or demonstrations might have taken place in relatively private locations to small audiences, others might have taken place in more public locations and consequently attracted large audiences. Rome's porticoes and public libraries frequently had rooms for just such purposes attached to them. [63] It is possible if not probable, that not just members of the senatorial and equestrian orders were present for some of these events, but also members of the plebeian orders.[64] Indeed, it has been suggested that this is how Asclepiades of Bithynia's approach to regimen and hydrotherapy became so popular and widely used.[65]

Second, oral transmission could occur informally through casual conversation, rumour or gossip, and even jokes (see Figure 4.2). Those employed in areas associated with healthcare presumably dispensed instructions to their customers along

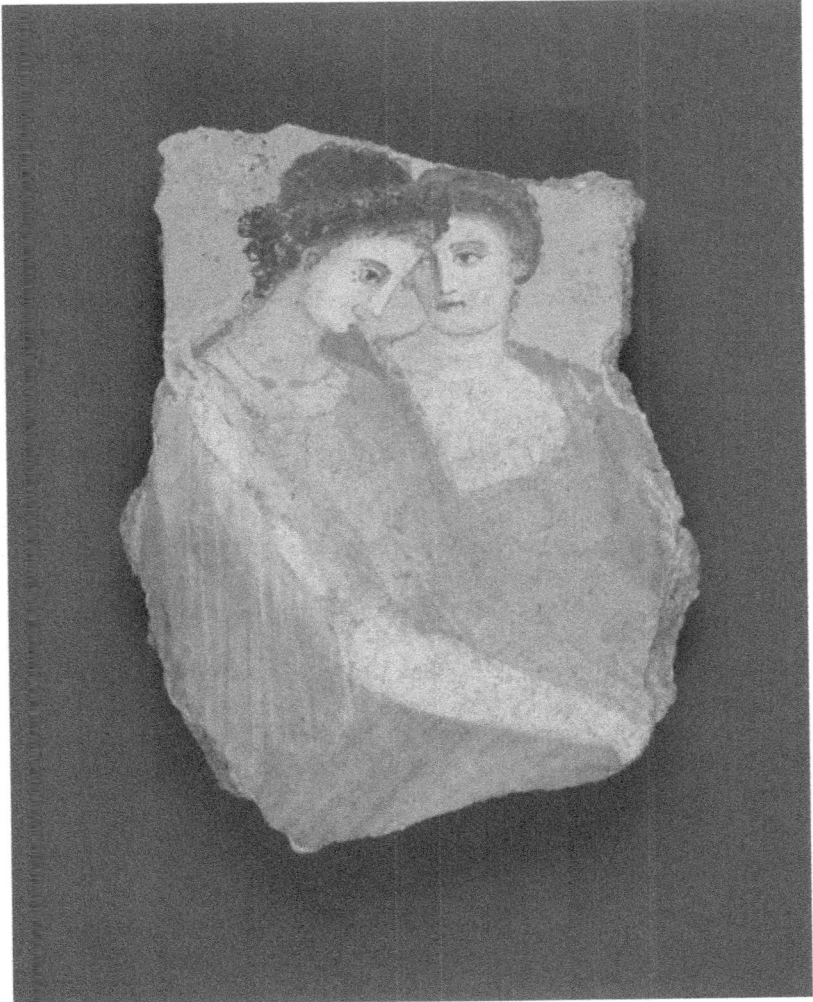

Figure 4.2 A fresco fragment depicting two women in conversation, first century CE.

Source: Image courtesy of the J. Paul Getty Museum, Open Content Program (J. Paul Getty Museum inv. 96.AG.302).

with their products, such as root-cutters and root sellers (*rhizopōlai*), perfume and unguent makers and sellers (*myrepsoi, myropōlai, myropolae, thurarii*), herbalists (*botanikoi*), pharmacists (*seplasarii*) and drug sellers (*pharmakopōlai, pharmacopolae*).[66] We see an ointment seller in Plautus' *Stichus* recommending a particular ointment for a hangover.[67] In such instances a vendor could give anything from minimal information concerning the remedy, its ingredients and preparation, to a detailed explanation of the entire process. The writers of botanical treatises such as Theophrastus, Dioscorides and Pliny the Elder state on numerous occasions that they obtained their information from vendors who were happy to speak to them, and there is no reason why consumers need not have had similarly enlightening conversations. Indeed, considering the prevalent anxieties about the potential of drugs to harm as well as heal, it would behove a vendor to set a consumer's mind at rest about the precise contents of their purchase and make sure that they did not accidentally poison themselves.[68] Certainly, individuals offered advice to their family members, friends and acquaintances: Martial recommends a variety of different remedies; to Phoebus, who suffers from constipation, he recommends lettuce and mallows, while to Severus, who suffers from a sore throat, he recommends eggs.[69] Marcus Aurelius writes a series of letters to Fronto in which he describes his step-by-step approach to dealing with a developing cold, including pouring oil on his head, having a lie in and gargling with honey water.[70] Many of the jokes included in the *Philogelos* poke fun at both physicians and their patients, but some listeners may have been tempted to try the remedies recommended, if not as a first resort, then as a last one.[71]

Related to both of these processes is the role of fashion as a means of transmitting medical knowledge. There are particular examples of members of the imperial family or prominent citizens setting trends. Augustus' physician Antonius Musa prescribed him lettuce, in direct contradiction to his previous physician Gaius Aemilius' instructions, and the subsequent popularity of lettuces led to the development of a new way of preserving them so as to make them readily available out of season.[72] Augustus' daughter Julia's daily tonic, made from elecampane with pepper or thyme, was recommended as being particularly beneficial for those suffering from weak digestion.[73] Additionally, practitioners attached famous names to their recipes as a means of marketing them.[74] Members of the lower orders do seem to have imitated the behaviour of the imperial family, senatorial and equestrian orders, albeit on a much smaller scale as their budgets allowed.[75]

Personal experience

As we have seen, individuals were expected to have comprehensive knowledge of their own bodies and their own needs, particularly in relation to any physical or mental weaknesses or deficiencies that they might possess. There were also particular conditions that would be experienced regularly enough for individuals to become familiar with them, even if they had not experienced them themselves, such as pregnancy and childbirth.

The role of informal education, formal education and training

The household and its occupants were central to Roman informal and formal education.[76] A child's education was in the first instance the responsibility of his or her parents. Tacitus offers an idealised version of education earlier in the history of Rome, but does include some significant historical figures as significant examples in support of his claims, which perhaps allows us to gauge how children were educated during the late Republic and early Principate:

> In the good old days, every man's son, born in wedlock, was brought up not in the chamber of some hireling nurse, but in his mother's lap, and at her knee. And that mother could have no higher praise than that she managed the house and gave herself to her children. Again, some elderly relative would be selected in order that to her, as a person who had been tried and never found wanting, might be entrusted the care of all the youthful scions of the same house; in the presence of such a one no base word could be uttered without grave offence, and no wrong deed done. Religiously and with the utmost delicacy she regulated not only the serious tasks of her youthful charges, but their recreations also and their games. It was in this spirit, we are told, that Cornelia, the mother of the Gracchi, directed their upbringing, Aurelia that of Caesar, Atia of Augustus: thus it was that these mothers trained their princely children. The object of this rigorous system was that the natural disposition of every child, while still sound at the core and untainted, not warped as yet by any vicious tendencies, might at once lay hold with heart and soul on virtuous accomplishments, and whether its bent was towards the army, or the law, or the pursuit of eloquence, might make that its sole aim and its all-absorbing interest.[77]

Thus we see that the mother and an older female relative, perhaps the paternal or even maternal grandmother, were considered to play important roles in the informal education of infants and children, an education that incorporated oversight of both health and well-being, and that involved a certain amount of personalisation. Indeed, despite the fact that Tacitus explicitly contrasts the process of educating children in the past with that of his present, Pliny the Younger discusses the family of Ummidia Quadratilla, and the details that he gives indicates that this family, at least, did as Cornelia, Aurelia and Atia had done.[78]

At some point, boys were passed from their mothers to their fathers to begin the process of formal education, and this seems to have combined book-learning with shadowing an older man, a father or perhaps a maternal uncle, and following his example.[79] Depending upon the social status of the family, the example set might include political activity, agricultural activity or a trade. Once boys set aside the *toga praetexta* and donned the *toga virilis*, they could embark upon preparation for public life through an apprenticeship to a worthy citizen (*tirocinium fori*) or a serving officer (*tirocinium militae*).[80] Likewise, girls shadowed their mothers and gradually learned the skills necessary to run a household of their own.[81]

Roman informal and formal education was essentially utilitarian, aiming to prepare children for the roles that they would perform in adulthood, and consequently both the body and the mind were attended to. Plutarch provides a lengthy description of Cato the Elder's approach to raising his elder son and, since his elder son was widely admired, if he had not died when his younger son was an infant, he would in all likelihood have repeated the process. While the fact that Plutarch covers the subject in such detail – he had, after all, had access to Cato's *To His Son* – indicates that Cato was somewhat atypical in this respect, it does give us an interesting insight into one particular Roman family and the fundamental role that health and well-being was considered by this family to play in preparation for adult life:

> After the birth of his son, no business could be so urgent, unless it had a public character, as to prevent him from being present when his wife bathed and swaddled the babe. For the mother nursed it herself, and often gave suck also to the infants of her slaves, that so they might come to cherish a brotherly affection for her son. As soon as the boy showed signs of understanding, his father took him under his own charge and taught him to read, although he had an accomplished slave, Chilo by name, who was a school-teacher, and taught many boys. Still, Cato thought it not right, as he tells us himself, that his son should be scolded by a slave, or have his ears tweaked when he was slow to learn, still less that he should be indebted to his slave for such a priceless thing as education. He was therefore himself not only the boy's reading-teacher, but his tutor in law, and his athletic trainer, and he taught his son not merely to hurl the javelin and fight in armour and ride the horse, but also to box, to endure heat and cold, and to swim lustily through the eddies and billows of the Tiber. His History of Rome, as he tells us himself, he wrote out with his own hand and in large characters, that his son might have in his own home an aid to acquaintance with his country's ancient traditions. He declares that his son's presence put him on his guard against indecencies of speech as much as that of the so-called Vestal Virgins, and that he never bathed with him. . . . So Cato wrought at the fair task of moulding and fashioning his son to virtue, finding his zeal blameless, and his spirit answering to his good natural parts. But since his body was rather too delicate to endure much hardship, he relaxed somewhat in his favour the excessive rigidity and austerity of his own mode of life.[82]

In turn, perhaps Cato's son adopted this approach to raising his own son.

The role of socialisation

The socialisation of Roman children played an important role in the transmission of medical knowledge from one generation to the next as a means of ensuring the survival of the family members, and through them the family itself. A child's domestic environment played an important role in socialisation, and this was reinforced by the religious, social and economic world around them, whether in an urban or rural context.[83] This domestic environment contained a wide range of individuals, members of the family, members of the household and members of the neighbourhood. According to Plautus, children, like buildings, required solid foundations.[84] From birth, Roman children would have been exposed to health-care theory, method and practice. A newborn baby was rubbed with salt, bathed, swaddled and fed water and honey.[85] Children were subjected to specific regimen, and it is likely that as they aged they came to question certain aspects of this regimen and seek explanation for them from their caregivers.[86] Roman children were often entrusted to wet nurses and pedagogues from soon after birth, following their parents' attempts to find the best caregiver possible (see Figure 4.3).[87] The wet nurse was subject to a regimen, too.

A caregiver did not just take care of the physical health and well-being of their charge. The caregiver also took care of their charge's mental and emotional health and well-being. They might sing a lullaby, give a cuddle, offer comfort, and attempt to distract them when they were ill or frightened.[88] A pedagogue not only oversaw childcare, illness, meals and educational activities, but also took his charge to the baths.[89]

The role of social networks

Friends might aid each other in times of illness and benefit themselves by adding to their store of medical knowledge and experience in the process.[90] The letters exchanged by Fronto and Marcus Aurelius are very informative regarding how involved close friends could be in each other's healthcare. On one occasion, Marcus writes to Fronto, who is suffering from a recurring foot complaint – possibly gout – and says that he wishes he were in a position to visit him at Baiae, where he is undergoing treatment, and assist him with it:

> This most hard necessity which keeps me a prisoner here with a heart so anxious and fettered with such great apprehension and does not let me run at once to my Fronto, to my most beautiful of souls, above all to be with him at a time when he is so unwell, to clasp his hands and in fine, as far as may be without pain, to massage the poor foot itself, foment it in the bath, and support him as he steps in?[91]

Considering that Marcus was Caesar at this point, the likelihood of him ever having behaved in such a way is debateable, but elsewhere in the correspondence Fronto writes to Lucius Verus regarding his friend Gavius Clarus, and describes the ministrations that Clarus offered him:

> He always devoted such attention to my health, was so unsparing, too, at all times of himself, that when I was sick he even sat up with me, and when rheumatism deprived me of the use of my hands he was wont to put the food to my mouth with his own hand.[92]

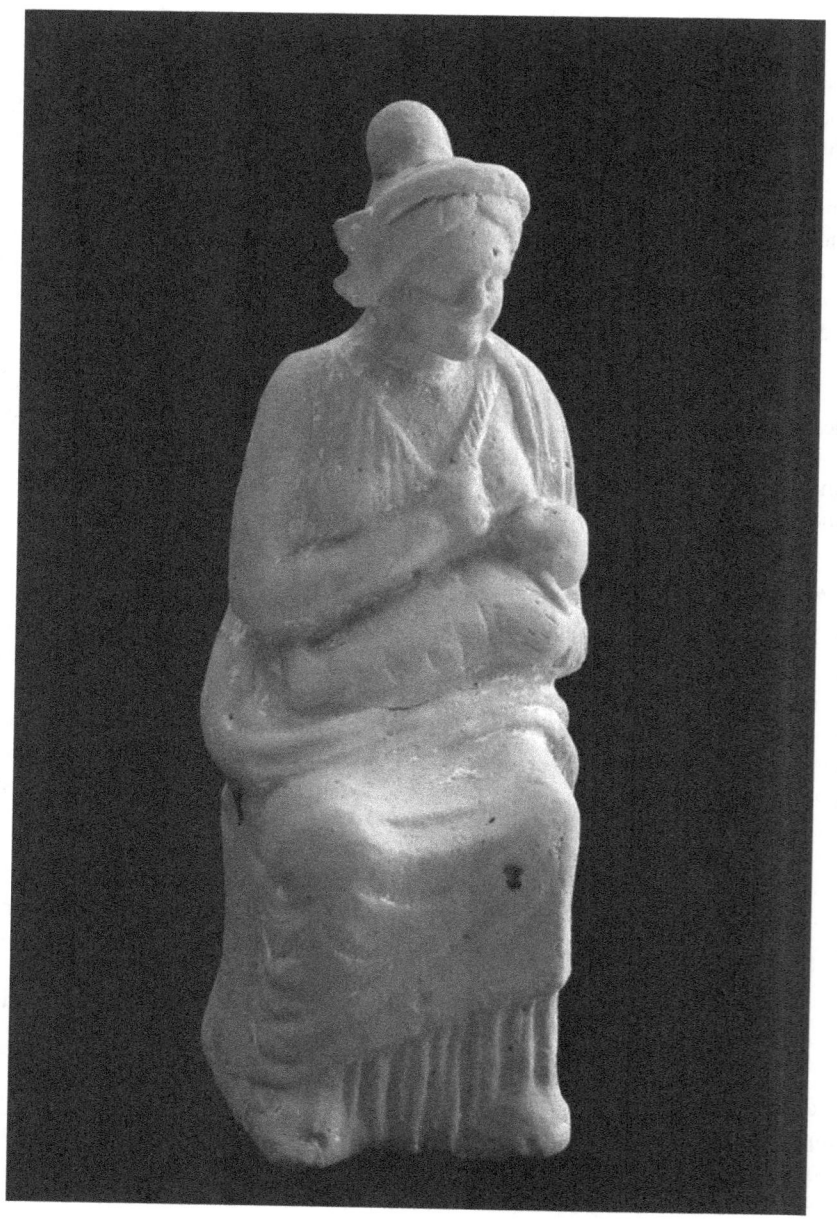

Figure 4.3 A terracotta figurine of a woman nursing a child, third century BCE–first century CE.

Source: Image courtesy of the Wellcome Library (Wellcome Collection/Science Museum A634990).

It seems that it was not necessarily the case that slaves were the ones who undertook such menial tasks, but presumably this level of intimacy, which involved a degree of debasement and required considerable trust, was reserved for family members and extremely close friends.

Cicero writes to his brother Quintus Tullius Cicero regarding the possibility of accommodating their mutual friend Marius during his illness, and that if his own home is not suitable he may resort to arranging accommodation with Anicius.[93] Seneca the Younger writes to Lucilius of his friends visiting him during an illness and not only keeping him entertained but also contributing to his recovery through their stimulating conversation.[94] Marcus Aurelius thanks Fronto for visiting Salvius Julianus during his illness, for cheering him up and making him more comfortable.[95] Aulus Gellius records conversations that took place between the philosopher Favorinus and Fronto, and between Julius Celsinus Numidius when Fronto was convalescing after an attack of gout, and was visited by many friends and acquaintances, and presumably these served a similar purpose, distracting Fronto from his discomfort if not actually contributing to his recovery.[96] Cicero's friends seem to have been happy to accommodate his slaves and freedmen during their illnesses and convalescences, and he did the same for them, and as we have seen Pliny the Younger made similar arrangements for his freedman Zosimus.[97] In extreme circumstances, people might open their homes to those who were ill or injured even if they were not friends or acquaintances; Tacitus records such an occurrence following the collapse of an amphitheatre in Fidenae in 27 CE that killed or maimed up to 50,000 people.[98]

The *salutatio* and the *deductio* provided an opportunity for patrons to see their clients and for clients to pay their respects to their patrons. Freedmen and freedwomen were the clients of their former masters and mistresses and consequently were expected to obey them, assist them and even potentially provide them with services, such as a specified number of days work, if that had been a condition of their manumission, even if the nature of the work was something they had learned after manumission.[99] For some clients, this might involve healthcare.[100] A patron with a client who was a physician could reasonably expect the provision of medical practice for himself or herself, and even friends and acquaintances.[101] Cicero refers to a woman named Sassia who established one of her freedmen, Strato, as a pharmacist, so it is not unreasonable to assume that she would have availed herself of his services.[102]

While not formalised like the patron–client relationship, it was expected that younger or socially inferior women would call on elder or socially superior women, and that women attend their sick or pregnant friends, and even assist with childbirth (see Figure 4.4).[103]

Finally, a Roman citizen's relationship with a non-citizen, guest-friendship or *hospitium*, might also involve healthcare. Livy records the case of the Roman Titus Quinctius Crispinus' guest-friendship with the Campanian Badius which originated when Badius fell ill in Rome and was looked after in Crispinus' house.[104] Livy also details much earlier cases of Etruscan prisoners of war being nursed back to heath in Roman households and becoming friendly to Rome as a result.[105]

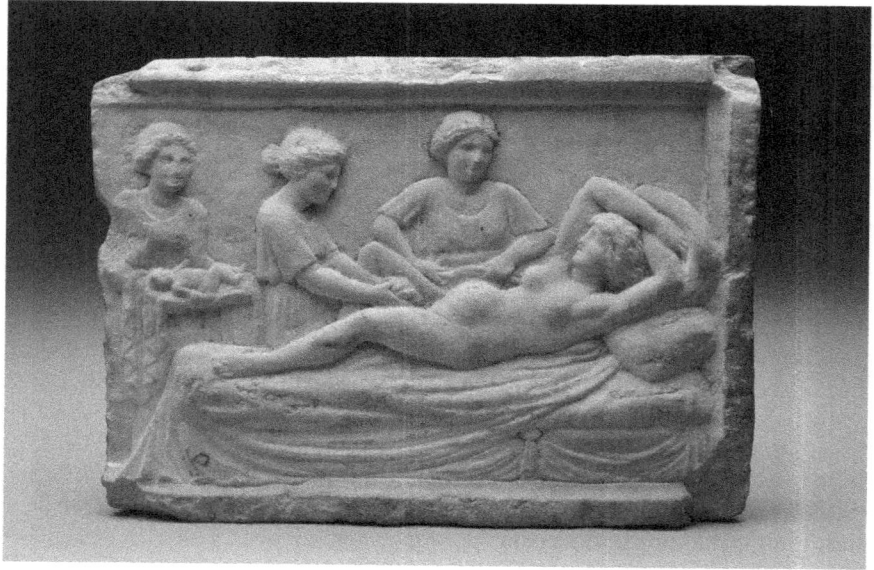

Figure 4.4 A marble plaque depicting a woman giving birth, second century CE.
Source: Image courtesy of the Wellcome Library (Wellcome Collection/Science Museum A129245).

The ambiguity of Roman domestic medical practice

The fundamental ambiguity of domestic medical practice and its practitioners is illustrated by an event that took place in 331 BCE during which many people died as a result of what was, depending on the account, either an epidemic or the first recorded case of a crime of poisoning.[106] A slave testified that a group of twenty Roman matrons, both patrician and plebeian, were preparing and administering *venena* that they claimed were remedies (*medicamenta salubria*) but were in fact poisons, and further investigation resulted in the attendants of another 170 matrons informing on their mistresses and leading to them being found guilty of the same crime. In Livy's *History of Rome*, he questions the veracity of the official account of the event and states that other authorities questioned it too. To the Romans, a *venenum* was anything that powerfully affected or changed the condition of the body –a remedy, poison or even magic – and so it was necessary for it to be qualified by good (*bonum*) or bad (*malum*). Consequently, there are several ways to read this story bearing in mind the variable meanings of the term *venenum*. The first is that the written record is entirely true, and the Roman matrons were guilty of poisoning people deliberately. The second is that the written record is partly true in that the Roman matrons produced remedies that poisoned people inadvertently. The third is that the written record is false and the Roman matrons were innocent, and their remedies were misidentified as poisons.

Accusations of poisoning were made frequently in the Roman Republic and Principate, with both men and women being accused of poisoning family members, friends and acquaintances, generally for the purposes of gaining some sort of advantage as a result of their deaths.[107] Additionally, poisoning appears in poetry and works of fiction, and as a scenario set for rhetorical practice exercises. The extent to which all or any of these accusations were true is impossible to know, but despite the sheer volume of episodes recorded, there are certain features common to many of them, and these common features can offer us an insight into the potential dangers of undertaking Roman domestic medical practice, whether it was successful or unsuccessful.

The negative tradition/stereotype of the Roman stepmother, considered to be at best hostile and at worst malevolent to her stepchildren, exemplifies the potential lack of trust between members of a newly blended household and its ramifications.[108] There are, however, indications that this was not just a tradition or a stereotype but an actual possibility. Surviving forensic speeches such as Cicero's *In Defence of Cluentius*, examples of rhetorical exercises such as Seneca the Elder's *Declamations* and Quintilian's *Institutes of Oratory* and sections of the Roman law codes offer examples of situations in which members of Roman households such as stepmothers were accused of poisoning those within their sphere of influence.

Conclusion

The three Roman agricultural treatises offer an insight into the ways in which these three different modes of transmission co-existed, overlapped and complemented each other. As we have seen, Cato the Elder was in possession of a notebook filled with medicinal remedies, and it is reasonable to assume that at least some on these survive in his *On Agriculture*.[109] These prescriptions and recipes indicate that, in addition to acting as a healer for the human members of his household, Cato also acted as a veterinarian for his livestock, and recommended that others do the same. Throughout the text the authority of the *dominus* which, it is made clear, results from a combination of knowledge and experience, is emphasised, as is the importance of drawing upon the resources immediately to hand. Of Cato's numerous prescriptions and recipes for the treatment of both humans and animals, the ingredients required are all those which he either explicitly states were cultivated on his estate, or were likely to have been, presumably at least in part with these specific uses in mind. While Cato emphasises the importance of knowledge and experience acquired by oneself, Varro defers to the knowledge and experience of others. He not only provides references to the works that he has utilised in the research and writing of his treatise *On Agriculture*, he also inserts real historical figures known to be authorities on these subjects as characters and allows them to present their theories and methods.[110] He does, nonetheless, use them to praise himself and his own theories, methods and practices:

> Did not our friend Varro here, when the army and fleet were at Corcyra, and all the houses were crowded with the sick and the dead, by cutting new

windows to admit the north wind, and shutting out the infected winds, by changing the position of doors, and other precautions of the same kind, bring back his comrades and his servants in good health?[111]

Unlike Cato, Varro is not necessarily averse to physicians.[112] Rather, he does not believe that they need to be present on an estate at all times, as not every medical situation requires their services.[113] As far as he is concerned, there are two types of knowledge with regard to the treatment of human beings, one of which is possessed by anyone and the other is possessed by a physician.[114] Thus, 'all directions for caring for the health of human beings and cattle, and all the sickness which can be treated without the aid of a physician, the head herdsman should keep in writing'.[115] He repeatedly emphasises the importance of having handbooks to refer to, while concurrently he promotes literacy in his staff.[116] This is perhaps an offshoot of his opinion that nothing should be bought, if it can be grown or made on the farm.[117] Columella, like Cato, emphasises the authority of the *dominus*, an authority acquired through knowledge and experience:

> But whoever is destined for this business must be very learned in it and very robust, so that he may both teach those under his orders and himself adequately carry out the instructions he gives; for indeed nothing can be taught or learned correctly without an example, and it is better that a bailiff should be the master, not the pupil, of his labourers. Cato, a model of old-time morals, speaking as head of a family, said: 'Things go ill with the master when his bailiff has to teach him'.[118]

Although it is the bailiff and the bailiff's wife that are responsible for healthcare, presumably they have been instructed by the *dominus* and the *domina*.[119] However, like Varro he emphasises the pedigree of his resources.[120]

Thus, the treatises of Cato, Varro and Columella set out a framework for healthcare theory and practice within the Roman household, requiring a combination of personal knowledge and expertise supplemented, perhaps even reinforced, by relevant medical literature. Both Cato and Varro were drawing on their personal experiences of owning agricultural estates in Italy, while Columella was drawing on his uncle's experiences of owning agricultural estates in Spain. However, it is important to remember that just because Cato, Varro and Columella recommended that lay medical practice be undertaken and provided guidance as to how individuals should go about doing it, it does not necessarily follow that anyone did as they suggested, either in Roman Italy or Spain, or anywhere else in the Roman Empire. It is important to remember that neither professional nor lay medical theories, methods and practices were standardised throughout the Roman world.[121] Yet, it is entirely possible, if not probable, that entirely independent traditions of lay medical practice developed simultaneously in different territories.

It would appear that no one person possessed all of the knowledge and experience necessary to fulfil all of the requirements of regimen on their own. Regimen was communal, a collective activity. This knowledge and experience was, however, easily accessible, whether you were based in the city of Rome or in a small town in Campania such as Pompeii or Herculaneum.

Notes

1 Pliny the Elder, *Natural History* 24.1.1–4 (trans. H. Rackham): *Ne silvae quidem horridiorque naturae facies medicinis carent, sacra illa parente rerum omnium nusquam non remedia disponente homini, ut medicina fieret etiam solitudo ipsa . . . haec sola neturae placuerat esse remedia parata vulgo, inventu facilia ac sine inpendio et quibus vivimus. postea fraudes hominum et ingeniorum capturae officinas invenere istas in quibus sua cuique homini venalis promittitur vita. statim compositiones et mixturae inexplicabiles decantantur, Arabia atque India remedia aestimantur, ulcerique parvo medicina a Rubro mari inputatur, cum remedia vera cotidie pauperrimus quisque cenet. nam si ex horto petantur, aut herba vel frutex quaeratur, nulla artium vilior fiat. ita est profecto, magnitudine populi R. periit ritus, vincendoque victi sumus. paremus externis, et una artium imperatoribus quoque imperaverunt. verum de his alias plura.*
2 See for example the empress Livia's well-attested interest in health and well-being, Barrett, 2002, pp. 108–112.
3 See for example recent attempts to recover the experience of slaves using material evidence: Thompson, 2003; George, 2013; Joshel and Peterson, 2014.
4 Blake, 2012.
5 Fitzgerald, 2000, p. 17.
6 Fitzgerald, 2000, p. 27.
7 Blake, 2016, p. 97, developing arguments initially made in Blake, 2012.
8 Blake, 2016, p. 97.
9 Cooper, 2007, p. 4. As noted by Saller, 1999, and as has been discussed above, since the designation *pater familias* was a legal one, in the eyes of the law, regarding property ownership, a woman could technically be a *pater familias*.
10 Cooper, 2007, p. 7.
11 Fitzgerald, 2000, p. 49.
12 Columella, *On Agriculture* 11.1.4.
13 Cicero, *On Duties* 1.150.
14 For a general summary of the process of the transmission of Greek medical knowledge to Italy, see Nutton, 2013, pp. 160–162.
15 Beagon, 1992, pp. 14–15.
16 See for example Varro, *On Agriculture* 1.1.7; Celsus, *On Medicine* preface; Pliny the Elder, *Natural History* 1. König and Woolf, 2013, pp. 35–37.
17 König and Woolf, 2013, p. 45.
18 Celsus, *On Medicine* preface 9.
19 For the legal view of what constituted a medical practitioner, see *Digest* 50.13.1.1–3.
20 Hardy and Totelin, 2016, p. 34. See for example Varro, *On Agriculture* 1.1.11 on agricultural knowledge; Dioscorides, *On Medical Materials* preface 5 on botanical knowledge. See also Bates, 1995 for discussion of the different ways of knowing, with emphasis on 'gnostic' knowing and 'epistemic' knowing.
21 Varro, *On Agriculture* 1.2.26–27.
22 For information on the Sasaernae, see Columella, *On Agriculture* 1.1.12; Pliny the Elder, *Natural History* 17.199; White, 1973, pp. 459–460.
23 Varro, *On Agriculture* 1.2.26.
24 Varro, *On Agriculture* 1.2.27. See Cato the Elder, *On Agriculture* 160 for a similar charm recommended for use against dislocation.
25 Varro, *On Agriculture* 1.2.28.
26 Galen, *Difficulties in Breathing.* 2.7; Cañizares, 2010, p. 87. See also König and Woolf, 2017.
27 Langslow, 2000.
28 Hillman, 2004, p. 2.
29 Langslow, 2000, p. 31.
30 Rawson, 1985.
31 Langslow, 2000.

32 Cicero, *Letters to Friends* 33.3 (VII.20.3) (trans. D. Shackleton Bailey): *Ego a Sex. Fadio, Niconis discipulo, librum abstuli Νίκωνος περὶ Πολυφαγίας. o medicum suavem meque docilem ad hanc disciplinam! sed Bassus noster me de hoc libro celavit, te quidem non videtur.*

33 Oribasius, *Epitome* preface. For the Classical Greek precedents of this type of work, see Hippocrates, *Affections*; Lloyd, 1979, pp. 228–229; Totelin, 2018.

34 Flemming, 2000, p. 59.

35 On the possible lay readers of collections of pharmacological recipes, see Totelin, 2009, p. 257.

36 However, see Houston, 2014, pp. 39–86, pp. 130–189 on specific book collections from Roman Egypt that give an insight into the breadth of individual book collectors' interests. The best evidence for private libraries comes from Roman Egypt and can be accessed through the CEDOPAL database.

37 Quintilian, *Institutes of Oratory* 1.8.19, 3.6.59.

38 Varro, *On Agriculture* 2.2.20, 2.3.8.

39 Varro, *On Agriculture* 2.5.18, 2.7.16, 2.10.10.

40 Pliny the Elder, *Natural History* 23.77.149; Totelin, 2004, p. 7.

41 See Vitruvius, *On Architecture* 6.4.1 and 6.5.2 for advice on how to build a room suitable for use as a private library.

42 Aemilius Paullus: Plutarch, *Aemilius Paullus* 28.6; Cornelius Sulla: Strabo, *Geography* 13.C609, Plutarch, *Sulla* 26; Lucius Licinius Lucullus: Cicero, *On Ends* 3.2.7, Plutarch, *Lucullus* 42, Isidore, *Origins* 6.5.1; Gnaeus Pompey: Pliny the Elder, *Natural History* 25.3.

43 Suetonius, *Divine Julius Caesar* 44.

44 Library of Asinius Pollio: Suetonius, *Grammarians* 20; Library on the Palatine: Ovid, *Tristia*, 3.1.71; Pliny the Elder, *Natural History* 7.115, 35.10; Isidore, *Origins* 6.5.2.

45 Pliny the Elder, *Natural History* 25.3; Suetonius, *Grammarians* 15. See also Mayor, 2010, pp. 240–241, 330–331.

46 Plutarch, *Pompey* 33 and 36–41.

47 Pliny the Elder, *Natural History* 23.77.

48 *CIL* VI 5639, 5638.

49 Ciaraldi, 2000.

50 Cicero, *On Ends* 3.7.

51 Rawson, 1985, p. 44.

52 Strabo, *Geography* 13.609; Diodorus Siculus, *Historical Library* 40.8.

53 Strabo, *Geography* 13.609; Varro, *On the Latin Language* 8.51; Pliny the Elder, *Natural History* 25.8.

54 Fronto, *Epistles* 1.7.4; Galen, *On Avoiding Grief* 6.

55 Catullus 14.17; Cicero, *Philippics* 2.21; Horace, *Epistles* 1.20.2, 2.3.345.

56 Starr, 1987, p. 214.

57 Marcus Cicero: Cicero, *Letters to Friends* 337.8 (XVI.21.8); Pliny the Elder: Pliny the Younger, *Letters* 3.5.

58 Horsfall, 2003, p. 31.

59 Horsfall, 2003, pp. 48–63 sees popular culture as not having been acquired through education or acculturation.

60 Suetonius, *Grammarians* 2.

61 Asclepiades: Cicero, *On Oratory* 1.62; Pliny the Elder, *Natural History* 26.12. Lucius Clodius: Cicero, *In Defence of Cluentius* 40.

62 Plutarch, *How to Tell a Flatterer* 71A; Dio Chrysostom, *Orations* 33.6; Athenaeus, *Dinner Sophists* 3.98C; Libanius, *Orations* 1.55.

63 In the late second century CE, Galen lectured and dissected live animals in public as part of the agonistic culture of the Second Sophistic, see Galen, *On his Own Books* 1–11.

64 Rawson, 1985, p. 53.

65 Fagan, 1999a, pp. 100–101.

66 On these, see Collard and Samama, 2006.

67 Plautus, *Stichus* 267.
68 Nutton, 1985; Totelin, 2016.
69 Martial, *Epigrams* 3.89, 7.49.
70 Fronto, *Correspondence* (Marcus Aurelius) iv.5, iv.6.
71 See for example *Philogelos* 22, in which a physician prescribes wine to a patient with a fever, much to his wife's disgust; see also *Philogelos* 222, in which a physician advises a glutton to add some pulses or oats to his drinks.
72 Pliny the Elder, *Natural History* 19.38.128.
73 Pliny the Elder, *Natural History* 19.29.92.
74 Flemming, 2007.
75 Cicero, *Laws* 3.30–31; Pliny the Elder, *Natural History* 33.32–33; Martial, *Epigrams* 12.70.
76 Indeed, it was recognised that the way that babies were treated during infancy was fundamental to their ability to develop as Roman citizens later in life in respect of their health and well-being, see Soranus, *Gynaecology* 2.9–10.
77 Tacitus, *A Dialogue on Oratory* 28.4–6 (trans. M. Hutton): *Nam pridem suus cuique filius, ex casta parente natus, non in cellula emptae nutricis, sed gremio ac sinu matris educabatur, cuius praecipua laus erat tueri domum et inservire liberis. Eligebatur autem maior aliqua natu propinqua, cuius probatis spectatisque moribus omnis eiusdem familiae suboles committeretur; coram qua neque dicere fas erat quod turpe dictu, neque facere quod inhonestum factu videretur. Ac non studia modo curasque, sed remissiones etiam lususque puerorum sanctitate quadam ac verecundia temperabat. Sic Corneliam Gracchorum, sic Aureliam Caesaris, sic Atiam Augusti [matrem] praefuisse educationibus ac produxisse principes liberos accepimus. Quae disciplina ac severitas eo pertinebat ut sincera et integra et nullis pravitatibus detorta unius cuiusque natura toto statim pectore arriperet artes honestas, et sive ad rem militarem sive ad iuris scientiam sive ad eloquentiae studium inclinasset, id solum ageret, id universum hauriret.* See Dixon, 1988 on the Roman mother.
78 Pliny the Younger, *Letters* 7.24.
79 Pliny the Younger, *Letters* 8.14.6; see also Plutarch, *Cato the Elder* 20 and *Aemilius Paullus* 6. See Eyben, 1993, pp. 124–127 on rhetorical education and *controversiae*, many of which included medical examples, and pp. 131–132 on medical education as part of the curriculum for young men.
80 Tacitus, *A Dialogue on Oratory* 34; Cicero, *On Friendship* 1; Cicero, *In Defence of Caelius* 11.
81 On Roman girlhood, see Caldwell, 2015; on Roman female education, see Hemelrijk, 1999.
82 Plutarch, *Cato the Elder* 20 (trans. B. Perrin): γενομένου δὲ τοῦ παιδὸς οὐδὲν ἦν ἔργον οὕτως ἀναγκαῖον, εἰ μή τι δημόσιον, ὡς μὴ παρεῖναι τῇ γυναικὶ λουούσῃ τὸ βρέφος καὶ σπαργανούσῃ. αὐτὴ γὰρ ἔτρεφεν ἰδίῳ γάλακτι· πολλάκις δὲ καὶ τὰ τῶν δούλων παιδάρια τῷ μαστῷ προσιεμένη κατεσκεύαζεν εὔνοιαν ἐκ τῆς συντροφίας πρὸς τὸν υἱόν. ἐπεὶ δὲ ἤρξατο συνιέναι, παραλαβὼν αὐτὸς ἐδίδασκε γράμματα, καίτοι χαρίεντα δοῦλον εἶχε γραμματιστὴν ὄνομα Χίλωνα, πολλοὺς διδάσκοντα παῖδας. οὐκ ἠξίου δὲ τὸν υἱόν, ὥς φησιν αὐτός, ὑπὸ δούλου κακῶς ἀκούειν ἢ τοῦ ὠτὸς ἀνατείνεσθαι μανθάνοντα βράδιον, οὐδέ γε μαθήματος τηλικούτου τῷ δούλῳ χάριν ὀφείλειν, ἀλλ᾽ αὐτὸς μὲν ἦν γραμματιστής, αὐτὸς δὲ νομοδιδάκτης, αὐτὸς δὲ γυμναστής, οὐ μόνον ἀκοντίζειν οὐδ᾽ ὁπλομαχεῖν οὐδ᾽ ἱππεύειν διδάσκων τὸν υἱόν, ἀλλὰ καὶ τῇ χειρὶ πὺξ παίειν καὶ καῦμα καὶ ψῦχος ἀνέχεσθαι καὶ τὰ δινώδη καὶ τραχύνοντα τοῦ ποταμοῦ διανηχόμενον ἀποβιάζεσθαι. καὶ τὰς ἱστορίας δὲ συγγράψαι φησιν αὐτὸς ἰδίᾳ χειρὶ καὶ μεγάλοις γράμμασιν, ὅπως οἴκοθεν ὑπάρχοι τῷ παιδὶ πρὸς ἐμπειρίαν τῶν παλαιῶν καὶ πατρίων ὠφελεῖσθαι· τὰ δ᾽ αἰσχρὰ τῶν ῥημάτων οὐχ ἧττον εὐλαβεῖσθαι τοῦ παιδὸς παρόντος ἢ τῶν ἱερῶν παρθένων, ἃς Ἑστιάδας καλοῦσι· συλλούσασθαι δὲ μηδέποτε . . . Οὕτω δὲ καλὸν ἔργον εἰς ἀρετὴν τῷ Κάτωνι πλάττοντι καὶ δημιουργοῦντι τὸν υἱόν, ἐπεὶ τὰ τῆς προθυμίας ἦν ἄμεμπτα καὶ δι᾽ εὐφυΐαν ὑπήκουεν ἡ ψυχή, τὸ δὲ σῶμα μαλακώτερον ἐφαίνετο τοῦ πονεῖν, ὑπανῆκεν αὐτῷ τὸ σύντονον ἄγαν καὶ κεκολασμένον τῆς διαίτης.

83 McWilliam, 2013, p. 264.
84 Plautus, *Mostellaria* 91–151.
85 Soranus, *Gynaecology* 2.11–17.
86 See for example Plutarch, *Consolation to his Wife* 2 on his daughter Timoxena's interactions with her nurse.
87 Soranus, *Gynaecology* 2.18.
88 Soranus, *Gynaecology* 2.38–40; Pseudo-Plutarch, *The Education of Children* 3; Oribasius, *Collections* 51.20.28; Dio Chrysostom, *Orations* 4.74.
89 Martial, *Epigrams* 11.39.1–2; Libanius, *Orations* 58.8–9, 10; Suetonius, *Nero* 36.2; Epictetus, *The Handbook* 3.19.5; Suetonius, *Divine Augustus* 44.2; Valerius Maximus, *Memorable Deeds and Sayings* 3.1.2.
90 Plutarch, *Advice on Keeping Well* 15.
91 Fronto, *Correspondence* (Marcus Aurelius) i.2 (trans. C. R. Haines): *Vel quomodo istam necessitatem meam durissimam condigne incusavero, quae me istic ita animo anxio tantaque sollicitudine praepedito adligatum adtinet, neque me sinit ad meum Frontonem, ad meam pulcherrimam animam confestim percurrere, praesertim in huiusmodi eius valetudine prope accedere, manus tenere, ipsum denique illum pedem, quantum sine incommodo fieri possit, adtrectare sensim, in balneo fovere, ingredienti manum subicere?*
92 Fronto, *Correspondence* (Lucius Verus) ii.7.3 (trans. C. R. Haines): *Valetudini meae curandae ita semper studuit, tantam omni tempore etiam operam dedit, ut excubaret etiam aegro mihi et, ubi meis ego uti manibus per valetudinem non possem, manu sua cibos ad os meum adferret*
93 Cicero, *Letters to Quintus* 12.2–3 (II.9.2–3).
94 Seneca the Younger, *Moral Epistles* 1.65, 78.
95 Fronto, *Correspondence* (Marcus Aurelius) iv.2.
96 Aulus Gellius, *Attic Nights* 2.26, 19.10.
97 See for example Cicero, *Letters to Atticus* 247 (XII.10); Pliny the Younger, *Letters* 5.19.
98 Tacitus, *Annals* 63; Suetonius, *Tiberius* 40 states that 20,000 people were killed.
99 *Digest* 38.1.1, 1.2, 1.16, 2.1, 31, 38. On *operae*, see Bradley, 1987, p. 81; Mouritsen, 2011, pp. 224–227.
100 *Digest* 38.1.26.
101 *Digest* 38.1.27.
102 Cicero, *In Defence of Cluentius* 178.
103 Lucilius 992, 1056; Ovid, *Art of Love* 3.641–642; Seneca the Younger, *Consolation to Marcia* 16.6; Juvenal, *Satires* 6.235.
104 Livy, *From the Founding of the City* 25.18.4.
105 Livy, *From the Founding of the City* 2.15.
106 Livy, *From the Founding of the City* 8.18; Valerius Maximus, *Memorable Deeds and Sayings* 2.5.3.
107 For a general overview of cases attested in ancient literature, see Kaufman, 1932.
108 On the ancient stepmother, see Watson, 1995; on the Roman stepmother, see Gray-Fow, 1988; on the blended Roman family, see Bradley, 1987.
109 Pliny the Elder, *Natural History* 29.8.15; Plutarch, *Cato the Elder* 23.4. See also Astin, 1978, pp. 183–184; Boscherini, 1993.
110 Varro, *On Agriculture* 2.5.18 (trans. W. D. Hooper and H. B. Ash). See also White, 1973.
111 Varro, *On Agriculture* 1.4.5 (trans. W. D. Hooper and H. B. Ash): *Non hic Varro noster, cum Corcyrae esset exercitus ac classis et omnes domus repletae essent aegrotis ac funeribus, immisso fenestris novis aquilone et obstructis pestilentibus ianuaque permutata ceteraque eius generis diligentia suos comites ac familiam incolumes reduxit?*
112 Nutton, 2013, p. 165.
113 Varro, *On Agriculture* 1.16.4.
114 Varro, *On Agriculture* 2.1.21.

115 Varro, *On Agriculture* 2.10.10 (trans. W. D. Hooper and H. B. Ash): *Quae ad valitudi-nem pertinent hominum ac pecoris et sine medico curari possunt, magistrum scripta habere oportet*. See for example 1.69.3, in which a man is stabbed and the physician called to deal with the situation.

116 Varro, *On Agriculture* 2.2.20; 2.3.8; 2.5.18; 2.7.16; 2.10.10.

117 Varro, *On Agriculture* 1.22.1.

118 Columella, *On Agriculture* 11.1.4 (trans. E. S. Forster and E. Heffner): *Quisquis autem destinabitur huic negotio, sit oportet idem scientissimus robustissimusque, ut et doceat subiectos, et ipse commode faciat quae praecipit. Siquidem nihil recte sine exemplo docetur, aut discitur praestatque villicum magistrum esse operariorum, non discipulum, cum etiam de patrefamiliae prisci moris exemplum Cato dixerit: 'Male agitur cum domino, quem villicus docet'*.

119 Columella, *On Agriculture* 11.1.22 and 12 preface 10.

120 Columella, *On Agriculture* 5.1.1.

121 Baker, 2002.

Conclusion

Bitterly chafing, Aeneas stood propped on his mighty spear, amid a great con-
course of warriors along with sorrowing Iülus, himself unmoved by their tears.
The aged healer [Iapyx], with robe rolled back, and girt in Paeonian fashion, with
healing hand and Phoebus' potent herbs works hard – in vain; in vain with his hand
he pulls at the arrow, and with gripping tongs tugs at the steel. No Fortune guides
his path, no help does Apollo's counsel give; and more and more the fierce alarm
swells over the plains, and disaster draws closer. Now they see the sky supported
on columns of dust; on come the horsemen, and shafts fall thick in the middle
of the camp. The dismal cry rises to heaven, of men that fight and men that fall
beneath the stern War God's hand. At this Venus, shaken by her son's cruel pain,
with a mother's care plucks from Cretan Ida dittany clothed with downy leaves and
purple flower; that herb is not unknown to wild goats, when winged arrows have
lodged in their flank. This Venus carried down, her face veiled in dim mist; this
she steeps with secret healing in river water poured into a bright-brimming ewer,
and sprinkles ambrosia's healing juices and fragrant panacea. With this water aged
Iapyx bathed the wound, unwitting; and suddenly, in truth, all pain fled from the
body, all blood was staunched deep in the wound. And now, following his hand,
with no force applied, the arrow fell out, and new strength returned, as it was
before.[1]

I opened this study into Roman domestic medical practice with a quotation from
Horace, and now I shall close it with one from his contemporary Virgil. At first
glance, this episode from the *Aeneid*, which is depicted in a fresco that was originally located in the triclinium of the House of Vedius Siricus and Vedius Nummianus from Pompeii (VII.1.47) but is now in the Naples National Archaeological
Museum (inv. 9009) (see Figure 5.1), seems to have little to do with domestic
medical practice. If it can be utilised in the service of reconstructing ancient
Roman medicine at all, surely what it offers insight into is military medicine, and
the rough-and-ready treatment that soldiers might receive on or adjacent to the
battlefield.[2] However, if we take a closer look, it becomes apparent that there is
much of relevance and significance to our purposes here, and if anything, this episode exemplifies for us, one final time, the plurality of Roman medical practice,
particularly Roman domestic medical practice.

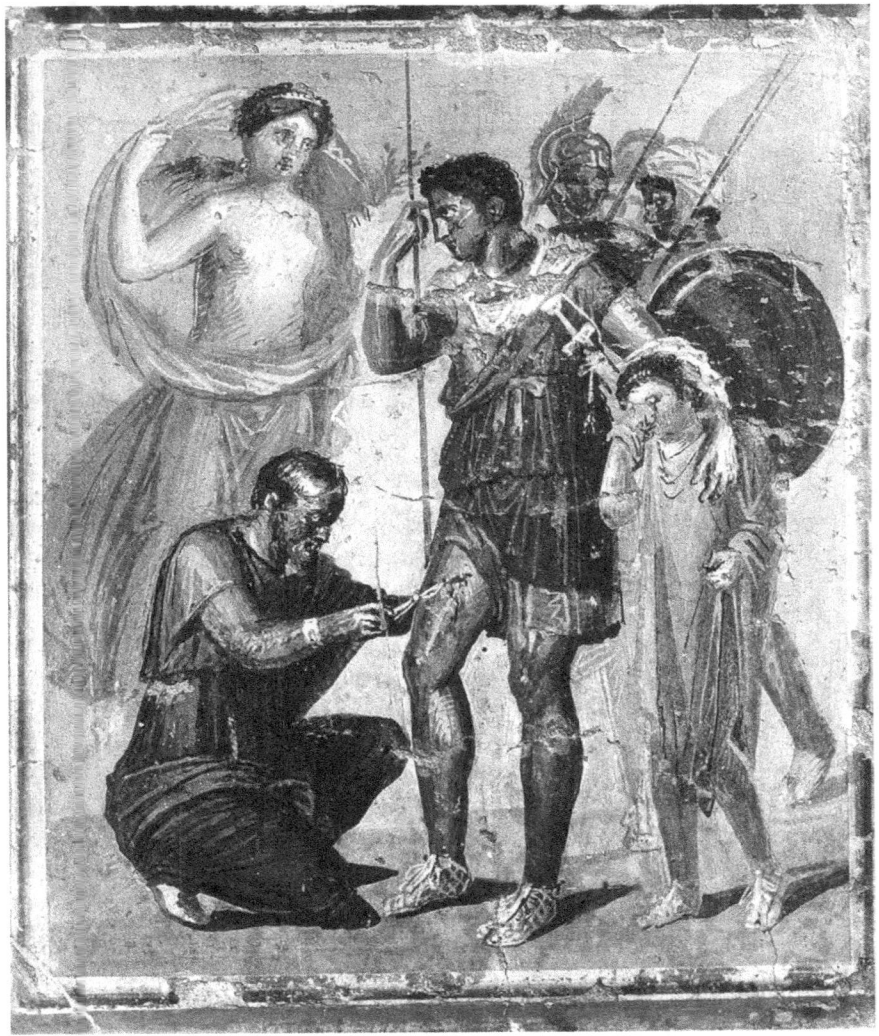

Figure 5.1 A fresco depicting Aeneas being treated by Iapyx, from the *triclinium* of the House of Vedius Siricus and Vedius Nummianus in Pompeii (VII.1.47), dating from the first century CE.

Source: Image courtesy of the Wellcome Library.

In the first instance, Iapyx is in possession of medical knowledge, skill and expertise because of a choice that he made regarding ensuring the health and well-being of a member of his family:

> Dearest beyond others to Phoebus, to whom once Apollo himself, smitten with love's sting, gladly offered his own arts, his own powers – his augury, his lyre, and his swift arrows. [Iapyx], to defer the fate of a father sick unto death, chose rather to know the virtues of herbs and the practice of healing, and to ply, inglorious, the silent arts.[3]

Presumably, once Apollo had bestowed his gifts, Iapyx proceeded to treat his father Iasus to the best of his newly acquired abilities, demonstrating a similar level of *pietas* to Aeneas in his care of Anchises. In this case, he demonstrates both pharmacological and surgical expertise, although to no avail. Since Iapyx's attempts at treatment meet with failure, Aeneas' mother Venus intervenes. She not only produces an exotic herb, dittany from Mount Ida on Crete, a simple remedy, but uses it as a base for creating a more complicated one with several ingredients, a compound remedy. This potion succeeds first in staunching and coagulating the blood pouring from Aeneas' wound, then in healing that wound entirely. While the healing event is miraculous rather than realistic, its components are informative.

Virgil takes care to attribute Venus' intervention to maternal feeling rather than to divine patronage; she is moved by Aeneas' cries of pain and the severity of his injury, just as we might expect any member of a Roman household or family to be when faced with a similar situation. Venus, who, as we have seen, was particularly connected with gardens and plants, acts as a Roman *mater familias* or *matrona* in utilising her knowledge of the medicinal properties of plants and of the way to prepare a medicinal remedy in tending to her son.[4] She and Iapyx work together (albeit unwittingly, on the part of Iapyx) to treat Aeneas, and so not only demonstrate how so-called professional and amateur medical practitioners might collaborate within a household to treat one of its members when sick or injured, but also how the knowledge, skill and expertise possessed by the amateur medical practitioner might ultimately prevail.

In the past, numerous scholars have acknowledged that domestic medical practice was a fundamental component of Roman medicine but their discussions have tended to go no further than this. What I have attempted to do in this monograph is shine a light on this understudied aspect not just of ancient medicine but also of ancient social and cultural history. I have argued that domestic medical practice was not just the foundation of the ancient medical marketplace but also represented the ancient medical marketplace in a microcosm.

In Chapter 1, I explored the social and cultural milieu in which domestic medical practice took place and argued that Romans were not only well-informed about what was necessary to attain good health and well-being but also, thanks to civic infrastructure and amenities such as public parks and bathhouses, and the ready availability of a wide range of local and exotic foodstuffs, able to access the tools necessary to enable them to do so, whether they were a member of the senatorial, equestrian or decurion orders or the plebeian order. In Chapter 2, I surveyed the ways in which the Roman house, whether *villa, domus, insula* or *casa*, and its garden were considered to contribute, both positively and negatively, to the health and well-being of its occupants. According to the sole surviving ancient architectural treatise, concerns over health were fundamental to planning and executing building programs, and further to this, certain areas of the house, the garden in particular, were thought to be both spaces and places that were particularly beneficial to health. Additionally, household produce could be utilised in the service of health and well-being in a variety of ways, as ingredients in food, drink and medicaments, as medical equipment and as a means of augmenting space through appearance and fragrance. In Chapter 3, I examined the people that would have been responsible for undertaking domestic medical practice, and explored how this practice affected the structure and organisation of the household. Finally, in Chapter 4 I assessed how medical knowledge was transmitted in Roman society, and suggested that there were a variety of formal and informal pathways by which medical knowledge was transmitted from outside the household to inside it, and once inside it between the members of the household, both free and slave.

Inevitably, the examples and evidence I have utilised throughout this study are not brand-new discoveries. However, the ways in which I have attempted to utilise them are something of a departure from their previous treatments. There is a considerable amount of circumstantial literary, documentary, archaeological and bioarchaeological evidence that can be integrated as a means of constructing a preliminary picture of Roman domestic medical practice, and thanks to the constant application of new techniques more is appearing all the time. It is my hope that this work will serve as encouragement to future historians, archaeologists and bioarchaeologists interested in exploring health and well-being in past societies.

Notes

1 Virgil, *Aeneid* 12.398–424 (trans. H. R. Fairclough, G. P. Goold): *Stabat acerba fremens ingentem nixus in hastam Aeneas magno iuvenum et maerentis Iuli concursu, lacrimis immobilis. ille retorto Paeonium in morem senior succinctus amictu multa manu medica Phoebique potentibus herbis nequiquam trepidat, nequiquam spicula dextra sollicitat prensatque tenaci forcipe ferrum. nulla viam Fortuna regit, nihil auctor Apollo subvenit, et scevus campis magis ac magis horror crebrescit propiusque malum est. iam pulvere caelum stare vident: subeunt equites et spicula castris densa cadunt mediis. it tristis ad aethera clamor bellantum iuvenum et duro sub Marte cadentum. Hic Venus indigno nati concussa dolore dictamnum genetrix Cretaea carpit ab Ida, puberibus caulem foliis et flore comantem purpureo; non illa feris incognita capris gramina, cum tergo volucres haesere sagittae. hoc Venus obscuro faciem circumdata nimbo detulit, hoc fusum labris splendentibus amnem inficit occulte medicans, spargitque salubris ambrosiae sucos et odoriferam panaceam. fovit ea vulnus lympha longaevus Iapyx ignorans, subitoque omnis de corpore fugit quippe dolor, omnis stetit imo vulnere sanguis. iamque secuta manum, nullo cogente, sagitta excidit, atque novae rediere in pristina vires.*
2 For full discussion of this, see Salazar, 2000.

3 Virgil, *Aeneid* 12.391–397 (trans. H. R. Fairclough, G. P. Goold): *Iamque aderat Phoebo ante alios dilectus Iapyx Iasides, acri quondam cui captus amore ipse suas artis, sua munera, laetus Apollo augurium citharamque dabat celerisque sagittas. ille, ut depositi proferret fata parentis, scire potestates herbarum usumque medendi maluit et mutas agitare inglorius artis.*

4 Varro, *On Agriculture* 1.1.6; Pliny the Elder, *Natural History* 19.19.50; Anonymous, *Venus' Rose Garden* 13.1–2.

Bibliography

Alföld, G. (1984) *Römische Sozialgeschichte* (Weisbaden: F. Steiner).

Alföld, G. (1986) *Die Römische Gesellschaft: Auswählte Beiträge* (Stuttgart: F. Steiner Verlag Wiesbaden).

Allbutt, T. C. (1921) *Greek Medicine in Rome* (London: Macmillan and Co.).

Allison, P. M. (1997) 'Artefact Distribution and Spatial Function in Pompeian Houses', in Rawson, B. and Weaver, P. (eds.) *The Roman Family in Italy: Status, Sentiment, Space* (Oxford: Clarendon Press), pp. 321–354.

Allison, P. M. (2004) *Pompeian Households: An Analysis of the Material Culture* (Los Angeles, CA: Cotsen Institute of Archaeology).

Allison, P. M. (2007) 'Engendering Roman Domestic Space', *British School at Athens Studies* 15, pp. 343–350.

Allison, P. M. (2011) 'Soldiers' Families in the Early Roman Empire', in Rawson, B. (ed.) *A Companion to Families in the Greek and Roman Worlds* (Malden, MA: Wiley-Blackwell), pp. 169–182.

Allison, P. M. (2013) *People and Spaces in Roman Military Bases* (Cambridge and New York, NY: Cambridge University Press).

Allison, P. M. (2015) ' "Everyday" Eating and Drinking in Roman Domestic Contexts', in Di Castro, A. A. and Hope, C. A. (eds.) *Housing and Habitat in the Ancient Mediterranear: Cultural and Environmental Responses* (Leuven, Paris and Bristol, CT: Peeters), pp. 267–281.

Amuncsen, D. W. (1974) 'Romanticizing the Ancient Medical Profession: The Characterization of the Physician in the Graeco-Roman Novel', *BHM* 48.3, pp. 320–337.

André, J. M. (1966) *L'otium dans la vie morale et intellectuale romaine, des origines à l'époque augustéenne* (Paris: Presses Universitaires de France).

André, J.-M. (1981) *L'alimentation et la Cuisine à Rome* (Paris: C. Klincksieck).

Argetsinger, K. (1992) 'Birthday Rituals: Friends and Patrons in Roman Poetry and Cult', *CA* 11.2, pp. 175–193.

Artelt, W. (1968) *Studien zur Geschichte der Begriffe 'Heilmittel' und 'Gift': Urzeit. Homer, Corpus Hippocraticum* (Darmstadt: Wissenschaftliche Buchgesellschaft).

Astin, A. E. (1978) *Cato the Censor* (Oxford and New York, NY: Oxford University Press).

Axtell, H. L. (1907) *The Deification of Abstract Ideas in Roman Literature and Inscriptions* (Chicago, IL: University of Chicago Press).

Baird, J. A. and Taylor, C. (2011) *Ancient Graffiti in Context* (London and New York, NY: Routledge).

Baker, P. A. (2002) 'Diagnosing Some Ills: The Archaeology, Literature and History of Roman Medicine', in Baker, P. A. and Carr, G. (eds.) *Practitioners, Practices and Patients: New Approaches to Medical Archaeology and Anthropology* (Oxford: Oxbow), pp. 16–29.

Baker, P. A. (2004) 'Roman Medical Instruments: Archaeological Interpretations of their Possible "Non-functional" Uses', *SHM* 71.1, pp. 3–21.

Baker, P. A. (2013) *The Archaeology of Medicine in the Greco-Roman World* (Cambridge: Cambridge University Press).

Bakker, J. T. (1994) *Living and Working with the Gods: Studies of Evidence for Private Religion and Its Material Environment in the City of Ostia (100–500 AD)* (Amsterdam: J. C. Gieben).

Barrett, A. A. (2002) *Livia: First Lady of Imperial Rome* (New Haven, CT and London: Yale University Press).

Barton, C. A. (1995) *Sorrows of the Ancient Romans: The Gladiator and the Monster* (Princeton, NJ: Princeton University Press).

Barton, I. M. (1996) *Roman Domestic Buildings* (Exeter: University of Exeter Press).

Bassani, M. and Ghedini, F. (2011) *Religionem Significare. Aspetti Storico-Religiosi, Strutturali, Iconografici e Materiali dei Sacra Privata: Atti dell'Incontro di Studio, Padova, 8–9 Giugno 2009* (Rome: Edizioni Quasar).

Basso, P. and Ghedini, F. (2003) *Subterranea e Domus: Ambienti Residenziali e di Servizio Nell'Edilizia Privata Romana* (Verona: Cierre Edizioni).

Bates, D. (1995) 'Scholarly Ways of Knowing: An Introduction', in Bates, D. (ed.) *Knowledge and the Scholarly Medical Traditions* (Cambridge: Cambridge University Press), pp. 1–22.

Baykan, D. (2008) *Allianoi Tip Aletleri = Studia ad Orientem Antiquum* (Istanbul: Institutum Turcicum Scientiae Antiquitas).

Beagon, M. (1992) *Roman Nature: The Thought of Pliny the Elder* (Oxford and New York, NY: Clarendon Press).

Becker, J. A. (2006) 'The Villa delle Grotte at Grottarossa and the Prehistory of Roman Villas', *JRA* 19, pp. 213–220.

Bendlin, A. (2000) 'Looking Beyond the Civic Compromise: Religious Pluralism in Late Republican Rome', in Bispham, E. and Smith, C. (eds.) *Religion in Archaic and Republican Rome and Italy: Evidence and Experience* (Edinburgh: Edinburgh University Press), pp. 115–135.

Bendlin, A. (2007) 'Purity and Pollution', in Ogden, D. (ed.) *A Companion to Greek Religion* (Malden, MA: Wiley-Blackwell), pp. 178–189.

Bergdolt, K. (2008) *Wellbeing: A Cultural History of Healthy Living* (Cambridge and Malden, MA: Polity).

Bergmann, B. (2002) 'Art and Nature in the Villa at Oplontis', in McGinn, T. A. (ed.) *Pompeian Brothels, Pompeii's Ancient History, Mirrors and Mysteries, Art and Nature at Oplontis & the Herculaneum "Basilica"* (Portsmouth, RI: *JRA* Supplement 47), pp. 87–121.

Bergmann, B. (2008) 'Staging the Supernatural: Interior Gardens of Pompeian Houses', in Mattusch, C. C. (ed.) *Pompeii and the Roman Villa: Art and Culture around the Bay of Naples* (New York, NY: Binocular), pp. 53–69.

Bernhardt, P. (2008) *Gods and Goddesses in the Garden: Greco-Roman Mythology and the Scientific Names of Plants* (New Brunswick, NJ and London: Rutgers University Press).

Bernstein, F. (2007) 'Pompeian Women', in Dobbins, J. J. and Foss, P. W. (eds.) *The World of Pompeii* (London and New York, NY: Routledge), pp. 526–537.

Berry, J. (1997) 'Household Artefacts: Towards a Reinterpretation of Roman Domestic Space', in Laurence, R. and Wallace-Hadrill, A. (eds.) *Domestic Space in the Roman World: Pompeii and Beyond* (Portsmouth, RI: *JRA* Supplement 22), pp. 183–195.

Berry, J. (2007) '*Instrumentum Domesticum* – A Case Study', in Dobbins, J. J. and Foss, P. W. (eds.) *The World of Pompeii* (London and New York, NY: Routledge), pp. 292–301.

Bettini, M. (2013) 'The *Lar Familiaris* of the Romans: A "Simple" God', in Katajala-Peltomaa, S. and Vuolanto, V. (eds.) *Religious Participation in Ancient and Medieval Societies: Rituals, Interaction and Identity* (Rome: Acta Instituti Romani Finlandiae), pp. 25–38.

Bisel, S. C. (1988) 'Nutrition in First Century Herculaneum', *Anthropologie* 26.1, pp. 61–66.

Bisel, S. C. and Bisel, J. F. (2002) 'Health and Nutrition at Herculaneum: An Examination of Human Skeletal Remains', in Jashemski, W. F. and Meyer, F. G. (eds.) *The Natural History of Pompeii* (Cambridge: Cambridge University Press), pp. 451–475.

Bivins, R., Marland, H. and Tomes, N. (2016) 'Histories of Medicine in the Household: Recovering Practice and "Reception"', *SHM* 29.4, pp. 669–675.

Blake, S. (2012) 'Now You See Them: Slaves and Other Objects as Elements of the Roman Master', *Helios* 39.2, pp. 193–211.

Blake, S. (2016) '*In Manus*: Pliny's Letters and the Arts of Mastery', in Keith, A. and Edmundson, J. (eds.) *Roman Literary Cultures: Domestic Politics, Revolutionary Poetics, Civic Spectacle* (Toronto, Buffalo, NY and London: University of Toronto Press), pp. 89–101.

Bliquez, L. J. (1994) *Roman Surgical Instruments and Other Minor Objects in the National Archaeological Museum of Naples* (Mainz: Verlag Philipp von Zabern).

Bliquez, L. J. (2015) *The Tools of Asclepius: Surgical Instruments in Greek and Roman Times* (Leiden: Brill).

Bodel, J. (2008) 'Cicero's Minerva, *Penates*, and the Mother of the *Lares*: An Outline of Roman Domestic Religion', in Bodel, J. and Olyan, S. M. (eds.) *Household and Family Religion in Antiquity* (Malden, MA and Oxford: Wiley-Blackwell), pp. 248–275.

Bond, S. E. (2015) '"As Trainers for the Healthy": Massage Therapists, Anointers, and Healing in the Late Latin West', *JLA* 8.2, pp. 386–404.

Borgognini Tarli, S. M. and Mazzotta, F. (1986) 'Physical Anthropology of Italy from the Bronze Age to the Barbaric Age', in Kandler-Palsson, B. (ed.) *Ethnogenese Europäischer Völker* (Stuttgart: F. Steiner Verlag Wiesbaden), pp. 147–172.

Borgongino, M. (2006) *Archeobotanica: Reperti Vegetali da Pompei e dal Territorio Vesuviano* (Rome: L'Erma di Bretschneider).

Boscherini, S. (1993) 'La Medicina in Catone e Varrone', *ANRW* II 37.1, pp. 729–755.

Boyce, G. K. (1937) 'Corpus of the Lararia of Pompeii', *MAAR* 14, pp. 5–112.

Bradley, K. R. (1986) 'Wet-nursing at Rome: A Study in Social Relations', in Rawson, B. (ed.) *The Family in Ancient Rome: New Perspectives* (Ithaca, NY: Cornell University Press), pp. 201–229.

Bradley, K. R. (1987) *Slaves and Masters in the Roman Empire: A Study in Social Control* (Oxford and New York, NY: Oxford University Press).

Bradley, K. R. (1991) *Discovering the Roman Family* (Oxford and New York, NY: Oxford University Press).

Bradley, K. R. (1994) *Slavery and Society at Rome* (Cambridge: Cambridge University Press).

Bradley, K. R. (2005) 'The Roman Child in Sickness and in Health', in George, M. (ed.) *The Roman Family in the Empire: Rome, Italy, and Beyond* (Oxford and New York, NY: Oxford University Press), pp. 67–92.

Bradley, M. (2002) "It All Comes Out in the Wash': Looking Harder at the Roman *fullonica*', *JRA* 15, pp. 20–44.

Bradley, M. (2009) *Colour and Meaning in Ancient Rome* (Cambridge and New York, NY: Cambridge University Press).

Bradley, M. (2012) 'Approaches to Pollution and Propriety', in Bradley, M. and Stow, K. (eds.) *Rome, Pollution and Propriety: Dirt, Disease and Hygiene in the Eternal City from Antiquity to Modernity* (Cambridge: Cambridge University Press), pp. 11–40.

Bradley, M. and Stow, K. (eds.) (2012) *Rome, Pollution and Propriety: Dirt, Disease and Hygiene in the Eternal City from Antiquity to Modernity* (Cambridge: Cambridge University Press).

Brand, N. (2008) 'The *Sanus Homo* in the *De Medicina* of Celsus', in Cilliers, L. (ed.) *Asklepios: Studies on Ancient Medicine* (Bloemfontein: Acta Classica: Proceedings of the Classical Association of South Africa Supplementum 2), pp. 29–48.

Brun, J.-P. (2000) 'The Production of Perfumes in Antiquity: The Cases of Delos and Paestum', *AJA* 104.2, pp. 277–308.

Caldwell, L. (2015) *Roman Girlhood and the Fashioning of Femininity* (Cambridge: Cambridge University Press)

Campbell, B. (2000) *The Writings of the Roman Land Surveyors: Introduction, Text, Translation and Commentary* (London: Roman Society).

Cañizares, P. P. (2010) 'The Importance of Having Medical Knowledge as a Layman. The Hippocratic Treatise Affections in the Context of the Hippocratic Corpus', in Horstmanshoff, M. (ed.) *Hippocrates and Medical Education: Selected Papers Read at the XIIth International Hippocrates Colloquium, Universiteit Leiden, 24–26th August 2005* (Leiden: Brill), pp. 87–100.

Carandini, A. (1985) *Settefinestre: Una Villa Schiavistica Nell'Etruria Romana* (Modena: Edizioni Panini).

Carlsen, J. (1993) 'The Vilica and Roman Estate Management', in De Neeve, P. W. and Sancisi-Weerdenburg, H. (eds.) *De Agricultura in Memoriam Pieter Willem De Neeve (1945–1990)* (Amsterdam: J. C. Gieben), pp. 197–205.

Carlsen, J. (1995) Vilici *and Roman Estate Managers Until AD 284* (Rome: L'Erma di Bretschneider).

Carlsen, J. (2011) 'Two Female Senatorial Households in Augustan Rome: Domitia Calvina and her Mother', in Whittaker, H. (ed.) *In Memoriam: Commemoration, Communal Memory and Gender Values in the Ancient Graeco-Roman World* (Newcastle Upon Tyne: Cambridge Scholars), pp. 78–90.

Carratelli, G. P. and Baldassarre, I. (1990) *Pompei: Pitture e Mosaici* (Rome: Istituto della Enciclopedia Italiana).

Carroll, M. (2003) *Earthly Paradises: Ancient Gardens in History and Archaeology* (Los Angeles, CA: J. Paul Getty Museum).

Carroll, M. (2012) 'Contextualising Art and Nature', in Borg, B. (ed.) *A Companion to Roman Art* (Malden, MA and Oxford: Wiley-Blackwell), pp. 533–552.

Carroll-Spillecke, M. (1989) *Kēpos: Der Antike Griechische Garten* (Munich: Deutscher Kunstverlag).

Carroll-Spillecke, M. (1992) 'The Gardens of Greece from Homeric to Roman Times', *JGH* 12, pp. 84–101.

Carroll, M. and Graham, E. J. (eds.) (2014) *Infant Health and Death in Roman Italy and Beyond* (Portsmouth, RI: JRA Supplement 96).

Catalano, P. and Minozzi, S. (2001) 'Le necropoli di Roma: Il Contributo dell'Antropologia', *RM* 108, pp. 353–381.

Ciaraldi, M. (2000) 'Drug Preparation in Evidence? An Unusual Plant and Bone Assemblage from the Pompeian Countryside, Italy', *VHA* 9.2, pp. 91–98.

Ciaraldi, M. (2002) 'The Interpretation of Medicinal Plants in the Archaeological Context: Some Case-Studies from Pompeii', in Arnott, R. (ed.) *The Archaeology of Medicine* (Oxford: Archaeopress) pp. 81–85.

Ciaraldi, M. (2007) *People and Plants in Ancient Pompeii: A New Approach to Urbanism from the Microscope Room: The Use of Plant Resources at Pompeii and in the Pompeian Area from the 6th Century BC to AD 79* (London: Accordia Research Institute).

Clarke, J. R. (1991) *The Houses of Roman Italy 100 BC – AD 250: Ritual, Space, and Decoration* (Berkeley, CA: University of California Press).

Clarke, J. R. (2003) *Art in the Lives of Ordinary Romans: Visual Representation and Non-Elite Viewers in Italy, 100 BC-AD 315* (Berkeley, CA: University of California Press).

Cokayne, K. (2003) *Experiencing Old Age in Ancient Rome* (London and New York, NY: Routledge).

Cokayne, K. (2007) 'Age and Aristocratic Self-Identity: Activities for the Elderly', in Harlow, M. and Laurence, R. (eds.) *Age and Aging in the Roman Empire* (Portsmouth, RI: *JRA* Supplement 65), pp. 209–220.

Collard, F. and Samama, E. (eds.) (2006) *Pharmacopoles et Apothicaires: Les 'Pharmaciens' de l'Antiquité au Grand Siècle* (Paris: L'Harmattan).

Cooper, K. (2007) 'Closely Watched Households: Visibility, Exposure and Private Power in the Roman "Domus" ', *P&P* 197.1, pp. 3–33.

Cova, E. (2013) 'Cupboards, Closets, and Shelves: Storage in the Pompeian House', *Phoenix* 67.3–4, pp. 373–391.

Craik, E. M. (1995) 'Diet, Diaita and Dietetics', in Powell, A. (ed.) *The Greek World* (London and New York, NY: Routledge), pp. 387–402.

Crook, J. (1967) '*Patria Potestas*', *CQ* 17.1, pp. 113–122.

Cruse, A. (2004) *Roman Medicine* (Stroud: Tempus).

Curtis, R. I. (1991) *Garum and Salsamenta: Production and Commerce in Materia Medica* (Leiden: Brill).

Curtis, R. I. (2008) 'Food Processing and Preparation', in Oleson, J. P. (ed.) *The Oxford Handbook of Engineering and Technology in the Classical World* (Oxford and New York, NY: Oxford University Press), pp. 369–392.

Cuvigny, H. (1996) 'The Amount of Wages Paid to the Quarry-Workers at Mons Claudianus', *JRS* 86, pp. 139–145.

Dalby, A. (1998, reissued 2010) *Cato On Farming De Agricultura: A Modern Translation with Commentary* (Totnes: Prospect Books).

Dalby, A. (2000) *Empire of Pleasures: Luxury and Indulgence in the Roman World* (London: Routledge).

Dalby, A. (2003) *Food in the Ancient World from A to Z* (London: Routledge).

D'Ambra, E. (2006) 'Imitations of Life: Style, Theme and a Sculptural Collection in the Iso a Sacra Necropolis, Ostia', in D'Ambra, E. and Métraux, G. P. R. (eds.) *The Art of Citizens, Soldiers and Freedmen in the Roman World* (Oxford: Archaeopress), pp. 73–89.

Daser, V. (ed.) (2004) *Naissance et Petite Enfance dans l'Antiquité: Actes de Colloque de Fribourg, 28 November – 1 Décember 2001* (Fribourg and Göttingen: Vandenhoeck and Ruprecht).

Daser, V, and Späth, T. (eds.) (2010) *Children, Memory and Family Identity in Roman Culture* (Oxford: Oxford University Press).

Davies, P. J. E. (2012) 'Pollution, Propriety and Urbanism in Republican Rome', in Bradley, M. and Stow, K. (eds.) *Rome, Pollution and Propriety: Dirt, Disease and Hygiene in the Eternal City from Antiquity to Modernity* (Cambridge: Cambridge University Press), pp. 67–80.

Day, J. (2013) *Making Senses of the Past: Towards a Sensory Archaeology* (Carbondale, IL: Southern Illinois University).

De Carolis, S. (ed.) (2009) *Ars Medica. I Ferri del Mestiere. La Domus 'del Chirurgo' di Rimini e la Chirurgia Nell'Antica Roma* (Rimini: Guaraldi).

DeLaine, J. (1999) 'Introduction: Bathing and Society', in DeLaine, J. and Johnson, D. E. (eds.) *Roman Baths and Bathing: Proceedings of the First International Conference on Roman Baths, held at Bath, England, 30 March - 4 April 1992* (Portsmouth, RI: *JRA* Supplement 37), pp. 7–16.

DeLaine, J. (2018) 'Gardens in Baths and Palaestras', in Jashemski, W. F., Gleason, K. L., Hartswick, K. J. and Malek, A.-A. (eds.) *Gardens of the Roman Empire* (Cambridge: Cambridge University Press), pp. 165–184.

de Ligt, L. and Northwood, S. (eds.) (2008) *People, Land and Politics: Demographic Developments and the Transformation of Roman Italy, 300 BC – AD 14* (Leiden: Brill).

de Marchi, A. (1896–1903) *Il Culto Private di Roma Antica: Volume 2* (Milan: Ulrico Hopeli).

Dewar, M. (2014) *Leisured Resistance: Villas, Literature and Politics in the Roman World* (London: Bloomsbury).

Dickmann, J.-A. (2011) 'Space and Social Relations in the Roman West', in Rawson, B. (ed.) *A Companion to Families in the Greek and Roman Worlds* (Malden, MA: Wiley-Blackwell), pp. 53–72.

Dilke, O. A. W. (1971) *The Roman Land Surveyors: An Introduction to the Agrimensores* (Newton Abbott: David and Charles).

Dixon, S. (1988) *The Roman Mother* (London: Croom Helm).

Dixon, S. (1991) 'The Sentimental Ideal of the Roman Family', in Rawson, B. (ed.) *Marriage, Divorce and Children in Ancient Rome* (Oxford: Clarendon Press), pp. 99–113.

Dixon, S. (1992) *The Ancient Roman Family* (Baltimore, MD and London: Johns Hopkins University Press).

Dixon, S. (1997) 'Conflict in the Roman Family', in Rawson, B. and Weaver, P. (eds.) *The Roman Family in Italy: Status, Sentiment, Space* (Canberra, New York, NY and Oxford: Clarendon Press), pp. 149–167.

Dixon, S. (2001) *Childhood, Class and Kin in the Roman World* (London and New York, NY: Routledge).

Dixon, S. (2011) 'From Ceremonial to Sexualities: A Survey of Scholarship on Roman Marriage', in Rawson, B. (ed.) *A Companion to Families in the Greek and Roman Worlds* (Malden, MA: Wiley-Blackwell), pp. 245–261.

Dolansky, F. (2011) 'Honouring the Family Dead on the Parentalia: Ceremony, Spectacle, and Memory', *Phoenix* 65.1/2, pp. 125–157.

Draycott, J. (2012) *Approaches to Healing in Roman Egypt* (Oxford: Archaeopress).

Draycott, J. (2015) 'Smelling Trees, Flowers and Herbs in the Ancient World', in Bradley, M. (ed.) *Smell and the Ancient Senses* (London: Routledge), pp. 60–73.

Draycott, J. (2016) 'Literary and Documentary Evidence for Lay Medical Practice in the Roman Republic and Empire', in Petridou, G. and Thumiger, C. (eds.) *Homo Patiens: Approaches to the Patient in the Ancient World* (Leiden: Brill), pp. 432–450.

Draycott, J. (2017) 'When Lived Ancient Religion and Lived Ancient Medicine Meet: The Household Gods, the Household Shrine and Regimen', *Religion in the Roman Empire* 3.2, pp. 164–180.

Dubourdieu, A. (1989) *Les origins et les développement du culte des Pénates à Rome* (Rome: École française de Rome).

Earle, S. (2007) 'Exploring Health', in Earle, S., Lloyd, C. E., Sidell, M., and Spurr, S. (eds.) *Theory and Research in Promoting Public Health* (London: Sage Publications), pp. 37–66.

Edlund-Berry, I. (2006) 'Healing, Health, and Well-being: Archaeological Evidence for Issues of Health Concerns in Ancient Italy', *ARG* 8.1, pp. 81–88.

Edwards, C. (1993) *The Politics of Immorality in Ancient Rome* (Cambridge and New York, NY: Cambridge University Press).

Edwards, M. (1997) 'Constructions of Physical Disability in the Ancient Greek World: The Community Concept', in Mitchell, D. T. and Snyder, S. L. (eds.) *The Body and Physical*

Difference: Discourses of Disability (Ann Arbor, MI: University of Michigan Press), pp. 35–50.

Erdkamp, P. (2005) *The Grain Market in the Roman Empire: A Social, Political, and Economic Study* (Cambridge and New York, NY: Cambridge University Press).

Eyben, E. (1993) *Restless Youth in Ancient Rome* (London and New York, NY: Routledge).

Fagan, G. G. (1999a) *Bathing in Public in the Roman World* (Ann Arbor, MI: University of Michigan Press).

Fagan, G. G. (1999b) 'Interpreting the Evidence: Did Slaves Bathe at the Baths?', in DeLaine, J. and Johnston, D. E. (eds.) *Roman Baths and Bathing* (Portsmouth, RI: *JRA* Supplement 37), pp. 25–34.

Fagan, G. G. (2006) 'Bathing for Health with Celsus and Pliny the Elder', *CQ* 56.1, pp. 190–207.

Farrar, L. (1998) *Ancient Roman Gardens* (Stroud: Sutton Publishing).

Farrar, L. (2016) *Gardens and Gardeners of the Ancient World: History, Myth and Archaeology* (Oxford: Oxbow).

Fears, J. R. (1981) 'The Cult of Virtues and Roman Imperial Ideology', *ANRW* II 17.2, pp. 827–948.

Fitzgerald, W. (2000) *Slavery in the Roman Literary Imagination* (Cambridge: Cambridge University Press).

Flemming, R. (2000) *Medicine and the Making of Roman Women: Gender, Nature, and Authority from Celsus to Galen* (Oxford: Oxford University Press).

Flemming, R. (2007) 'Women, Writing, and Medicine in the Classical World', *CQ* 57.1, pp. 257–279.

Flohr, M. (2012) 'Working and Living Under One Roof: Workshops in Pompeian Atrium Houses', in Anguissola, A. (ed.) *Privata Luxuria: Towards an Archaeology of Intimacy* (Munich: Herbert Utz Verlag), pp. 51–72.

Flory, M. B. (1984) 'Where Women Precede Men: Factors Influencing the Order of Names in Roman Epitaphs', *CJ* 79.3, pp. 216–224.

Flower, H. I. (1996) *Ancestor Masks and Aristocratic Power in Roman Culture* (Oxford: Clarendon Press).

Flower, H. I. (2017) *The Dancing Lares and the Serpent in the Garden: Religion at the Roman Street Corner* (Princeton, NJ: Princeton University Press).

Förtsch, R. (1993) *Archäologischer Kommentar zu den Villenbriefen des Jüngeren Plinius* (Mainz: Philipp von Zabern).

Foss, P. W. (1994) *Kitchens and Dining Rooms at Pompeii: The Spatial and Social Relationship of Cooking to Eating in the Roman Household* (Ann Arbor, MI: University of Michigan Unpublished PhD Thesis).

Foss, P. W. (1997) 'Watchful Lares: Roman Household Organisation and the Rituals of Cooking and Eating', in Laurence, R. and Wallace-Hadrill, A. (eds.) *Domestic Space in the Roman World: Pompeii and Beyond* (Portsmouth RI: *JRA* Supplement 22), pp. 197–218.

Frayn, J. M. (1979) *Subsistence Farming in Roman Italy* (Fontwell: Centaur Press).

Frayn, J. M. (1993) *Markets and Fairs in Roman Italy: Their Social and Economic Importance from the Second Century BC to the Third Century AD* (Oxford and New York, NY: Clarendon Press).

French, R. (1994) *Ancient Natural History: Histories of Nature* (London and New York, NY Routledge).

Fröhlich, T. (1991) *Lararien und Fassadenbilder in den Vesuvstädten: Untersuchungen zur 'Volkstümlichen' Pompejanischen Malerei* (Mainz: Philipp von Zabern).

Frost, F. (1999) 'Sausage and Meat Preservation in Antiquity', *GRBS* 40, pp. 241–252.

Gardner, J. F. (1995) 'Gender-Role Assumptions in Roman Law', *Echos du Monde Classique/Classical Views* 39, pp. 377–400.

Gardner, J. F. (1998) *Family and* Familia *in Roman Law and Life* (Oxford: Clarendon Press).

Garland, A. (1992) 'Cicero's *Familia Urbana*', *G&R* 39.2, pp. 163–172.

Garnsey, P. D. A. (1979) 'Where did Italian Peasants Live?', *CCJ* 25, pp. 1–25.

Garnsey, P. (1991) 'Child Rearing in Ancient Italy', in Kertzer, D. I. and Saller, R. P. (eds.) *The Family in Italy from Antiquity to the Present* (New Haven, CT and London: Yale University Press), pp. 48–65.

Garnsey, P. (1998) *Cities, Peasants and Food in Classical Antiquity: Essays in Social and Economic History* (Cambridge and New York, NY: Cambridge University Press).

Garnsey, P. (1999) *Food and Society in Classical Antiquity* (Cambridge: Cambridge University Press).

Gautherie, A. (2014) 'Medical Dialogue in the Books on Dietetics in the *De Medicina*: Celsus Taking Account of the Patient as a Friend and Individual', in Michaelides, D. (ed.) *Medicine and Healing in the Ancient Mediterranean World* (Oxford and Havertown, PA: Oxbow), pp. 118–121.

Gentilcore, D. (1998) *Healers and Healing in Early Modern Italy* (Manchester: Manchester University Press).

George, M. (ed.) (2005) *The Roman Family in the Empire: Rome, Italy, and Beyond* (Oxford and New York, NY: Oxford University Press).

George, M. (ed.) (2013) *Roman Slavery and Roman Material Culture* (Toronto, Buffalo, NY and London: University of Toronto Press).

Giacobello, F. (2008) *Larari Pompeiani: Iconografia e Culto dei Lari in Ambito Domestico.* Università Degli Studi di Milano, Pubblicazioni della Facoltà di Lettere e Filosofia 251 (Milan: LED).

Giannecchini, M. and Moggi-Cecchi, J. (2008) 'Stature in Archeological Samples from Central Italy: Methodological Issues and Diachronic Changes', *AJPA* 135.3, pp. 284–292.

Giesecke, A. L. (2007) *The Epic City: Urbanism, Utopia, and the Garden in Ancient Greece and Rome* (Washington, DC Cambridge MA and London: Harvard University Press).

Giesecke, A. L. (2014) *The Mythology of Plants: Botanical Lore from Ancient Greece and Rome* (Los Angeles, CA: J. Paul Getty Museum Publications).

Giesecke, A. L. (2016) 'Autopsy and Empire: Temporal Collapse in the Designed Landscapes of Ancient Rome', *Studies in the History of Gardens and Designed Landscapes* 36.4, pp. 225–244.

Gill, C. (2013) 'Philosophical Therapy as Preventative Psychological Medicine', in Harris, W. V. (ed.) *Mental Disorders in the Classical World* (Leiden: Brill), pp. 339–360.

Gill, C. (2018) 'Philosophical Psychological Therapy: Did It Have any Impact on Medical Practice?' in Thumiger, C. and Singer, P. (eds.) *Mental Illness in Ancient Medicine: From Celsus to Paul of Aegina* (Leiden: Brill), pp. 365–380.

Gleason, K. L. (1990) 'The Garden Portico of Pompey the Great: An Ancient Public Park Preserved in the Layers of Rome', *Expedition* 32.2, pp. 4–14.

Gleason, K. L. (1994) 'Porticus Pompeiana: A New Perspective on the First Public Park of Ancient Rome', *JGH* 14.1, pp. 13–27.

Gleason, K. L. (2013) 'Design', in Gleason, K. (ed.) *A Cultural History of Gardens in Antiquity* (London: Bloomsbury), pp. 15–40.

Gleason, K. L. and Palmer, M. A. (2018) 'Constructing the Ancient Roman Garden' in Jashemski, W. F., Gleason, K. L., Hartswick, K. J. and Malek, A.-A. (eds.) *Gardens of the Roman Empire* (Cambridge: Cambridge University Press), pp. 369–401.

Gleason, K. L., Hartswick, K. J., Malek, A.-A. and Palmer, M. A. (2018) 'Conclusions: New Perspectives on the Roman Garden', in Jashemski, W. F., Gleason, K. L., Hartswick, K. J. and Malek, A.-A. (eds.) *Gardens of the Roman Empire* (Cambridge: Cambridge University Press), pp. 481–494.

Glinister, F. (2014) 'Festus and Ritual Foodstuffs', *Eruditio Antiqua* 6, pp. 215–227.

Gobbo, B. (2009) 'Casa VI, 13, 13', in Verzar Bass, M. and Oriolo, F. (eds.) *Rileggere Pompei 2: L'insula 13 della Regio IV* (Rome: L'Erma di Bretschneider), pp. 29–102.

Godlee, F. (2011) 'What Is Health?', *BMJ* 343, p. 4817.

Gordon, R. (1995) 'The Healing Event in Graeco-Roman Folk Medicine', in van der Eijk, P. J., Horstmanshoff, H. F. J. and Schrijvers, P. H. (eds.) *Ancient Medicine in its Socio-Cultural Context: Volume 2* (Amsterdam and Atlanta, GA: Rodopi), pp. 363–376.

Gourevitch, D. (2010) 'The Sick Child in his Family: A Risk for the Family Tradition', in Dasen, V. and Späth, T. (eds.) *Children, Memory, and Family Identity in Roman Culture* (Oxford: Oxford University Press), pp. 273–297.

Gowers, E. (2011) 'Trees and Family Trees in the *Aeneid*', *CA* 30.1, pp. 87–118.

Gowland, R. and Garnsey, P. (2010) 'Skeletal Evidence for Health, Nutritional Status and Malaria in Rome and the Empire', in Eckardt, H. (ed.) *Roman Diasporas: Archaeological Approaches to Mobility and Diversity in the Roman World* (Portsmouth, RI: *JRA* Supplement 78), pp. 131–156.

Graf, F. (2006) 'New Interpretive Approaches to Ancient Healing Sanctuaries: Antike Heilheiligtümer: Neue Deutungszugänge: Einführung', *ARG* 8.1, p. 3.

Graham, E.-J. and Carroll, M. (2012) 'Introduction: Infant Health and Death in Roman Italy and Beyond', in Carroll, M. and Graham, E.-J. (eds.) *Infant Health and Death in Roman Italy and Beyond* (Portsmouth, RI: *JRA* Supplement 96), pp. 9–22.

Graham, E.-J. (2013) 'Disparate Lives or Disparate Deaths? Post-mortem Treatment of the Body and the Articulation of Difference', in Laes, C., Goodey, C. F. and Rose, M. L. (eds.) *Disabilities in Roman Antiquity: A Capite ad Calcem* (Leiden: Brill), pp. 249–274.

Gray-Fow, M. J. G. (1988) 'The Wicked Stepmother in Roman Literature and History: An Evaluation', *Latomus* 47.4, pp. 741–757.

Green, F. M. (2015) 'Cooking Class', in Tuori, K. and Nissi, L. (eds.) *Public and Private in the Roman House and Society* (Portsmouth, RI: *JRA* Supplement 102), pp. 133–147.

Green, R. M. (1955) *Asclepiades: His Life and Writings* (New Haven, CT: Licht).

Grimal, P. (1969) *Les Jardins Romains* (Paris: Presses Universitaires de France).

Gruen, E. S. (1992) *Culture and National Identity in Republican Rome* (Ithaca, NY: Cornell University Press).

Hales, S. (2003) *The Roman House and Social Identity* (Cambridge: Cambridge University Press).

Hanninen, M.-L. (2013) 'Domestic Cult and the Construction of an Ideal Roman Family', in Katajala-Peltomaa, S. and Vuolanto, V. (eds.) *Religious Participation in Ancient and Medieval Societies: Rituals, Interaction and Identity* (Rome: Acta Instituti Romani Finlandiae 41), pp. 39–49.

Hanson, A. E. (1991) 'Continuity and Change: Three Case Studies in Hippocratic Gynecological Therapy and Theory', in Pomeroy, S. B. (ed.) *Women's History and Ancient History* (Chapel Hill, NC and London: University of North Carolina Press), pp. 73–110.

Hanson, A. E. (1992) 'The Logic of the Gynecological Prescriptions', in López Férez, J. A. (ed.) *Tratados Hipocráticos (Estudios Acerca de su Contenido, Forma e Influencia): Actas del VIIe Colloque International Hippocratique (Madrid, 24–29 de Septiembre de 1990)* (Madrid: Universidad Nacional de Educación a Distancia), pp. 235–250.

Hardy, G. and Totelin, L. (2016) *Ancient Botany* (London: Routledge).

Harlow, M. and Laurence, R. (2002) *Growing Up and Growing Old in Ancient Rome: A Life Course Approach* (London and New York, NY: Routledge).

Harmon, D. P. (1978) 'The Family Festivals of Rome', *ANRW* II.16.2, pp. 1592–1603.

Harris, W. V. (1986) 'The Roman Father's Power of Life and Death', in Bagnall, R. S. and Harris, W. V. (eds.) *Studies in Roman Law in Memory of A. Arthur Schiller* (Leiden: Brill), pp. 81–95.

Harris, W. V. (ed.) (2013a) *Mental Disorders in the Classical World* (Leiden: Brill).

Harris, W. V. (2013b) 'Thinking About Mental Disorders in Classical Antiquity', in Harris, W. V. (ed.) *Mental Disorders in the Classical World* (Leiden: Brill), pp. 1–23.

Harris, W. V. (ed.) (2016a) *Popular Medicine in Graeco-Roman Antiquity: Explorations* (Leiden: Brill).

Harris, W. V. (2016b) 'Popular Medicine in the Classical World', in Harris, W. V. (ed.) *Popular Medicine in Graeco-Roman Antiquity: Explorations* (Leiden: Brill), pp. 1–64.

Hartnett, J. (2017) *The Roman Street: Urban Life and Society in Pompeii, Herculaneum, and Rome* (Cambridge and New York, NY: Cambridge University Press).

Hasegawa, K. (2005) *The Familia Urbana During the Early Empire: A Study of* Columbaria *Inscriptions* (Oxford: Archaeopress).

Hemelrijk, E. A. (1999) Matrona Docta: *Educated Women in the Roman Elite from Cornelia to Julia Domna* (London and New York, NY: Routledge).

Henderson, J. (2004) *The Roman Book of Gardening* (London: Routledge).

Henneberg, M. and Henneberg, R. J. (2002) 'Reconstructing Medical Knowledge in Ancient Pompeii from the Hard Evidence of Bones and Teeth', in Renn, J. and Castagnetti, G. (eds.) *Homo Faber: Studies on Nature, Technology, and Science at the Time of Pompeii* (Rome: L'Erma di Bretschneider), pp. 169–187.

Hermansen, G. (1982) *Ostia: Aspects of Roman City Life* (Edmonton: University of Alberta Press).

Hersch, K. (2010) *The Roman Wedding: Ritual and Meaning in Antiquity* (Cambridge: Cambridge University Press).

Hillman, D. C. (2004) *Representations of Pharmacy in Roman Literature from Cato to Ovid* (Madison, WI: University of Wisconsin-Madison Unpublished PhD Thesis).

Hirt Raj, M. (2006) *Médecins et Maladies de l'Egypte Romaine. Étude Socio-Légale de la Profession Médicale et de ses Praticiens du Ier au IVe Siècle ap. J.-C.* (Leiden: Brill).

Holland, L. A. (1937) 'The Shrine of the Lares Compitales', *TAPA* 68, pp. 428–441.

Holleran, C. (2011) 'The Street Life of Ancient Rome', in Laurence, R. and Newsome, D. J. (eds.) *Rome, Ostia, Pompeii: Movement and Space* (Oxford: Oxford University Press), pp. 245–261.

Holleran, C. (2012) *Shopping in Ancient Rome: The Retail Trade in the Late Republic and the Principate* (Oxford: Oxford University Press).

Holleran, C. and Pudsey, A. (2011) *Demography and the Graeco-Roman World: New Insights and Approaches* (Cambridge: Cambridge University Press).

Holmes, B. (2010) 'Marked Bodies: Gender, Race, Class, Age, Disability, and Disease', in Garrison, D. H. (ed.) *A Cultural History of the Human Body in Antiquity* (London: Bloomsbury), pp. 159–183.

Hopkins, K. (1966) 'On the Probable Age Structure of the Roman Population', *Population Studies* 20.2, pp. 245–264.

Hopkins, K. (1983) *Death and Renewal: Sociological Studies in Roman History* (Cambridge: Cambridge University Press).

Horden, P. (2005) 'Travel Sickness: Medicine and Mobility in the Mediterranean from Antiquity to the Renaissance', in Harris, W. V. (ed.) *Rethinking the Mediterranean* (Oxford: Oxford University Press), pp. 179–199.

Horden, P. and Purcell, N. (2000) *The Corrupting Sea: A Study of Mediterranean History* (Oxford and Malden, MA: Wiley-Blackwell).

Horsfall, N. (2003) *The Culture of the Roman Plebs* (London: Bristol Classical Press).

Horstmanshoff, M. (1999) 'Ancient Medicine Between Hope and Fear: Medicament, Magic and Poison in the Roman Empire', *ER* 7.1, pp. 37–51.

Houston, G. W. (2014) *Inside Roman Libraries: Book Collections and Their Management in Antiquity* (Chapel Hill, NC: University of North Carolina Press).

Hsu, E. (2002) 'Medical Anthropology, Material Culture, and New Directions in Medical Archaeology, in Baker, P. A. and Carr, G. (eds.) *Practitioners, Practices and Patients: New Approaches to Medical Archaeology and Anthropology* (Oxford: Oxbow), pp. 1–15.

Huebner, S. R. (2017) 'A Mediterranean Family? A Comparative Approach to the Ancient World', in Huebner, S. R. and Nathan, G. (eds.) *Mediterranean Families in Classical Antiquity: Households, Extended Families, and Domestic Space* (Oxford and Malden, MA: Wiley-Blackwell), pp. 3–26.

Huebner, S. R. and Ratzan, D. (eds.) (2009) *Growing up Fatherless in Antiquity* (Cambridge and New York, NY: Cambridge University Press).

Hughes, J. D. (1994) *Pan's Travail: Environmental Problems of the Ancient Greeks and Romans* (Baltimore, MD: Johns Hopkins University Press).

Hulskamp, M. (2012) 'Space and the Body: Uses of Astronomy in Hippocratic Medicine', in Baker, P., Nigdam, H. and van't Land, K. (eds.) *Medicine and Space: Body, Surroundings and Borders in Antiquity and the Middle Ages* (Leiden: Brill), pp. 149–168.

Israelowich, I. (2015) *Patients and Healers in the High Roman Empire* (Baltimore, MD: Johns Hopkins University Press).

Jackson, M. (2008) '"Home Sweet Home": Historical Perspectives on Health and the Home', in Jackson, M. (ed.) *Health and the Modern Home* (London and New York, NY: Routledge), pp. 1–17.

Jackson, R. (1988) *Doctors and Diseases in the Roman Empire* (London: British Museum Press).

Jansen, G. C. M. (1991) 'Water Systems and Sanitation in the Houses of Herculaneum', *Papers of the Netherlands Institute in Rome* 50, pp. 145–166.

Jansen, G. C. M., Kolowski-Ostrow, A. O. and Moormann, E. (eds.) (2011) *Roman Toilets: Their Archaeology and Cultural History* (Leuven, Paris and Walpole, MA: Peeters).

Jashemski, W. F. (1974) 'The Discovery of a Market-garden Orchard at Pompeii: The Garden of the "House of the Ship Europa"', *AJA* 78.4, pp. 391–404.

Jashemski, W. F. (1977) 'The Excavation of a Shop-house Garden at Pompeii (I.xx.5)', *AJA* 81.2, pp. 217–227.

Jashemski, W. F. (1979a) '"The Garden of Hercules at Pompeii" (II.viii.6): The Discovery of a Commercial Flower Garden', *AJA* 83.4, pp. 403–411.

Jashemski, W. F. (1979b) *The Gardens of Pompeii, Herculaneum and the Villas Destroyed by Vesuvius: Volume 1* (New Rochelle, NY: Caratzas Brothers).

Jashemski, W. F. (1993) *The Gardens of Pompeii, Herculaneum and the Villas Destroyed by Vesuvius: Volume 2* (New Rochelle, NY: Aristide Caratzas).

Jashemski, W. F. (1996) 'Ancient Roman Gardens in Campania and Tunisia: A Comparison of the Evidence', *JGH* 16.4, pp. 231–243.

Jashemski, W. F. (1999) *A Pompeian Herbal: Ancient and Modern Medicinal Plants* (Austin, TX: University of Texas Press).

Jashemski, W. F. (2018a) 'Produce Gardens', in Jashemski, W. F., Gleason, K. L., Hartswick, K. J. and Malek, A.-A. (eds.) *Gardens of the Roman Empire* (Cambridge: Cambridge University Press), pp. 121–151.

Jashemski, W. F. (2018b) 'Gardening Practices and Techniques', in Jashemski, W. F., Glea-son, K. L., Hartswick, K. J. and Malek, A.-A. (eds.) *Gardens of the Roman Empire* (Cambridge: Cambridge University Press), pp. 432–454.

Jashemski, W. F., Gleason, K. L., Hartswick, K. J. and Malek, A.-A. (eds.) (2018) *Gardens of the Roman Empire* (Cambridge: Cambridge University Press).

Jashemski, W. F., Gleason, K. L. and Hertenbach, M. (2018) 'Plants of the Roman Garden', in Jashemski, W. F., Gleason, K. L., Hartswick, K. J. and Malek, A.-A. (eds.) *Gardens of the Roman Empire* (Cambridge: Cambridge University Press), pp. 455–480.

Jashemski, W. F. and Meyer, F. G. (eds.) (2002) *The Natural History of Pompeii* (Cambridge: Cambridge University Press).

Jashemski, W. F., Meyer, F. G. and Ricciardi, M. (2002) 'Plants: Evidence from Wall Paint-ings, Mosaics, Sculpture, Plant Remains, Graffiti, Inscriptions, and Ancient Authors', in Jashemski, W. F. and Meyer, F. G. (eds.) *The Natural History of Pompeii* (Cambridge: Cambridge University Press), pp. 80–180.

Johansson, L. (2010) 'The Roman Wedding and the Household Gods: The Genius and the Lares and their Different Roles in the Rituals of Marriage', in Larsson Lovén, L. and Strömberg, A. (eds.) *Ancient Marriage in Myth and Reality* (Newcastle upon Tyne: Cambridge Scholars), pp. 136–147.

Joshel, S. R. (1992) *Work, Identity and Legal Status at Rome: A Study of the Occupational Inscriptions* (Norman, OK and London: University of Oklahoma Press).

Joshel, S. R. and Peterson, L. H. (2014) *The Material Life of Roman Slaves* (Cambridge and New York, NY: Cambridge University Press).

Jouanna, J. (2015) 'Regimen in the Hippocratic Corupus: Diaita and its Problems', in Dean-Jones, L. and Rosen, R. M. (eds.) *Ancient Concepts of the Hippocratic: Papers Pre-sented at the XIIIth International Hippocrates Colloquium, Austin, Texas, August 2008* (Leiden: Brill), pp. 209–241.

Kastenmeier, P. (2007) *Luoghi del Lavoro Domestico Nella Casa Pompeiana* (Rome: L'Erma di Bretschneider).

Kaufmann, D. B. (1932) 'Poisons and Poisoning Among the Romans', *CP* 27.2, pp. 156–167.

Kellum, B. A. (1994) 'The Construction of Landscape in Augustan Rome: The Garden Room at the Villa ad Gallinas', *The Art Bulletin* 76.2, pp. 211–224.

Kertzer, D. I. and Saller, R. P. (eds.) (1991) *The Family in Italy from Antiquity to the Pre-sent* (New Haven, CT and London: Yale University Press).

Killgrove, K. (2013) Bioarchaeology in the Roman Empire, *Encyclopedia of Global Archaeology* (New York, NY: Springer), pp. 876–882.

Killgrove, K. and Montgomery, J. (2016) 'All Roads Lead to Rome: Exploring Human Migration to the Eternal City Through Biochemistry of Skeletons from Two Imperial-Era Cemeteries (1st-3rd Centuries AD)', *PLoS ONE* 11.2, pp. 1–30.

Killgrove, K. and Tykot, R. (2013) 'Food for Rome: A Stable Isotope Investigation of Diet in the Imperial Period (1st-3rd Centuries AD), *Journal of Anthropological Archaeology* 32.1, pp. 28–38.

King, A. C. (1999) 'Diet in the Roman World. A Regional Inter-Site Comparison of the Mammal Bones', *JRA* 12, pp. 168–202.

King, H. (1995) 'Self-Help, Self-Knowledge: In Search of the Patient in Hippocratic Gynaecology', in Hawley, R. and Levick, B. (eds.) *Women in Antiquity: New Assess-ments* (London and New York, NY: Routledge), pp. 135–148.

King, H. (1997) 'Review: Beyond the Medical Market-Place: New Directions in Ancient Medicine', *Early Science and Medicine* 2.1, pp. 88–97.

King, H. (1998) *Hippocrates' Women: Reading the Female Body in Ancient Greece* (London and New York, NY: Routledge).

King, H. (2005) 'Introduction: What is Health?', in King, H. (ed.) *Health in Antiquity* (London and New York, NY: Routledge), pp. 1–11.

Kleinman, A. (1980) *Patients and Healers in the Context of Culture: An Exploration of the Borderland Between Anthropology, Medicine, and Psychiatry* (Berkeley, CA: University of California Press).

Knapp, C. (1914) 'Horace, *Sermones*, I, I', *TPAPA* 45, pp. 91–109.

Koloski-Ostrow, A.-O. (2015) *The Archaeology of Sanitation in Roman Italy: Toilets, Sewers and Water Systems* (Chapel Hill, NC: University of North Carolina Press).

König, J. (2005) *Athletics and Literature in the Roman Empire* (Cambridge: Cambridge University Press).

König, J. and Woolf, G. (eds.) (2013) *Encyclopaedism from Antiquity to the Renaissance* (Cambridge and New York, NY: Cambridge University Press).

König, J. and Woolf, G. (eds.) (2017) *Authority and Expertise in Ancient Scientific Culture* (Cambridge and New York, NY: Cambridge University Press).

Köpke, N. and Baten, J. (2003) 'The Biological Standard of Living in Europe During the Last Two Millennia', *European Review of Economic History* 9.1, pp. 61–95.

Korpela, J. (1995) '*Aromatarii, Pharmacopolae, Thurarii et Ceteri*. Zur Sozialgeschichte', in van der Eijk, P. J., Horstmanshoff, H. F. J. and Schrijvers, P. H. (eds.) *Ancient Medicine in its Socio-Cultural Context: Volume 1* (Amsterdam and Atlanta, GA: Rodopi), pp. 101–118.

Kron, G. (2005) 'Anthropometry, Physical Anthropology, and the Reconstruction of Ancient Health, Nutrition, and Living Standards', *Historia* 54.1, pp. 68–83.

Kron, G. (2012) 'Nutrition, Hygiene and Mortality. Setting Parameters for Roman Health and Life Expectancy Consistent with our Comparative Evidence', in Lo Cascio, E. (ed.) *L'impatto della "Peste Antonina"* (Bari: Edipuglia), pp. 193–252.

Kron, G. (2014) 'Comparative Evidence and the Reconstruction of the Ancient Economy: Greco-Roman Housing and the Level and Distribution of Wealth and Income', in De Callataÿ, F. (ed.) *Quantifying the Greco-Roman Economy and Beyond* (Bari: Edipuglia), pp. 123–146.

Kron, G. forthcoming, 'Comparative Perspectives on Nutrition and Social Inequality in the Roman World', in Erdkamp, P. and Holleran, C. (eds.) *Diet and Nutrition in the Roman World* (London: Routledge).

Künzel, H. (1974) *Der Römische Genius* (Heidelberg: F. H. Kerle).

Künz, E. (1983) *Medizinische Instrumente aus Sepulkralfunden der Römischen Kaiserzeit* (Bonn and Köln: Rheinland Verlag).

Kuttner, A. (1999) 'Looking Outside Inside: Ancient Roman Garden Rooms', *Studies in the History of Gardens and Designed Landscapes* 19.1, pp. 7–35.

Laes, C. (2010) 'The Educated Midwife in the Roman Empire: An Example of "Differential Equations"', in Horstmanshoff, H. J. F. (ed.) *Hippocrates and Medical Education: Selected Papers Read at the XIIth International Hippocrates Colloquium, Universiteit Leiden, 24–26 August 2005* (Leiden: Brill), pp. 261–286.

Landgren, L. (2004) *Lauro, Myrto et Buxo Frequentata: A Study of the Roman Garden Through its Plants* (Lund: Lund University Unpublished PhD Thesis).

Landgren, L. (2013) 'Plantings', in Gleason, K. L. (ed.) *A Cultural History of Gardens in Antiquity* (London: Bloomsbury), pp. 75–98.

Langslow, D. R. (2000) *Medical Latin in the Roman Empire* (Oxford: Clarendon Press).

Larsson Lovén, L. and Strömberg, A. (eds.) (2009) *Ancient Marriage in Myth and Reality* (Newcastle Upon Tyne: Cambridge Scholars).

Laurence, R. and Strömberg, A. (2012) *Families in the Greco-Roman World* (London and New York, NY: Continuum).

Laurence, R. and Wallace-Hadrill, A. (eds.) (1997) *Domestic Space in the Roman World: Pompeii and Beyond* (Portsmouth RI: *JRA* Supplement 22).

Lazer, E. (2008) *Resurrecting Pompeii* (London and New York, NY: Routledge).

Lazer, E. (2016) 'Skeletal Remains and the Health of the Population at Pompeii', in Flohr, M. and Wilson, A. (eds.) *The Economy of Pompeii* (Oxford: Oxford University Press), pp. 135–160.

Lefebvre, H. (1991) *The Production of Space* (Oxford: Wiley-Blackwell).

Lennon, J. J. (2012) 'Pollution, Religion and Society in the Roman World', in Bradley, M. and Stow, K. (eds.) *Rome, Pollution and Propriety: Dirt, Disease and Hygiene in the Eternal City from Antiquity to Modernity* (Cambridge: Cambridge University Press), 43–58.

Lennon, J. J. (2014) *Pollution and Religion in Ancient Rome* (Cambridge: Cambridge University Press).

Linderski, J. (2001) '*Imago hortorum*: Pliny the Elder and the Gardens of the Roman Poor', *CP* 96.3, pp. 305–308.

Littlewood, A. R. (1987) 'Ancient Literary Evidence for the Pleasure Gardens of Roman Country Villa', in MacDougall, E. B. (ed.) *Ancient Roman Villa Gardens* (Cambridge, MA: Harvard University Press), pp. 9–30.

Littlewood, A. R. (1992) 'Gardens of Byzantium', *JGH* 12, pp. 126–153.

Littlewood, A. R. (2002) 'The Scholarship of Byzantine Gardens', in Littlewood, A. R., Maguire, H., and Wolschke-Bulmahn, J. (eds.) *Byzantine Garden Culture* (Washington DC: Dumbarton Oaks), pp. 13–22.

Littlewood, A. R. (2018) 'Greek Literary Evidence for Roman Gardens', in Jashemski, W. F., Gleason, K. L., Hartswick, K. J. and Malek, A.-A. (eds.) *Gardens of the Roman Empire* (Cambridge: Cambridge University Press), pp. 245–257.

Lloyd, G. E. R. (1979) *Magic, Reason, and Experience: Studies in the Origin and Development of Greek Science* (Cambridge: Cambridge University Press).

Lo Cascio, E. (1999) 'Canon Frumentarius, Suarius, Vinarius: Stato e Private Nell'Approvvigionamento dell'Urbs', in Harris, W. V. (ed.) *The Transformation of the Urbs Roma in Late Antiquity* (Portsmouth, RI: *JRA* Supplement 33), pp. 163–182.

Lo Cascio, E. (2006) 'Did the Population of Imperial Rome Reproduce Itself?', in Storey, G. R. (ed.) *Urbanism in the Pre-Industrial World: Cross-Cultural Approaches* (Tuscaloosa, AL: University of Alabama Press), pp. 52–68.

Lo Presti, R. (2012) 'Shaping the Difference: The Medical Inquiry into the Nature of Places and the Early Birth of Anthropology in the Hippocratic Treatise *Airs Waters Places*', in Baker, P., Nigdam, H. and van't Land, K. (eds.) *Medicine and Space: Body, Surroundings and Borders in Antiquity and the Middle Ages* (Leiden: Brill), pp. 169–195.

Lowe, J. C. B. (1985) 'Cooks in Plautus', *CA* 4.1, pp. 72–102.

Lucas, K. and Lloyd, B. (2005) *Health Promotion: Evidence and Experience* (London: Sage Publications).

Macaulay-Lewis, E. (2006) 'The Role of *Ollae Perforatae* in Understanding Horticulture, Planting Techniques, Garden Design, and Plant Trade in the Roman World', in Morel, J. P., Juan, J. T. and Matamala, J. C. (eds.) *The Archaeology of Crop Fields and Gardens: Proceedings from 1*st *Conference on Crop Fields and Gardens Archaeology, University of Barcelona, Spain, June 1–3rd 2006* (Bari: EdiPuglia), pp. 207–220.

Macaulay-Lewis, E. (2008) 'The Fruits of Victory: Generals, Plants, and Power in the Roman World', in Bragg, E., Hau, L. I. and Macaulay-Lewis, E. (eds.) *Beyond the Battlefields: New Perspectives on Warfare and Society in the Graeco-Roman World* (Newcastle upon Tyne: Cambridge Scholars), pp. 205–224.

MacKinnon, M. (2001) 'High on the Hog: Linking Zooarchaeological, Literary, and Artistic Data for Pig Breeds in Roman Italy', *AJA* 105.4. pp. 649–673.

MacKinnon, M. (2007) 'Osteological Research in Classical Archaeology', *AJA* 111.3, pp. 473–504.

Maiuri, A. (2013) *Sacra Privata. Rituali Domestici e Istituti Giuridici in Roma Antica.* (Rome: L'Erma di Bretschneider).

Manniche, L. (1986) *An Ancient Egyptian Herbal* (London: British Museum Press).

Manniche, L. (2006) *An Ancient Egyptian Herbal* (London: British Museum Press).

Mantle, I. C. (2002) 'The Roles of Children in Roman Religion', *G&R* 49.1, pp. 89–106.

Marganne-Mélard, M.-H. (1996) 'La Médecine dans l'Égypte Romaine: Les Sources et les Méthodes', *ANRW* II 37.3, pp. 2709–2740.

Marquardt, J. (1886) *Das Privatleben der Römer* (Leipzig: S. Hirzel).

Martin, R. (1985) 'Em Présent des Etudes sur Columelle', *ANRW* II 32.3, pp. 1959–1979.

Marwood, M. A. (1988) *The Roman Cult of Salus* (Oxford: Archaeopress).

Marzano, A. (2007) *Roman Villas in Central Italy: A Social and Economic History* (Leiden: Brill).

Mattero, S. (1992) 'The Gluttonous Genius: Yearning for Vitality and Fertility', *Arctos* 26, pp. 85–96.

Mayer, E. (2012) *The Ancient Middle Classes* (Cambridge, MA: Harvard University Press).

Mayor, A. (2010) *The Poison King: The Life and Legend of Mithridates: Rome's Deadliest Enemy* (Princeton, NJ: Princeton University Press).

McCreight, T. D. (2006) 'Psyche's Sisters as *Medicae*? Allusions to Medicine in *Cupid and Psyche*', in Zimmerman, M., Nauta, R. R., and Panayotakis, S. (eds.) *Lectiones Scrupulosae: Essays on the Text and Interpretation of Apuleius'* Metamorphoses *in Honour of Maaike Zimmerman* (Groningen: Barkhuis), pp. 123–167.

McDonnell, M. (2006) *Roman Manliness: Virtus and the Roman Republic* (Cambridge and New York, NY: Cambridge University Press).

McNamara, L. (2003–04) ' "Conjurers, Purifiers, Vagabonds and Quacks"? The Clinical Roles of the Folk and Hippocratic Healers of Classical Greece', *Iris* 16–17, pp. 2–25.

McWilliam, J. (2013) 'The Socialisation of Roman Children', in Grubbs, J. E. et al. (eds.) *The Oxford Handbook of Childhood and Education in the Classical World* (Oxford: Oxford University Press), pp. 264–285.

Meiggs, R. (1982) *Trees and Timber in the Ancient Mediterranean World* (Oxford: Clarendon Press).

Miller, J. I. (1969) *The Spice Trade in the Roman Empire, 29 BC – AD 641* (Oxford: Clarendon Press).

Milnor, K. (2005) *Gender, Domesticity, and the Age of Augustus: Inventing Private Life* (Oxford: Oxford University Press).

Mols, S. T. A. M. (1999) *Wooden Furniture in Herculaneum: Form, Technique and Function* (Amsterdam: J. C. Gieben).

Morello, R. and Morrison, A. D. (2007) *Ancient Letters: Classical and Late Antique Epistolography* (Oxford and New York, NY: Oxford University Press).

Morford, M. (1987) 'The Stoic Garden', *JGH* 7.2, pp. 151–175.

Morley, N. (1996) *Metropolis and Hinterland: The City of Rome and the Italian Economy 200 B.C. – A.D. 200* (Cambridge and New York, NY: Cambridge University Press).

Morley, N. (2005) 'The Salubriousness of the Roman City', in King, H. (ed.) *Health in Antiquity* (London: Routledge), pp. 192–204.

Morley, N. (2006) 'The Poor in the City of Rome', in Atkins, M. and Osborne, R. (eds.) *Poverty in the Roman World* (Cambridge: Cambridge University Press), pp. 21–39.

Morvillez, E. (2018) 'The Garden in the *Domus*', in Jashemski, W. F., Gleason, K. L., Hartswick, K. J. and Malek, A.-A. (eds.) *Gardens of the Roman Empire* (Cambridge: Cambridge University Press), pp. 17–71.

Mouritsen, H. (2011) *The Freedman in the Roman World* (Cambridge and New York, NY: Cambridge University Press).

Mudry, P. (1980) '*Medicus Amicus*: Un Trait Romaine de la Médecine Antique', *Gesnerus* 37.1–2, pp. 17–20.

Myers, K. S. (2005) '*Docta Otia*: Garden Ownership and Configurations of Leisure in Statius and Pliny the Younger', *Arethusa* 38.1, pp. 103–129.

Myers, K. S. (2018) 'Representations of Gardens in Roman Literature' in Jashemski, W. F., Gleason, K. L., Hartswick, K. J. and Malek, A.-A. (eds.) *Gardens of the Roman Empire* (Cambridge: Cambridge University Press), pp. 257–277.

Nevett, L. C. (2015) 'Understanding Variation in Ancient House-Forms: A Preliminary Discussion', in Di Castro, A. and Hope, C. A. (eds.) *Housing and Habitat in the Ancient Mediterranean: Cultural and Environmental Responses* (Leuven, Paris and Bristol, CT: Peeters), pp. 143–149.

Nielsen, I. (2013) 'Types of Gardens', in Gleason, K. L. (ed.) *A Cultural History of Gardens in Antiquity* (London: Bloomsbury), pp. 41–74.

Nijhuis, K. (1995) 'Greek Doctors and Roman Patients: A Medical Anthropological Approach', in van der Eijk, P. J., Horstmanshoff, H. F. J. and Schrijvers, P. H. (eds.) *Ancient Medicine in its Socio-Cultural Context: Volume 1* (Amsterdam and Atlanta, GA: Rodopi), pp. 49–67.

Noy, D. (2000) *Foreigners at Rome: Citizens and Strangers* (London: Duckworth and the Classical Press of Wales).

Noy, D. (2010) 'Epigraphic Evidence for Immigrants at Rome and in Roman Britain', in Eckardt, H. (ed.) *Roman Diasporas: Archaeological Approaches to Mobility and Diversity in the Roman World* (Portsmouth, RI: *JRA* Supplement 78), pp. 13–26.

Nutton, V. (1985) 'The Drug Trade in Antiquity', *JRSM* 78.2, pp. 138–145.

Nutton, V. (1992) 'Healers in the Medical Market Place: Towards a Social History of Graeco-Roman Medicine', in Wear, A. (ed.) *Medicine in Society* (Cambridge and New York, NY: Cambridge University Press), pp. 1–58.

Nutton, V. (1993) 'Roman Medicine: Tradition, Confrontation, Assimilation', *ANRW* II 37.1, pp. 49–78.

Nutton, V. (2000) 'Medical Thoughts on Urban Pollution', in Hope, V. M. and Marshall, E. (eds.) *Death and Disease in the Ancient City* (London and New York, NY: Routledge), pp. 65–73.

Nutton, V. (2013) *Ancient Medicine* (London: Routledge).

Oberhelman, S. M. (2013) 'Introduction: Medical Pluralism, Healing, and Dreams in Greek Culture', in Oberhelman, S. M. (ed.) *Dreams, Healing, and Medicine in Greece: From Antiquity to the Present* (Farnham and Burlington, VT: Ashgate), pp. 1–32.

Olson, K. (2008) *Dress and the Roman Woman: Self-Presentation and Society* (Abingdon and New York, NY: Routledge).

Olson, K. (2009) 'Cosmetics in Roman Antiquity: Substance, Remedy, Poison', *CW* 102.3, pp. 291–310.

Olson, K. (2017) *Masculinity and Dress in Roman Antiquity* (Abingdon and New York, NY: Routledge).

Orr, D G. (1973) *Roman Domestic Religion: A Study of the Roman Household Deities and their Shrines at Pompeii and Herculaneum* (Ann Arbor, MI: University of Michigan Unpublished PhD Thesis).

Orr, D G. (1978) 'Roman Domestic Religion: The Evidence of the Household Shrines', *ANRW* II 16.2, pp. 1557–1591.

Osborne, R. (1992) 'Classical Greek Gardens: Between Farm and Paradise', in Dixon Hunt, J. (ed.) *Garden History: Issues, Approaches, Methods* (Washington D. C.: Dumbarton Oaks), pp. 373–391.

O'Sullivan, T. M. (2011) *Walking in Roman Culture* (Cambridge: Cambridge University Press).

Pagán, V. E. (2006) *Rome and the Literature of Gardens* (London: Bloomsbury).

Parker H. (1997) 'Women Physicians in Greece, Rome, and the Byzantine Empire', in Furst, L. R. (ed.) *Women Physicians and Healers* (Lexington, KY: University of Kentucky Press), pp. 131–150.

Parker H. (2012) 'Galen and the Girls: Sources for Women Medical Writers Revisited', *CQ* 62.1, pp. 359–386.

Parker, R. (1983) *Miasma: Pollution and Purification in Early Greek Religion* (Oxford: Clarendon Press).

Parkin, T. (1992) *Demography and Roman Society* (Baltimore, MD: Johns Hopkins University Press).

Parkin, T. (1997) 'Out of Sight, Out of Mind: Elderly Members of the Roman Family', in Rawson, B. and Weaver, P. (eds.) *The Roman Family in Italy: Status, Sentiment, Space* (Oxford: Clarendon Press), pp. 123–148.

Parkin, T. (2003) *Old Age in the Roman World* (Baltimore, MD: Johns Hopkins University Press).

Perry, M. (2015) 'The *Paterfamilias* and the Family Council in Roman Public Law', in Tuori, K. and Nissi, L. (eds.) *Public and Private in the Roman House and Society* (Portsmouth, RI: *JRA* Supplement 102), pp. 77–86.

Peterson, L. H. (2012) 'Collecting Gods in Roman Houses: The House of the Gilded Cupids (VI.16.7, 38) at Pompeii', *Arethusa* 45.3, pp. 319–332.

Petridou, G. and Thumiger, C. (eds.) (2016) Homo Patiens: *Approaches to the Patient in the Ancient World* (Leiden: Brill).

Pirson, F. (1997) 'Rented Accommodations at Pompeii: The Evidence of the Insula Arianna Polliana VI.6', in Laurence, R. and Wallace-Hadrill, A. (eds.) *Domestic Space in the Roman World: Pompeii and Beyond* (Portsmouth, RI: *JRA* Supplement 22), pp. 161–185.

Pollard, E. A. (2009) 'Pliny's *Natural History* and the Flavian *Templum Pacis*: Botanical Imperialism in First-Century C.E. Rome', *JWH* 20.3, pp. 309–338.

Pollini, J. (2008) 'A New Bronze Lar and the Role of the Lares in the Domestic and Civic Religion of the Romans', *Latomus* 67.2, pp. 391–398.

Porter, R. (1985a) 'The Patient's View: Doing Medical History from Below', *Theory and Society* 14.2, pp. 175–198.

Porter, R. (1985b) (ed.) *Patients and Practitioners: Lay Perceptions of Medicine in Pre-Industrial Society* (Cambridge: Cambridge University Press).

Prell, M. (1997) *Sozialökonomische Untersuchungen zur Armut im Antiken Rom. Von den Gracchen bis Kaiser Diokletian* (Stuttgart: In Kommission bei Franz Steiner).

Prescendi, F. (2010) 'Children and the Transmission of Religious Knowledge', in Dasen, V, and Späth, T. (eds.) *Children, Memory and Family Identity in Roman Culture* (Oxford: Oxford University Press), pp. 73–94.

Prowse, T. L. (2011) 'Diet and Dental Health through the Life Course in Roman Italy', in Agarwai, S. and Glencross, B. A. (eds.) *Social Bioarchaeology* (Oxford and Malden, MA: Wiley-Blackwell), pp. 410–437.

Prowse, T., Saunders, S., Schwarcz, H. P., Macchiarelli, R., and Bondioli, L. (2004) 'Isotopic Paleodiet Studies of Skeletons from the Imperial Roman-Age Cemetery of Isola Sacra, Rome, Italy', *JAS* 31.3, pp. 259–272.

Prowse, T., Saunders, S., Schwarcz, H. P., Garnsey, P., Macchiarelli, R. and Bondioli, L. (2008) 'Isotopic and Dental Evidence for Infant and Young Child Feeding Practices in an Imperial Roman Skeletal Sample', *AJPA* 137.3, pp. 294–308.

Purcell, N. (1987) 'Town in Country and Country in Town', in MacDougall, E. B. (ed.) *Ancient Roman Villa Gardens* (Cambridge, MA: Harvard University Press), pp. 187–203.

Purcell, N. (1995) 'The Roman *Villa* and the Landscape of Production', in Cornell, T. J. and Lomas, K. (eds.) *Urban Society in Roman Italy* (London: UCL Press), pp. 151–179.

Purcell, N. (1996) 'The Roman Garden as a Domestic Building', in Barton, I. M. (ed.) *Roman Domestic Buildings* (Exeter: University of Exeter Press), pp. 121–151.

Rawson, B. (1966) 'Family Life Among the Lower Classes at Rome in the First Two Centuries of the Empire', *CP* 61.2, pp. 71–83.

Rawson, B. (ed.) (1986) *The Family in Ancient Rome: New Perspectives* (Ithaca, NY: Cornell University Press).

Rawson, B. (ed.) (1991) *Marriage, Divorce and Children in Ancient Rome* (Oxford: Clarendon Press).

Rawson, B. (ed.) (1992) *The Family in Ancient Rome: New Perspectives* (Ithaca, NY: Cornell University Press).

Rawson, B. (ed.) (2011) *A Companion to Families in the Greek and Roman Worlds* (Malden, MA: Wiley-Blackwell).

Rawson, B. and Weaver, P. (eds.) (1997) *The Roman Family in Italy: Status, Sentiment, Space* (Oxford: Clarendon Press).

Rawson, E. D. (1982) 'The Life and Death of Asclepiades of Bithynia', *CQ* 32.2, pp. 358–370.

Rawson, E. D. (1985) *Intellectual Life in the Late Roman Republic* (London: Duckworth).

Ray, N. M. (2016) 'Consumer Behaviour in Pompeii', in Flohr, M. and Wilson, A. (eds.) *The Economy of Pompeii* (Oxford: Oxford University Press), pp. 87–110.

Reay, B. (2005) 'Agriculture, Writing, and Cato's Aristocratic Self-Fashioning', *CA* 24.2, pp. 331–361.

Renberg, G. H. (2006/2007) 'Public and Private Places of Worship in the Cult of Asclepius at Rome', *MAAR* 51/52, pp. 87–172.

Retief, F. P. and Cilliers, L. (2000) 'Poisons, Poisoning and the Drug Trade in Ancient Rome', *Akroterion* 45.1, pp. 80–100.

Riddle, C. A. (2013) 'The Ontology of Impairment: Rethinking How We Define Disability', in Wappett, M. and Arndt, K. (eds.) *Emerging Perspectives on Disability Studies* (New York, NY: Palgrave Macmillan), pp. 23–40.

Riddle, J. M. (1992) *Contraception and Abortion from the Ancient World to the Renaissance* (Cambridge, MA and London: Harvard University Press).

Riddle, J. M. (1996) 'High Medicine and Low Medicine in the Roman Empire', *ANRW* II 37.1, pp. 79–101.

Robinson, O. F. (1994) *Ancient Rome: City Planning and Administration* (London: Routledge).

Robinson, M. and Rowan, E. (2015) 'Roman Food Remains in Archaeology and the Contents of a Sewer at Herculaneum', in Wilkins, J. and Nadeau, R. (eds.) *Companion to Food in the Ancient World* (Oxford and Malden, MA: Wiley-Blackwell), pp. 105–115.

Roller M. (2001) *Constructing Autocracy: Aristocrats and Emperors in Julio-Claudian Rome* (Princeton, NJ: Princeton University Press).

Ross, S. (1998) *What Gardens Mean* (Chicago, IL: University of Chicago Press).

Roth, U. (2004) 'Inscribed Meaning: The *Vilica* and the Villa Economy', *PBSR* 72, pp. 101–124.

Roth, U. (2007) *Thinking Tools: Agricultural Slavery Between Evidence and Models* (London: Institute of Classical Studies).

Rousselle, A. (1988) *Porneia: On Desire and the Body in Antiquity* (Oxford and New York, NY Basil Blackwell).

Rowan, E. (2014) *Roman Diet and Nutrition in the Vesuvian Region: A Study of the Bioarchaeological Remains from the Cardo V Sewer at Herculaneum* (University of Oxford Unpublished MPhil. Thesis).

Rowan, E. (2016) 'Sewers, Archaeobotany and Diet at Pompeii and Herculaneum', in Flohr, M. and Wilson, A. (eds.) *The Economy of Pompeii* (Oxford: Oxford University Press), pp. 111–134.

Rüpke, J. (ed.) (2007) *A Companion to Roman Religion* (Malden, MA: Wiley-Blackwell).

Salazar, C. F. (2000) *The Treatment of War Wounds in Graeco-Roman Antiquity* (Leiden: Brill).

Saller R. P. (1984) ' "*Familia, Domus*" and the Roman Conception of the Family', *Phoenix* 38.4, pp. 336–355.

Saller R. P. (1987) 'Men's Age at Marriage and its Consequences in the Roman Family', *CP* 82.1, pp. 21–34.

Saller R. P. (1994) *Patriarchy, Property and Death in the Roman Family* (Cambridge: Cambridge University Press).

Saller R. P. (1999) '*Pater Familias, Mater Familias*, and the Gendered Semantics of the Roman Household', *CP* 94.2, pp. 182–197.

Saller R. P. (2003) 'Women, Slaves, and the Economy of the Roman Household', in Balch, D. L. and Osiek, C. (eds.) *Early Christian Families in Context: An Interdisciplinary Dialogue* (Grand Rapids, MI: William B. Eerdmans), pp. 185–204.

Saller R. P. (2011) 'The Roman Family as a Productive Unit', in Rawson, B. (ed.) *A Companion to Families in the Greek and Roman Worlds* (Malden, MA: Wiley-Blackwell), pp. 116–128.

Saller R. P. and Shaw, B. (1984) 'Tombstones and Roman Family Relations in the Principate: Civilians, Soldiers and Slaves', *JRS* 74, pp. 124–156.

Samama, É. (2003) *Les Médecins Dans le Monde Grec: Sources Epigraphiques Sur la Naissance d'un Corps Médical* (Geneva: Droz).

Samter, E. (1901) *Familienfeste der Griechen und Römer* (Berlin: G. Reimer).

Sartorio, G. P. (1988) 'Compita Larum. Edicole sacre nei crocicchi di Roma antica', *Bollettino della Unione storia ed arte* 31, pp. 23–34.

Scarborough, J. (1969) *Roman Medicine* (Ithaca, NY: Cornell University Press).

Scarborough, J. (1993) 'Roman Medicine to Galen', *ANRW* II 37.1, pp. 3–48.

Scarborough, J. (2002) 'Herbs of the Field and Herbs of the Garden in Byzantine Medicinal Pharmacy', in Littlewood, A. R., Maguire, H., and Wolschke-Bulmahn, J. (eds.) *Byzantine Garden Culture* (Washington D. C.: Dumbarton Oaks), pp. 177–188.

Scheid, J. (2007) 'Sacrifices for Gods and Ancestors', in Rüpke, J. (ed.) *A Companion to Roman Religion* (Malden, MA: Wiley-Blackwell), pp. 263–271.

Scheidel, W. (2001a) 'Roman Age Structure: Evidence and Models', *JRS* 91, pp. 1–26.

Scheidel, W. (ed.) (2001b) *Debating Roman Demography* (Leiden: Brill).

Scheidel, W. (2003) 'Germs for Rome', in C. Edwards and G. Woolf (eds.) *Rome the Cosmopolis* (Cambridge and New York, NY: Cambridge University Press), pp. 158–176.

Scheidel, W. (2006) 'Stratification, Deprivation and Quality of Life', in Atkins, M. and Osborne, R. (eds.) *Poverty in the Roman World* (Cambridge: Cambridge University Press), pp. 40–59.

Scheidel, W. (2007) 'A Model of Real Income Growth in Roman Italy', *Historia* 56.3, pp. 322–346.

Scheidel, W. (2012) 'Physical Well-being', in Scheidel, W. (ed.) *The Cambridge Companion to the Roman Economy* (Cambridge: Cambridge University Press), pp. 321–333.

Schmidt, O. E. (1990) 'Ciceros Villen', in Reutti, F. (ed.) *Die römische Villa* (Darmstadt: Wissenschaftliche Buchgesellschaft), pp. 13–40.

Scobie, A. (1986) 'Slums, Sanitation, and Mortality in the Roman World', *Klio* 68, pp. 399–433.

Scullard, H. H. (1981). *Festivals and Ceremonies of the Roman Republic* (London: Thames and Hudson).

Severy, B. (2003) *Augustus and the Family at the Birth of the Roman Empire* (London and New York, NY: Routledge).

Shaw, B. D. (1987) 'The Age of Roman Girls at Marriage: Some Reconsiderations', *JRS* 77, pp. 30–46.

Shaw, B. D. (2001) 'Raising and Killing Children: Two Roman Myths', *Mnemosyne* 54.1, pp. 31–77.

Shelton, J. A. (1990) 'Plinius the Younger and the Ideal Wife', *CM* 41, pp. 163–186.

Simelius, S. (2015) 'Activities in Pompeii's Private Peristyles: The Place of the Peristyle in the Public/Private Dichotomy', in Tuori, K. and Nissin, L. (eds.) *Public and Private in the Roman House and Society* (Portsmouth, RI: *JRA* Supplement 102), pp. 119–132.

Smith, R. H. (1992) '"Bloom of Youth": A Labelled Syro-Palestinian Unguent Jar', *JHS* 112, pp. 163–167.

Spencer, W. G. (1935) *Celsus: On Medicine: Volume 1, Books 1–4* (Cambridge, MA: Harvard University Press).

Spencer, D. (2010) *Roman Landscape and Identity* (Cambridge: Cambridge University Press).

Starr, R. J. (1987) 'The Circulation of Literary Texts in the Roman World', *CQ* 37.1, pp. 213–223.

Stafford, E. (2000) *Worshipping Virtues: Personification and the Divine in Ancient Greece* (Swansea: Duckworth and the Classical Press of Wales).

Stafford, E. (2005) 'Without you No-one is Happy': The Cult of Health in Ancient Greece', in King, H. (ed.) *Health in Antiquity* (London: Routledge), pp. 120–135.

Storey, G. R. (2004) 'The Meaning of "Insula" in Roman Residential Terminology', *MAAR* 49, pp. 47–84.

Tacoma, L. E. (2016) *Moving Romans: Migration to Rome in the Principate* (Oxford: Oxford University Press).

Taub, L. (2002) 'Ancient Meteorology: Astronomy and Weather Prediction', in Renn, J. and Castagnetti, G. (eds.) *Homo Faber: Studies on Nature, Technology, and Science at the Time of Pompeii* (Rome: L'Erma di Bretschneider), pp. 143–152.

Taub, L. (2004) *Ancient Meteorology* (London and New York, NY: Routledge).

Taylor R. (2003) *Roman Builders: A Study in Architectural Process* (Cambridge and New York, NY: Cambridge University Press).

Temkin, O. and Temkin, C. L. (ed.) (1967) *Ancient Medicine: Selected Papers of Ludwig Edelstein* (Baltimore, MD: John Hopkins University Press).

Terrenato, N. (2001) 'The Auditorium Site in Rome and the Origins of the Villa', *JRA* 14, pp. 5–32.

Thompson, F. H. (2003) *The Archaeology of Greek and Roman Slavery* (London: Duckworth).

Thumiger, C. and Singer, P. (eds.) (2018) *Mental Illness in Ancient Medicine: From Celsus to Paul of Aegina* (Leiden: Brill).

Thurmond, D. L. (2006) *A Handbook of Food Processing in Classical Rome: For Her Bounty No Winter* (Leiden: Brill).

Thüry, G. E. and Walter, J. (1997) *Condimenta: Gewürzpflanzen in Koch- und Backrezepten aus de Römischen Antike: Begleitbuch zur Pflanzenschau < Altrömische Gewürze >* (Vienna: Institut für Botanik und Botanischer Garten der Universität Wien).

Toner, J. (1995) *Leisure in Ancient Rome* (Cambridge: Polity).

Totelin, L. M. V. (2004) 'Mithridates' Antidote: A Pharmacological Ghost', *ESM* 9.1, pp. 1–19.

Totelin, L. M. V. (2009) *Hippocratic Recipes: Oral and Written Transmission of Pharmacological Knowledge in Fifth- and Fourth-Century Greece* (Leiden: Brill).

Totelin, L. M. V. (2012) 'Botanizing Rulers and their Herbal Subjects: Plants and Political Power in Greek and Roman Literature', *Phoenix* 66.1–2, pp. 122–144.

Totelin, L. M. V. (2016) 'Pharmokopōlai: A Re-Evaluation of the Sources', in Harris, W. V. (ed.) *Popular Medicine in Graeco-Roman Antiquity: Explorations* (Leiden: Brill), pp. 65–85.

Totelin, L. M. V. (2018) 'Gone with the Wind: Laughter and the Audience of the Hippocratic Treastises', in Bouras-Vallianatos, P. and Xenophontos, S. (eds.) *Greek Medical Literature and its Readers from Hippocrates to Islam and Byzantium* (London and New York, NY: Routledge), pp. 30–47.

Treggari, S. (1975a) 'Family Life among the Staff of the Volusii', *TAPA* 105, pp. 393–402.

Treggari, S. (1975b) 'Jobs in the Household of Livia', *PBSR* 43, pp. 48–77.

Treggari, S. (1976) 'Jobs for Women', *AJAH* 1, pp. 76–104.

Treggari, S. (1991) *Roman Marriage: Iusti Coniuges from the Time of Cicero to the Time of Ulpian* (Oxford: Clarendon Press).

Vallance, J. T. (1990) *The Lost Theory of Asclepiades of Bithynia* (Oxford: Clarendon Press).

Vallance, J. T. (1993) 'The Medical System of Asclepiades of Bithynia', *ANRW* II 37.1, pp. 693–727.

Vanacore, S. (2005) 'Il larario della Villa 6 di Terzigno. Distacco, interventi, materiali, musealizzazione', in Biscontin, G. and Driussi, G. (eds.) *Sulle pitture murali: riflessione, coroscenze, interventi. Atti del convegno di studi, Bressanone, 12–15 July 2005* (Venice: Edizioni Arcadia Ricerche), pp. 1205–1212.

van Tilburg, C. (2015) 'A Good Place to Be: Meteorological and Medical Conditions in Ancient Cities', *Mnemosyne* 68.5, pp. 794–813.

Viitaren, E.-M. (2010) Locus Bonus: *The Relationship of the Roman Villa to its Environment in the Vicinity of Rome* (Helsinki: Helsinki University Print).

von Stackelberg, K. T. (2009) *The Roman Garden: Space, Sense and Society* (London and New York, NY: Routledge).

von Staden, H. (1996) 'Liminal Perils: Early Roman Receptions of Greek Medicine', in Ragep, F. J. and Ragep, S. (eds.) *Tradition, Transmission, Transformation: Proceedings of Two Conferences on Pre-modern Science* (Leiden: Brill) pp. 369–409.

Waites, M. C. (1920) 'The Nature of the Lares and Their Appearance in Roman Art', *AJA* 24.3, pp. 241–261.

Wallace-Hadrill, A. (1988) 'The Social Structure of the Roman House', *PBSR* 56, pp. 43–97.

Wallace-Hadrill, A. (1994) *Houses and Society in Pompeii and Herculaneum* (Princeton, NJ: Princeton University Press).

Wallace-Hadrill, A. (1998) 'The Villa as a Cultural Symbol', in Frazer, A. (ed.) *The Roman Villa: Villa Urbana* (Philadelphia: University Museum, University of Pennsylvania), pp. 43–53.

Wallace-Hadrill, A. (2008) *Rome's Cultural Revolution* (Cambridge and New York, NY: Cambridge University Press).

Warwick-Booth, L., Cross, R., and Lowcock, D. (2012) *Contemporary Health Studies: An Introduction* (Cambridge: Polity).

Watson, A. (1987) *Roman Slave Law* (Baltimore, ML: Johns Hopkins University Press).

Watson, P. A. (1995) *Ancient Stepmothers: Myth, Misogyny and Reality* (Leiden: Brill).

Webster, J. (2010) 'Routes to Slavery in the Roman World: A Comparative Perspective on the Archaeology of Forced Migration', in Eckardt, H. (ed.) *Roman Diasporas: Archaeological Approaches to Mobility and Diversity in the Roman World* (Portsmouth, RI: *JRA* Supplement 78), pp. 45–65.

White, K. D. (1973) 'Roman Agricultural Writers I: Varro and his Predecessors', *ANRW* I.4, pp. 439–497.

WHO (1948) and WHO (2006) www.who.int/about/mission/en/ (accessed August 2018).

Wilkins, J. (2000) *The Boastful Chef: The Discourse of Food in Ancient Greek Comedy* (Oxford and New York, NY: Oxford University Press).

Wilkins, J. (2005) 'Hygieia at Dinner and at the Symposium', in King, H. (ed.) *Health in Antiquity* (London: Routledge), pp. 136–159.

Winkler, L. (1995) *Salus: Vom Staatskult Zur Politischen Idee: Eine Archäologische Untersuchung* (Heidelberg: Verlag Archäologie und Geschichte).

Wissowa, G. (1902) *Religion und kultus der Römer* (Munich: C. H. Beck).

Woods, R. (2003) 'Urban-Rural Mortality Differentials: An Unresolved Debate', *Population and Development Review* 29.1, pp. 29–46.

Woolf, G. (2006) 'Writing Poverty in Rome', in Atkins, M. and Osborne, R. (eds.) *Poverty in the Roman World* (Cambridge: Cambridge University Press), pp. 83–99.

Xenophontos, S. (2014) 'Psychotherapy and Moralising Rhetoric in Galen's Newly Discovered *Avoiding Distress (Peri Alypias)*', *Medical History* 58.4, pp. 585–603.

Yegül, F. (1992) *Baths and Bathing in Classical Antiquity* (Cambridge, MA: Harvard University Press).

Yegül, F. (2009) *Bathing in the Roman World* (Cambridge: Cambridge University Press).

Zarmakoupi, M. (2014) *Designing for Luxury on the Bay of Naples: Villas and Landscapes (c. 100 BCE-79 CE)* (Oxford: Oxford University Press).

Index

Note: Page numbers in *italics* indicate figures on the corresponding page.

ad unguentum 3
ad valetudinarium 3–4, 105
Aeneas 154, *155*, 156, 157n1
Agrippa, Marcus Vipsanius 35–36, 46n83; Baths of 35–36, 46n83; Gardens of 35; Portico of 35
Amerimnus, Marcus Ulpius: funerary relief of 5, *6*
ancient Greece 4, 6, 96, 104; medicine in 4, 19n31
ancient Rome 6, 96, 104; daily life in 10; health in 15, 20n69; poverty in 47n111; pollution in 130n178; street life of 83n8
Antonius, Marcus 105
Aphrodite *see* Venus
Apollo 52, 154, 156, 157n1, 158n3; Oracle at Delphi 52
Appendix Vergiliana 66, 87n119; *Moretum* 63, 66, 87n119
Apuleius (Lucius Apuleius Madaurensis) 102, 126n64; *The Golden Ass* 102
Arbiter, Gaius Petronius *see* Petronius
Archagathus 28, 31
Ariphron 24; *Hymn to Health* 24–25
Aristotle 54, 137–138
Asclepiades of Bithynia 30, 32, 45n67, 138–139
Asklepios/Aesculapius 10, 51, 76, rod of *11*
astronomy 50, 83n14
Athens 28, 30, 69; gardens of 69
atrium 52, 61, 64–65, 67–68, 77, 79
Attica, Scribonia: funerary relief of 5, *5*
Augustan Principate 79, 94–95, 97
Augustus Caesar 4, 35, 42n5, 83n17, 95, 100–103, 105, 126n66, 137, 140–141
Aurelius, Marcus *see* Marcus Aurelius

bathhouses/baths 32, 34–36, 46n86, 46n94, 65–66, 118, 143; of Agrippa 35–36, 46n83; Central Baths 35; Forum Baths 35; private 66; public 35–37, 50, 66, 156; Republican Baths 35; Stabian Baths 35; Suburban Baths 37
Bay of Naples 13, 15–16, 40, 44n46, 58, 69, 73, 89n185
bioarchaeology 13, 39
Britain (Roman province) 4

Caesar, Gaius Julius *see* Julius Caesar
Campania 15, 21n84, 35, 54, 62, 69, 123, 137–138, 145, 148
Carus, Titus Lucretius *see* Lucretius
casa 61, 63, 82
Cato the Elder (Marcus Porcius Cato) 30–31, 53, 76, 92n246, 98–99, 105, 129n161, 133–134, 136, 142, 147; *To His Son* (*Ad filium*) 30–31, 136, 142; *On Agriculture* 30–31, 53–54, 76, 136
Cato the Younger (Marcus Porcius Cato Uticensis) 138
Celsus, Aulus Cornelius 12, 32–37, 51, 72, 84n22, 120, 133; *Arts* 136; *On Medicine* 21n72, 32–37, 45n66, 45n77, 45n78, 83n7
cemeteries: Casal Bertone 15, 40; Castellaccio Europarco 15, 40; Gabii 15; Isola Sacra 5, *5*, *6*, 15, 40; Saint Callixtus 15; Saints Peter and Marcellinus 15; suburban 40; Velia 15
Ceres 55, 122
China 6
Cicero, Marcus Tullius 2–4, 8, 37, 40, 57, 69, 79, 86n79, 89n183, 101, 107, 121, 127n96, 136, 138, 145; *Against Piso*

130n183; *In Defence of Cluentius* 147;
  On His House 75, 91n229; *Letters to
  Friends* 150n32; *On Old Age* 46n106;
  Tusculan Disputations 29, 44n50
Cicero, Quintus Tullius 57, 145
Cilicia (province) 56
Cincinnatus, Lucius Quinctius 68
Civil Wars 55, 95
cleanliness 120–121; pollution 129n177,
  130n178; purity 120, 129n177
coemptio 100–101
Colosseum 36
columbaria/columbarium 3–4, 12,
  42n4, 109
Columella, Lucius Junius Moderatus
  32–33, 37, 54, 56–58, 62, 66, 76, 102,
  105, 109–110, 116–118, 121, 148; *On
  Agriculture* 33, 53, 56, 70–71, 85n67,
  85–86n68, 98, 102
confarreatio 100
cosmeticus 8
Crispinus, Titus Quinctius 145

deductio 145
Diocles of Carystus 27
Dioscorides 136, 140; *On Medical
  Materials* 136
dipinti 12–13
disease 20n72, 24, 37, 48, 76, 89n166,
  118; definition 29
domina 65, 99, 103, 132, 148
dominus 58, 65, 68, 92n246, 100, 103,
  131–132, 147–148
Domitian 36, 46n94, 128n136
domus 57–58, 60–61, 63–64, 66, 69,
  82, 83n6, 86n69, 96–97, 126n71, 132,
  152n111, 157; *atrium* house 61, 67;
  atrium/peristyle house 61; definition
  96–97

early modern period 18n6
education 33, 118, 141–143, 150n59;
  female 151n81; formal 17, 134,
  141–142; informal 17, 141–142; liberal
  arts 136; medical 151n79; philosophical
  69; rhetorical 151n79
Egypt (Roman province) 4, 12, 14, 20n67,
  49, 113, 150n36

familia 31, 76–77, 82, 104, 123, 124n16;
  definition 96–97; *see also familia
  rustica; familia urbana; mater familias;
  pater familias*
familia rustica 104–105

familia urbana 3–4, 8, 104
feast days 73, 120, 122; *Ides* 73, 120;
  Kalends 73, 120; *Nones* 73, 120
Flaccus, Quintus Horatius *see* Horace
flowers 62, 73–74, 110, 122; properties of
  73–74; garlands 73–74, *73*, 77, 82, 113,
  114, 120–122
fomentum 8
foodstuffs 8, 14–16, 36, 40, 62, 66, 68, 70,
  73, 111, 114–116, 122–123, 156
freedmen 8, 18n16, 50, 71, 93n266,
  94–95, 105, 107, 114, 137–138, 145
freedwomen 8, 71, 95, 105, 107, 114,
  138, 145
Fronto, Marcus Cornelius 4, 140, 143, 145,
  152n91, 152n92

Galen 136, 150n63
Genius 76, 79, *80, 81,* 93n266
Gentilcore, David 6–7
graffiti 12–13
Greece 14; Classical 69; *see also* ancient
  Greece

health: definition 24–29; infant 47n125;
  mental 29, 38, 42n8, 43n34, 44n49, 48,
  99, 103, 120; physical 29, 38, 42n8,
  43n34, 48, 99, 103, 120, 143; *see also*
  disease, healthcare practitioner
healthcare practitioner 3, 7–8, 41, 44n49;
  domestic 7; external 3, 71; internal 3;
  professional 7–8; slave 105
Hellenisation 44n56; 58 of Italian
  peninsula 28
Hellenistic period 69, 138
Hemina, Lucius Cassius 28
Herculaneum 13, 15–16, 20n59, 36, 40,
  52–53, 65, 67, 76, 78, 88n147, 96,
  121–122, 148; Insula Orientalis II 16
heredium 62, 76
Herodicus of Selymbria 27
Hippocrates 27
Hippocratic Corpus 18n8, 25, 27, 51
Hippocratic humoral theory 25, 32, 36
Hippocratic treatises 27; *On Airs, Waters,
  Places* 27, 50–51, 83n11, 83n14; *On
  Ancient Medicine* 27; *On the Nature of
  Man* 27, 50; *On Regimen* 27; *Regimen
  in Health* 27; *On Regimen in Acute
  Diseases* 27
Horace (Quintus Horatius Flaccus) 1, 7–8,
  18n1, 75, 83n3, 91n230, 109, 117, 121,
  130n184, 154; *Odes* 75, 91n230
Hortensius 109

hydrotherapy 32, 139
Hygiea/Salus 10, *26*, 29, 51

insula (*insulae*) 57–58, 61, 63–65, 71, 82,
    86n77, 86n95, 157; *cenacula* 61, 65–66,
    71, 86n95; *taberna* (*tabernae*) 16, 58, 61
Iron Age 15, 21n78
Ischomachus 101
Italy 15, 28, 35, 39, 55–56, 58, 85n58,
    96, 112, 133, 148, 149n14; central 2,
    10, 12–13, 23, 32, 39, 52, 57, 133, 137;
    early modern 6–7; Greek colonies in 28;
    Italian peninsula 28; Roman 15, 123,
    130n199, 148; southern 35; *see also*
    ancient Rome

Janus 22
Julia (daughter of Augustus) 140
Julius Caesar 105
Juno (goddess) 122
Juno 76, 79, *80*
Jupiter 68, 101, 122
Juvenal (Decimus Junius Juvenalis) 65,
    121 130n185

Kleinman, Arthur 6–7

Largus, Scribonius 12, 32, 136;
    Compositions 32, 136
Latium 15, 53–54, 69, 137–138
libraries 35, 136–139; of Apellicon of
    Teos 137–138; of Macedonian kings
    137 of Mithridates 137; on Palatine
    137 private 137, 150n36, 150n41;
    public 137, 138–139; in Temple of
    Liberty 137; in Temple of Peace 137
Livia Drusilla (Julia Augusta) 3–4, 8, 22,
    42n4, 42n8, 105–106, 127n90, 149n2;
    Portico of 35
Livy (Titus Livius Patavinus) 102, 116,
    145 *History of Rome* 146
Lucretius (Titus Lucretius Carus) 68

Madaurensis, Lucius Apuleius *see*
    Apuleius
Maecenas, Gaius Cilnius 1, 8
Magnus, Gnaeus Pompeius *see* Pompey
Mago the Carthaginian 55, 137
manus 91n230, 98–101, 126n64, 152n91
Marcus Aurelius 140, 143, 145
Maro, Publius Vergilius *see* Virgil
Mars 122
Martial (Marcus Valerius Martialis) 20n48,
    34, 64, 71, 109, 128n149, 140

mater familias 17, 76, 79, 95, 103, 156;
    and marriage 100–103
medical marketplace 2–3, 6, 12, 16, 18n8,
    104, 156; Roman 3
medical pluralism 5–10
medicamen 8, 20n45
medicamentum 8
medici (physician) 3–4
medicine from below 4, 7
medicus chirurgicus (surgeon) 4, 7–8
medicus ocularius (eye doctor) 3, 8
Medieval period 15, 18n6, 21n78
Mediterranean 14, 18n6, 70, 110; ancient
    19n40
meteorology 50
Methodist system of medicine 32
miasma 56, 120, 129n177
midwife/midwives *see obstetrix*
Mithridates VI of Pontus 45n67, 137;
    Mithridatium 137
Mnesistheos of Athens 27
Moretum 63, 66, 87n119
mosaicist approach 12, 14, 20n50

Naso, Publius Ovidius *see* Ovid
Nature 68, 131
negotium 28–29, 34, 89n183
Nepos, Cornelius 53–54; *Cato* 53; *On
    Great Generals* 54
Nero (Lucius Domitius Ahenobarbus) 36,
    53, 137
nutrix 105, 129n170, 143, *144*

Oberhelman, Steven 7
obstetrices see obstetrix
obstetrix 3–5, 7–8, 19n42, 103, 105, *146*
Octavius, Gaius 105; *see also* Augustus
    Caesar
osteoarchaeology 20n60
Ostia *5, 6*, 13, *26*, 36, 52–53, 61, 64, 76,
    86n95
otium 28–29, 34, 64, 86n88, 89n183
Ovid (Publius Ovidius Naso) 65, 71, 118

Patavinus, Titus Livius *see* Livy
pater familias 17, 31, 68, 76, 79, 95,
    97–101, 103, 125n47, 131–132, 149n9
patria potestas 98, 101
patricians 100, 146
pedagogues 103, 143
peristyle 61, 64–65, 69, 71–72, 77,
    89n181
Petronius (Gaius Petronius Arbiter) 72, 104,
    120, 128n128; *Satyricon* 72, 120, 128n128

pharmakon 8, 20n45
Phoebus 140, 154, 156
Phylotimos and Diphilos of Siphos 27
physical intimacy 33–34
Plato 27, 51; *Laws* 51
Plautus, Titus Maccius 79, 102, 115–116,
    120, 143; *The Pot of Gold* 77, 92n252,
    122; *Pseudolus* 116, 128–129n150;
    Stichus 140
plebeians 12, 14, 28–29, 50, 69, 139,
    146, 157
Pliny the Elder (Gaius Plinius Secundus)
    12, 23, 28, 30, 32–33, 37, 54, 68,
    71–72, 75–76, 98, 122, 131, 133,
    137–138, 140; *Natural History* 33,
    44n53, 44n55, 83n7, 89n169, 90n207,
    90n212, 130n189, 136, 149n1
Pliny the Younger (Gaius Plinius Caecilius
    Secundus) 4, 37–38, 49, 57, 59, 64,
    102–103, 127n113, 141, 145; *Letters*
    46–47n107, 47n108, 83n6, 86n91;
    marriage of 125n59; wife of 126n83
Plutarch (Lucius Mestrius Plutarchus) 23,
    30–31, 98, 118, 137, 142; *Advice on
    Keeping Well* 23, 42n6, 42–43n11; *Cato
    the Elder* 44n59, 53, 98, 151n82
poison/poisonings 22, 137, 140, 146–147
Pollio, Gaius Asinius 137
Pollio, Marcus Vitruvius *see* Vitruvius
pollution: urban 20n72; *see also*
    cleanliness
Pompeii *10*, *11*, 13, 15–16, 21n91, 35–37,
    40, 47n122, 47n123, 52–53, 61, 64–67,
    76, 78, 87n98, 89n177, 96, *106*, 107,
    113–114, 121–123, 137, 148; Garden of
    Hercules 74; House of Aufidius Primus
    123; House of Julius Polybius *80*; House
    of Octavius Primus 123; House of Pansa
    123; House of Sutoria Primigenia 123;
    House of the Ephebe 66; House of the
    Faun 64, 66; House of the Labyrinth
    66; House of the Pork 123; House of
    the Sarno Lararium 123; House of the
    Surgeon 64; House of Vedius Siricus
    and Vedius Nummianus 154, *155*; *Insula*
    of Arriana Paulina 61; Praedia of Julia
    Felix 61, 64; shrine of Marcus Epidius
    Rufus 93n266
Pompey (Gnaeus Pompeius Magnus) 137;
    Portico of 35, 88n123
Praxagoras of Cos 27
Priapus 122
Principate 14–15, 17, 20n51, 44n45, 147;
    Augustan 79, 94–95, 97; early 15,

20n65, 41, 76, 83n17, 95–96, 113, 131,
    133, 137, 141; health in 22–42
Pseudo-Dioscorides 136
Psyche 102, *113*
public parks 156

Quintilian (Marcus Fabius Quintilianus)
    32–33, 37, 54; *Institutes of Oratory* 33,
    84n22, 147

regimen 16, 27–29, 38–42, 44n48, 45n60,
    46n102, 46n106, 47n108, 47n125, 49,
    66, 70, 99, 103–104, 106, 115, 122,
    127n103, 139, 143, 148; definition 25,
    27–28; in Principate 32–38; in Roman
    Republic 29–32
Roman domestic religion 74–82, 85n52,
    121–122; *Compitalia* 75–76; *Genius*
    76, 79, *80*, *81*, 93n266; household gods
    75–76, 82, 122; *Juno* 76, 79, *80*, 122;
    Lar 77–78, *78*, 92n248, 122; *Lares*
    75–79, 91n231, 93n266, 130n197; *Lar
    compitalis* 78; *Lar familiaris* 75, 77–78;
    Parentalia festival 82; *Penates* 75–76,
    79; Vesta 76, 79, 82, 122
Roman Empire 70, 89n169, 148; early 2
Roman garden 16, 50, 53, 69–70, 74,
    82, 87n99, 87n102, 87n122; design of
    61–64, 87n103; *hortus* 63–64, 69, 76;
    peristyle 61, 64, 69, 72, 89n181; use of
    68–74; *viridarium* 64, 72
Roman house 50, 53–54, 74, 82; design
    of 51–61; use of 64–68; *see also casa*;
    domus; *insula*; *villa*
Roman household 94–123, 131, 133,
    145, 147–148, 156; *see also domina*;
    dominus; foodstuffs; *mater familias*;
    pater familias; Roman domestic
    religion; wine
Roman Republic 16–17, 20n51, 23, 39,
    100, 127n99, 133, 147; late 3, 133;
    middle 2; regimen in 29–32
Rome, city of 1, 3, 12–15, 19n40, 28,
    30, 36, 39–40, 71, 104, 133, 137, 148;
    healthiness of 23, 83n2, 84n37; *see
    also* Principate; ancient Rome; Roman
    Republic
Romulus 62, 76

sacra privata 75, 91n229
sacra publica 91n229
salutatio 34, 65, 68, 89n164, 145
Saserna the Elder and Younger 134
Second Punic War 53–54

Second Sophistic 150n63
Secuncus, Gaius Plinius *see* Pliny
　the Elder
Secuncus, Gaius Plinius Caecilius *see*
　Pliny the Younger
Seneca the Elder (Lucius [Marcus]
　Annaeus Seneca): *Declamations* 147
Seneca the Younger (Lucius Annaeus
　Seneca) 4, 22–23, 40, 48, 62, 65, 117,
　130n181, 145; *Moral Epistles* 82–83n1,
　89n 66, 126n82, 128n145, 129n160
seplasarius (pharmacist) 8, 107, *108*, 134,
　140–145
Servius Tullius 65, 75
sexual activity 27, 33, 36–37
Sicily 35
Silvanus 122
slaves 7–8, 10; health and well-being
　of 32, 34, 36, 83n7, 109, 118; in
　house and garden 50, 54, 60, 65, 68,
　71; household 90n206, 95–100, 102,
　104–105, 107, 109, 114–115, *115*, 118,
　120–121, 126n84, 127n105, 127n113,
　129n165; old 127n107; sick 127n107;
　and transmission of medical knowledge
　132–133, 138, 142, 145, 149n3
socialisation 17, 134, 142–143
Soranus 43n32, 136; *Gynaecology* 136
Spain (Roman province) 56, 88n131, 148
Spurinna, Titus Vestricius 37–38
Statius, Publius Papinius 59
Suetorius (Gaius Suetonius
　Tranquillus) 22
Superbus, Tarquinius 68
supra medicos (chief physician) 3, 105
Syria (Roman province) 56

Tacitus, Publius Cornelius 22, 53, 141,
　145 *Annals* 22, 42n1, 42n5, 84n39; *A
　Dialogue on Oratory* 151n77
Tellus 55
Temple of Tellus 55, 134
Themison of Laodicea 32
Theophrastus 54, 137–138, 140
Tiber 35, 142
Tiberius Caesar 4, 22–23, 32, 42n4,
　42n5, 137
Titus 36, 46n94
Trajan 36
Tranquillus, Gaius Suetonius *see* Suetonius

transmission of medical knowledge
　131–134, 146–148; literary 134–138;
　oral 138–140; personal experience
　140–145
Twelve Tables 63, 76; *Law of the Twelve
　Tables* 98

unctores 3–4
unctrix 3, 106, 118
unguentarius 8, 118
usus 100–101

Varro, Marcus Terentius 53–58, 62,
　64–66, 76, 107, 109–110, 133–134,
　136–138, 147–148; *Disciplines* 136;
　On Agriculture 18n11, 53–57, 85n58,
　85n59, 85n60, 85n61, 85n62, 86n69, 98,
　105, 121, 127n98, 153n115
Venus 25, 74, 154, 156, 157n1
Vesta 76, 79, 82, 122
Vestal Virgins 142
veterinary medicine 119
vilicus/vilica 103
villa 44n46, 48, 55, 57–60, *59*, 63–65,
　69, 82, 84n42, 109, 130n189, 137, 157;
　pars fructaria 58; *pars rustica* 58; *pars
　urbana* 58; of Pliny the Younger 64,
　88n125; Villa 6 at Terzigno 123; Villa
　della Pisanella at Boscoreale 66; *villa
　maritima* 29, *59*; Villa of Numerius
　Popidius Florus, Boscoreale *67*; Villa of
　Poppidius Florus at Pisanella 66; Villa
　of Publius Fannius Synistor, Boscoreale
　73, *119*; Villa Regina at Boscoreale 64,
　66; *villa rustica* 58, 63; *villa suburbana*
　29; *villa urbana* 29, 58
Virgil (Publius Vergilius Maro) 65, 154,
　156; *Aeneid* 154, 157n1, 158n3
Vitruvius (Marcus Vitruvius Pollio) 35,
　51–53, 56–57, 66, 72, 83n17; *On
　Architecture* 53, 83n17, 84n28, 84n29,
　88n158, 90n209, 150n41

wet nurses *see nutrix*
wine 14, 16, 32, 45n66, 54, 61–62, 66, 68,
　74, 77, 116–118, 121–122, 129n149,
　151n71
World Health Organisation 24

Xenophon 101